Gateway to
Operative
Surgery

Gateway to
Operative Surgery

MD Ray

MBBS, MS (Surgery) DU, Oncosurgery (Safdarjang Hospital, New Delhi), Fellow (Oncosurgery),
Senior Researcher (Oncosurgery) ICMR, FICS (Surgical oncology), FAIS

Consultant, Surgical Oncology
All India Institute of Medical Sciences (AIIMS)
New Delhi, India

Forewords

Chintamani
Sanjay Kapoor

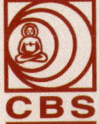

CBS Publishers & Distributors Pvt Ltd

New Delhi • Bengaluru • Chennai • Kochi • Mumbai • Pune
Hyderabad • Kolkata • Nagpur • Patna • Vijayawada

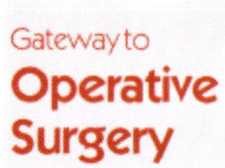

Gateway to
Operative Surgery

ISBN: 978-81-239-2591-2

Copyright © Author and Publisher

First Edition: 2015

Published by Satish Kumar Jain and Produced by Varun Jain for

CBS Publishers & Distributors Pvt Ltd

4819/XI Prahlad Street, 24 Ansari Road, Daryaganj, New Delhi 110 002, India.

Ph: 23289259, 23266861, 23266867   Fax: 011-23243014   Website: www.cbspd.com
e-mail: delhi@cbspd.com; cbspubs@airtelmail.in.

Corporate Office: 204 FIE, Industrial Area, Patparganj, Delhi 110 092

Ph: 4934 4934   Fax: 4934 4935   e-mail: publishing@cbspd.com; publicity@cbspd.com

Branches

- **Bengaluru:** Seema House 2975, 17th Cross, K.R. Road,
  Banasankari 2nd Stage, Bengaluru 560 070, Karnataka
  Ph: +91-80-26771678/79   Fax: +91-80-26771680   e-mail: bangalore@cbspd.com
- **Chennai:** No. 7, Subbaraya Street, Shenoy Nagar, Chennai 600 030, Tamil Nadu
  Ph: +91-44-42032115   Fax: +91-44-42032115   e-mail: chennai@cbspd.com
- **Kochi:** 36/14 Kalluvilakam, Lissie Hospital Road, Kochi 682 018, Kerala
  Ph: +91-484-4059061-65   Fax: +91-484-4059065   e-mail: kochi@cbspd.com
- **Mumbai:** 83-C, Dr E Moses Road, Worli, Mumbai-400018, Maharashtra
  Ph: +91-22-24902340/41   Fax: +91-22-24902342   e-mail: mumbai@cbspd.com
- **Pune:** Bhuruk Prestige, Sr. No. 52/12/2+1+3/2 Narhe, Haveli
  (Near Katraj-Dehu Road Bypass), Pune 411 041, Maharashtra
  Ph: +91-20-64704058/59, 32392277   Fax: +91-20-24300160   e-mail: pune@cbspd.com

Representatives

- **Hyderabad** 0-9885175004   • **Kolkata** 0-9831437309, 0-9051152362
- **Nagpur** 0-9021734563   • **Patna** 0-9334159340   • **Vijayawada** 0-9000660880

Printed at

to

---

my parents, teachers, guide, friends, followers
and
students— present, past and future

Foreword

If you are really thankful, what do you do? You share.

W. Clement Stone

There is no better way than writing a book to share both one's knowledge and ignorance.

It indeed is a great pleasure to be writing a Foreword for such an outstanding book that will go a long way in making learning of various procedures in surgery enjoyable and simple. The book has a vivid and step-by-step description of procedures that are well illustrated and range from very basic to the advanced. The science and art of surgery is best learnt by following the instructions from some one with excellence as a motto in life, a quality that Dr Ray has in abundance. This book would serve well for all surgery residents including those going for MS, MRCS, DNB, MCh examinations, and also for those that are training to excel including younger surgeons in practice.

The book covers a wide range of topics and also issues relating to X-rays, specimens, instruments, and tips regarding various examinations. The book is strongly recommended for all and especially for those with a dream to excel in the field of surgery.

Having written a few books myself, I understand the hard work required to write such a book and I must complement Dr Ray for such an excellent masterpiece that he has put together for the benefit of all. I wish him and his book a great success and would recommend the reader to be part of this experience.

God bless us all

Prof. Chintamani

MS, FRCS (Ed.), FRCS (Eng.), FRCS (Glas.), FRCS (Irel.), FACS, FICS (Surg Oncol), FIMSA
President, The Association of Breast Surgeons of India
Chairman/Editor in Chief, *Indian Journal of Surgery*
President-Elect, Association of Surgeons of India (Delhi Chapter)
Governing Council Member, Association of Surgeons of India
Hon. Secretary, The Association of Surgeons of India (2012)
Fellow, The Royal Society of Medicine, UK
Editor in Chief, *Surgical Clinics of India*
Joint Editor, *Indian Journal of Surgical Oncology*
Professor, Department of Surgery, Vardhman Mahavir Medical College and Safdarjang Hospital, New Delhi

Foreword

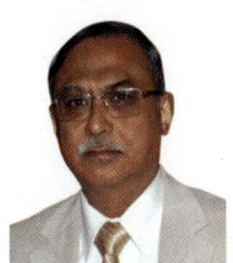

It gives me immense pleasure to see that after the great success of his debut book, *Gateway to Success in Surgery*, Dr MD Ray has now compiled his second book *Gateway to Operative Surgery* for all the surgery residents (MS, DNB and MCh) and MBBS students of course. It is a great moment of my life, to see my favorite student launching his second book, and I am really feeling proud. Even at this young age, he has done what many of us want to do, but do not, since we suffer from the 'writer's block'.

Academics has three stages, learning, teaching and writing and it is great to see him reach the third and the final stage so soon and am sure that this book, meant to help the surgery residents and medical students, will be as useful as the first one.

Residency in surgery is multitasking where we have to learn many things. To asses a patient and reach a diagnosis, to study for passing examinations, and to learn operative skills. Working gives experience but that is never enough. To pass examinations and even for assessing patient, one need to know theory, studies are mandatory; as the 'eyes do not see what the mind does not know'. There are innumerable books that but much of what we need in practice are not mentioned in these books, and much of what are written are not practised, hence a balanced blend of work and reading is essential to pass examinations and to be a good surgeon.

Knowing theory is like making a skeleton, practices add flesh, but it is only experience that puts the soul. So, learning is an ongoing process. First we learn when and how to operate, but we become good surgeons only when we can also decide when not to operate.

Besides learning the operative skills, something that a surgeon needs to learn is to trust the faith of his patients in him for handing over his body and life to him and under his knife.

I wish Dr MD Ray, the book and all the budding surgeons, who read this, all the best.

Brigadier Sanjay Kapoor VSM
Senior Consultant and Professor
Surgery and Surgical Oncology
Indian Army

Preface

"Hardwork is like a staircase and luck is like a lift; lift may fail many times but staircase takes us to the top often"

Most people, the vast majority in fact, lead the lives that circumstances have thrust upon them, and though some repine, looking upon themselves as round pegs in square holes and think that if things had been different they might have made a much better showing, the greater part accept their lot, if not with serenity, at all events with resignation. I think they are like tram cars traveling forever on the self same rails. They go backward and forward inevitably, till they can go no longer and then are sold as a scrap iron.

My sincere effort to write the book is to make the student an exceptional personality in the field of surgery through this *Gateway to Operative Surgery*. I feel the book will help all the medical students, both undergraduate and postgraduate, to face *viva voce* tables and to get through in examination, which is very important gateway to enter the field of operative surgery.

I have tried to include surgical anatomy and pitfalls of each operation. The main thing is the step-by-step approach of each operation. I know many good surgeons and students of surgery; they do the surgery reasonably well but very much are unable to describe the procedure step-by-step which is very much important in teaching as well as professional front, specially for students of surgery to get through the examination door. I have also included common complications and their management, and lastly very common instruments, X-rays, specimen along with viva tips to complete the viva aspect of any kind of surgery examination. Towards the end, I will mention that there is no alternative to hard work. So keep studying standard textbooks, and try to understand the subject and learn a little but learn accurately forever. As far as the skill of surgery is concerned, I would say the same "practice makes you perfect". Until or unless you do the surgery, you would not be able to do it by watching or assisting alone. So, the dictum is "see thrice, do twice and teach once", then only you would be confident enough to do the surgery.

Lastly, I will say, prove William Shakespeare's words in Macbeth wrong "it (life) is a tale told by an idiot, full of sound and fury, signifying nothing".

Say with me, life is a tale told by a wise, full of joy and merry, signifying many things. I will like to welcome constructive criticism from the readers.

All the best

MD Ray
majordrmdray@aiims.ac.in
dr_mdray@yahoo.com

Acknowledgments

I am ever grateful to the following personalities for this book and for my career forever:

1. Brigadier (Dr) Prof Sanjay Kapoor is a great oncosurgeon. He is overall a superb human being and my research guide in oncosurgery under ICMR, New Delhi, and he will remain my teacher always. His valuable lecture notes are included in the book. Without his guidance, the book would have never been completed. He is a man of confidence in his professional as well as personal front of life too. He knows how to become an ideal guide always in life. I am ever grateful to you Sir.

2. Prof Chintamani is a malty talented academician. In academic field I feel not a single person is there who does not know Prof Chintamnai. I cannot express his level. During my senior residency in Safdarjang Hospital, I have learnt a lot from him. He is so kind to write a foreword of my book without little hesitation. He is so broad minded fellow and he arranged to release this book in front of 7000 surgeons in ASICON 2014 Hyderabad, really I am grateful to you sir. Prof GK Rath, truly speaking, I have never seen such a humble person in my life. Initially, I could not recognize him that he is the chief of the Cancer Center, AIIMS. He is always my inspiration not only to become a big doctor but also become a superb human being. Now, he is the Director of National Cancer Institute but I know him as my senior colleague and guide only. Thank you very much Sir.

3. Prof NK Shukla, Head, Department of Surgical Oncology, All India Institute of Medical Sciences, New Delhi, is not only a great oncosurgeon, but also an exemplary person of sober gentleness and a great example of patience. To tell the truth, I have never seen such a big man as such a kind, simple and sober person, who established the onco-center at All India Institute of Medical Sciences, New Delhi. I feel most lucky person to get such a kind of senior colleague in my life. Long live Sir.

4. Prof SVS Deo, Senior Surgical Oncologist at All India Institute of Medical Sciences, New Delhi. To tell the truth, I have never seen such an extraordinary humble professional man. He is a man of quality, perfection and remodeling in every aspect on oncosurgery. He is just like my elder brother. With or without reason, I always like to take his sincere guidance in my path of career.

5. Prof (Dr) AN Sinha, Senior Consultant Surgeon, and former Head, Department of Surgery, VMMC and Safdarjung Hospital, New Delhi, my big guide and well-wisher all the way.

6. Brig (Dr) CK Jakhmola, GI Surgeon, the principal editor of my previous book, who took a great pain to correct all the aspects of the book. The way he encouraged me for my writing showed his greatness and great heartedness. As a surgeon as well as a human, he is really a big man. I will always be grateful to him.

7. Dr Gopal Chandra Bhattacharya: A couple of years back, surprisingly a fatherly figure joined the list of my friends and became my friend, philosopher and guide. He is a renowned pathologist, a young man of 85 years who loves to encourage with all his versatile experiences in all field of life to all the talented persons he meets. His constant companionship was a welcome help to me in the publication of the book.

8. Prof (Maj Gen) RP Choubey, GI Surgeon, my MS guide and teacher. He was literally excited to see the publishing of my book. I am very much grateful to him too.

9. Dr Abdul Motin Molla: Very enthusiastic doctor keeps on encouraging me constantly to complete the book. It is more than sufficient for a writer to hold the patience to do the tough jobs. I am really grateful to him too.

10. Dr (Prof) PK Dutta: A retired Army Professor, offers constant mental support to me, not only in writing for the medical profession but also in different fields of literature too. He is really a man of principle and a real well wisher always. I am really grateful to him.

11. Dr Sanjeev Kumar Gupta, laparoscopic surgeon, is my batchmate and friend always. He edited the book very sincerely within his busy scheduled of private practice. Thanks a lot SK.

12. Dr Durgatosh Pandey, a highly talented surgical oncologist. His knowledge in literature and general aspects is beyond imagination. His kind editing of this book made this book better. His guidance in my professional front is really remarkable. I am very much thankful to him always.

13. Dr Sachidanand Jee Bharati: My friend, philosopher and guide not only in perioperative care of patient but also on personal front.

I am grateful to all of my friends for their ever encouragements in all of my social and academic activities in life.

OTHERS

AIIMS, New Delhi

AIIMS faculty colleagues: Dr (Prof.) Lalit Kumar, Prof Sameer Bakhshi, Prof Sanjay Thulkar, Prof PK Julka, Dr Pranay Tanwar, Dr Sanjeev Gupta, Dr Ritu Gupta, Dr Suman Bhaskar, Dr Sushmita Pathy, Dr Rambha Pandey, Dr Prabhat Malik and Dr Ahitagni Biswas.

Dr Sunil Kumar, my colleague in Surgical Oncology, for his unconditional support and time editing of the book. Dr (Prof) Sushma Bhatnagar, HOD, Anesthesia, Dr BRA, IRCH, Dr Seema Mishra, Dr Sachidanand Jee Bharati, Rakesh Garg, Nishkarsh Gupta and Vinod Kumar are my competent anesthetist colleagues at AIIMS. Dr Haresh, Subhash Gupta, Dr DN Sharma, Dr Chandrashekhara SH, Dr Deva, Dr Manisha, Dr Amar Ranjan, Dr Ajay Gogia, Dr Ranjit and all MCh residents Dr Ashish, Dr Dilip, Dr Pankaj Garg, Dr Vinay, Dr Sandeep, Dr Mahesh, Dr Jyoti, Dr Manju, Dr Paras, Dr Palani, Dr Ashutosh, Seema, Tapan, Niju Shibam, Barart Parmesh, Raja Pramani K, Praveen.

Special thanks to Dr Pankaj Kumar Garg for his contribution in specimen, and editing of this book. Dr Manju Govil for her kind editing of the book in general aspects and Dr Kiran Ruhil for her kind editing the book in structural aspect and Mr Anand Kumar Sharma my most sincere guide always.

Dr Sanjeev Kumar Gupta and Dr Himanshu, Laparoscopic Surgeons.

Lt. Col. D Bandopadhyaya, Dr S Mata, Army College of Medical Sciences, Dr Sujay Singh Tomar, VK Mishra, Lt. Col. (Dr) Abhijit Basu, Dr Mohan, Dr Narayyan Bhattachaya, Dr Pinaki Debnath.

Dr Sanjay, Dr Biswajit (Bishu), other encouraging people in my life Mukul Da — a man of quality of thoughts and English. Arun Sanyal Da too. All of my elder and younger sisters: Archana, Bandana, Kavita, Suparna, Alpana, Chandrima, Munni, Dada Amit, Boudi Seema and Meghasrita, Munai, Uttam, U Das mother-in-law, Santu, Subho Toya. Biswjit Sansanka and D Bhattacharya.

I am very much thankful to my loving father late Mahim Chandra Ray, mother Smt Sarala Shree Ray and my beloved wife Anisha Ray, graded classical artist, All India Radio, for their constant support in making this hard work possible. I am also very much thankful to my 11 years old, very sweet son Mayukhraj, who is my astrologer, friend, philosopher and guide all the time. He always gives a positive astrology to get my every hard work done.

I am also ever thankful to all of my patients—present, past and future without their supports, this book would never have been brought into light.

My sincere thanks to Sunil Gothwal, an enthusiastic boy in our department, who typed this book very sincerely. He also modified structural aspects of the book. Without his sincere efforts, the book could not have been handed over to the publisher. Thanks to Praveen Sharma, Subhash and Pradeep Kumar also in our department, for their unconditional help.

Lastly, I am definitely thankful to CBS Publishers and Distributors Pvt Ltd for their kind efforts in bringing out the book, namely Mr SK Jain (CMD), Mr YN Arjuna (Sr VP, Publishing) and Mr PG Bandhu.

MD Ray

Contents

For undergraduate and postgraduate students, the operations marked as stars (*) are enough to learn for the examinations.

Suggestions for Success

"Winner's are not those who never fail but never quit"

- Marry/keep constant relation with the right person. This one decision will determine 90% of your happiness or misery
- Give people more than they expect and do it cheerfully
- Be forgiving to yourself and others
- Be generous
- Have a grateful heart
- Persistent
- Discipline yourself to save money on even the most modest salary
- Treat everyone you meet like you want to be treated
- Commit yourself to quality
- Be loyal
- Be honest
- Be a self-starter
- Stop blaming others. Take responsibility in every area of your life
- Take good care of those you love.

The basic triad of success:

1. Exercise
2. Meditation
3. Study

It is very very important to realize that valuable man is always far better than a successful man. Always try to be a valuable man in life.

General Principles of Surgery

Concept and Strategy

Success in surgical discipline requires clear anatomical knowledge, good planning, clear picturing of the operation and definitely technical skill.

To develop the concept, we should know anatomy, pathophysiology and pathology of the concerned disease.

Think about the merits of alternative treatment options before putting the knife.

If you decide the surgery, you know preoperative preparation including nutritional upliftment is a very important aspect. Before any major surgery see the following things and calculate the risk of the operation. High-risk factors: (1) age more than 65 years, (2) body mass index (BMI) less than 18 years or more than 30 years; (3) Hb% less than 10 g%; (4) *total leukocyte count* (TLC) less than 4,000/cumm or more than 12,000/cumm; (5) *prothrombin time* (PT), *international normalized ratio* (INR); (6) albumin less than 3 g%; (7) comorbidities, like *ischemic heart disease* (IHD), *chronic obstructive pulmonary disease* (COPD), *hypertension* (HTN), *tuberculosis* (TB) and specially diabetes; (8) history of smoking and alcohol intake; (9) ascites and (10) patient's mental status and consent—is last but not at all least.

Now, reflect on the personal experience or concept with complications, morbidity, and possibility of mortality.

Review postoperative complications and poor results or mortality of the patients. Criticize yourself, analyze the happenings sincerely and attempt to make an objective appraisal of what went wrong. Think about the poor judgment regarding the selection of the case for the operation.

Please, keep official as well as personal records for the future references, i.e. go through the records before going for the operation of the same type of case. It helps a lot to improve surgeon rapidly.

And persist in a lifetime study of the published literature in basic science and in clinical surgery.

As per the "strategy" is concerned, it is advisable that advanced planning of the technical steps of the operation is essentially vital for the safety and efficiency of difficult surgical procedures.

In a word, the operative strategy is that, what the surgeon discusses the day before or ponders the night before the operation.

Anticipating the potential problems and danger points before the operation is the keyword for the success than the handling of an awkward situation, in the operation theater after both the surgeon and patient are in a thick soup.

Remember: The main goal of any successful operation strategy is to make the operation easy. Good preoperative preparation, good exposure, very good light, expert assistants are the essential part of the successful surgery.

If the surgeon is in difficulty, should stop cutting and start thinking why the operation steps seem to be difficult—poor exposure, wrong position, bad light or bloody field, etc.?

The best surgeon makes always the operation easy, just because of a good operation strategy. And lastly I say, when the surgeon is in real trouble, should call for a help from a more expert colleague.

Remember the proverb "asking for a help is not weakness, rather it is strength". I do not know how much it is practical in our day-to-day life but I know it is more appropriate proverb during a difficult surgery.

And believe me, in surgical discipline, try to be honest, always confess the wrong thing/mistakes you have inadvertently done and be a great critic of yourself.

I personally believe, whatever you try to convince your assistants or colleagues to cover up your mistake or wrong technique, it is you and your conscience will be echoing the fact to you.

Your inner happiness is more important after the surgery than the outer smile. Is not it?

MD Ray

What is Surgery?

1. Surgery is an art of learning not only when to cut but it is more important to learn when not to cut.
2. Surgery is such an act which once done, cannot be reversed.
3. All surgeries are major; there is no minor surgery.
4. Surgery is a science as well as an art. Try to be artistic in surgery and life too.
5. Surgical triad
   - Measure thrice
   - Think twice
   - Cut once.
6. Doing the surgery may be easier, but it is managing the patient which counts finally.
7. The lesser the indication, the greater the complication.
8. In surgery as well as life too there is no question of "Short Cut".
9. A surgeon carries success or failure with in self. It does not depend at all on outside conditions or sayings.
10. Many skilled operators are not good surgeons.
11. Attitude for a surgeon may be a small thing, but it makes a very big difference—all the time! Learn to say 'Sorry' on mistake and never forget of sa 'thank you' and please even without credit. These three words are really magic words discovered till day.
12. Remember Mahatma Gandhi's famous word, for the patients.

"A patient is the most important visitor on our premises. He is not dependent on us. We are dependent on him. He is not an interuption in our work. He is the purpose of it. He is not an out sider in our buisness. He is the part of it. We are not doing him a favor by serving him. He is doing us a favor by giving us an opportunity to do so."

Lastly believe me, never get irritated with the patient or party in anyway, they will nerver go against you. Just talk nicely always thats the need and your too.

1. Proper dressing, simple, sober clothes, full sleeve apron—well written examination Roll No. over it, and do not forget to wear *Smile and Confidence always*. Think at the examination hall "I tried my level best—nothing to get tense. I know better than anyone else". Take long breathe frequently to avoid anxiety and fear.

2. Take the following things in examination hall:
   - Two pens
   - Stethoscope, sphygmomanometer
   - Measuring tape
   - Torch
   - Gloves and lignocaine gel
   - Roll made X-ray film
   - Four tourniquets
   - Hammer.

3. Be gentle and polite in examination hall. Never argue with the examiners never and never. Not only in examination, it is applicable in all the fields of life too.

4. When you are given a case, go to the patient smiling and introduce yourself. Give him/her a packet of biscuit and tell "this is my very important examination, cooperate me and do not get annoyed please". Make him/her comfortable and friendly. Take relevant history. Request him/her; tell the same story/words to the examiner also, if he/she is asked by the examiner please.

5. Take proper history. You know perfect history taking will take you through the *Gateway to Surgery*. Remember the points for the specific case and write down the long case till case summery and provisional/differential diagnosis.

6. Examination of patient and its findings should be perfect. Do not try to make it as per book, make it whatever it is. Examiners like the truth, not the book knowledge or the manipulation. You know he is more than hundred times experience than you.

7. Be confident to see the examiners. Say "good morning sir", thank you sir, etc.

8. If examiner asks to tell history, always better to speak history without seeing case sheet. Have eye to eye contact with examiner. If he asks the summary or diagnosis tell that thing only. First you listen what examiner is asking you. Take a pause then start speaking—speak in proper speed, not very fast, not too slow. Give a common diagnosis first. Remember diagnosis a rare disease will be rarely correct.

9. Always avoid speaking uncommon words, uncommon terms or syndromes.

10. Think for a second which you are going to tell. In examination hall, each word is important which makes you through or may not through the "Gateway".

11. Maintain basic things. If you do not know the answer, say, "I do not know sir". Never stand dumb. And never try to make examiner fool by giving irrelevant answers. If required quote a standard textbook not any guide book or note please.

12. Lastly, I would say the same, "practice makes perfect". Practice case presentation in Clinical Meeting, in front of teachers, friends and above all at home in front of a mirror repeatedly.

Wish you easy overcome the "Gateway" to Surgery

All the best—ever and always

MD Ray

In OPD: Advice for
  i. Hygiene
  ii. Nutrition
  iii. Spirometry
  iv. Stop smoking or any form of tobacco intake.

In Ward
  i. Antiseptic bath regularly with chlorhexidine/Savlon soap, specially evening before surgery and morning at the day of surgery.
  ii. Shaving at the incisional site/sites only. Clipping and depilatory cream for hair removal are acceptable at the morning of the day of surgery.
  iii. Bowel preparation for colorectal surgery to start 48 hours prior to surgery (not 24 hours). Oral tinidazole 1 gm + Erythromycin 1 gm to be given at 13:00 hrs (1 pm), 16:00 hrs (4 pm) and 23:00 hrs (11 pm).
  iv. Clean hand before touching each patient
  v. Check Hb%, albumin, any infection at any site, TLC, sugar level, age, BMI, consent, special consent, etc.

In OT
  i. Ensure prophylactic antibiotics to be given 30 minutes before making incision. Antibiotics prophylaxis as follow, 2nd dose after 6 hours and 16 hours after surgery. In clean surgery, single dose is enough.

Site	First name	Step-up
Breast	Cefazolin	Cefoperazone-sulbactam/Ceftazidime/Cefipime 1–2 gm 12 hourly
STS	Cefazolin	Cefoperazone-sulbactam/Ceftazidime/Cefipime 1–2 gm 12 hourly
RP tumor	Cefazolin	Cefoperazone-sulbactam/Ceftazidime/Cefipime 1–2 gm 12 hourly
Nonoral H&N	Cefazolin	Cefazolin/Ceftazidine
Oral	Cefuroxime+metro	Cefaperazon/ Ceftadizine+Amikacin
Upper GI	Cefazolin+sulbacum	Ceftadizine /Piperacillin/Tazobactum+Metro+Amikacin
Lower GI	Cefaperazone+sulbacum+metrogyl	Ceftadizine /Piperacillin/Tazobactum+Metro+Amikacin
Hepatobiliary	Cefaperazone+sulbacum	Piperacillin/Tazobactum +Amikacin
Thoracic	Cefuroxime	Levofloxacin/ceftazidine/Cefipime
Genitourinary	Cefazolin+metro	Cefaperazone + Sulbactam/Piperacillin+Tazobactum+ Amikacin

Note

Pulmonary complications	Levofloxacin 750 mg OD (In renal insufficiency 250 mg OD)	

Lymphangitis: Roxithromycin 150 BD. In renal insufficiency, dose modification is not required in the following drugs—cefazolin, cefipime, piperacillin,tazobactam, metrogyl. Only ceftazidine and cefaperazon up to 2 gram/day is acceptable.

  ii. Wash hand with chlorhexidine minimum for 2–5 minutes
      Soap cleaning for 2 minutes and chlorhexidine washing for 3 minutes minimum
      And pay attention to other people's handwashing including nursing staff.
  iii. Cleaning and draping
      Chlorhexidine and alcohol based antiseptics are the recommendation. Minimum contact period is 3 minutes.

iv. Wear always double gloves

Change surgical gloves at 3 hours, if the surgery is long.

Torn/burnt gloves to change immediately

v. Surgical technique: Good wash with NS before closing. In case of obese patients/high-risk patient, use topical antibiotics—gentamycin/amikacin/metrogyl. Place a suction drain.

Postoperative

- Open sterile dressing after 48 hours
- Clean hand with sterillium before touching each patient
- Send routine investigations including electrolytes on 1st POD, 3rd POD and 6th/7th POD
- Blood transfusion/when Hb% only <8 gm
- Early mobilization, chest physiotherapy, spirometry at the earliest
- Remove drains, catheter as early as possible. Usually Breast drain <40 ml, ICD <100 ml, neck drain <30 ml, abdominal drain <50 ml, groin drain <30 ml
- Discharge certificate would be in details including advice and medicine and next follow-up date and time. Document SSI on follow-up pl.

My colleagues in Surgical Oncology

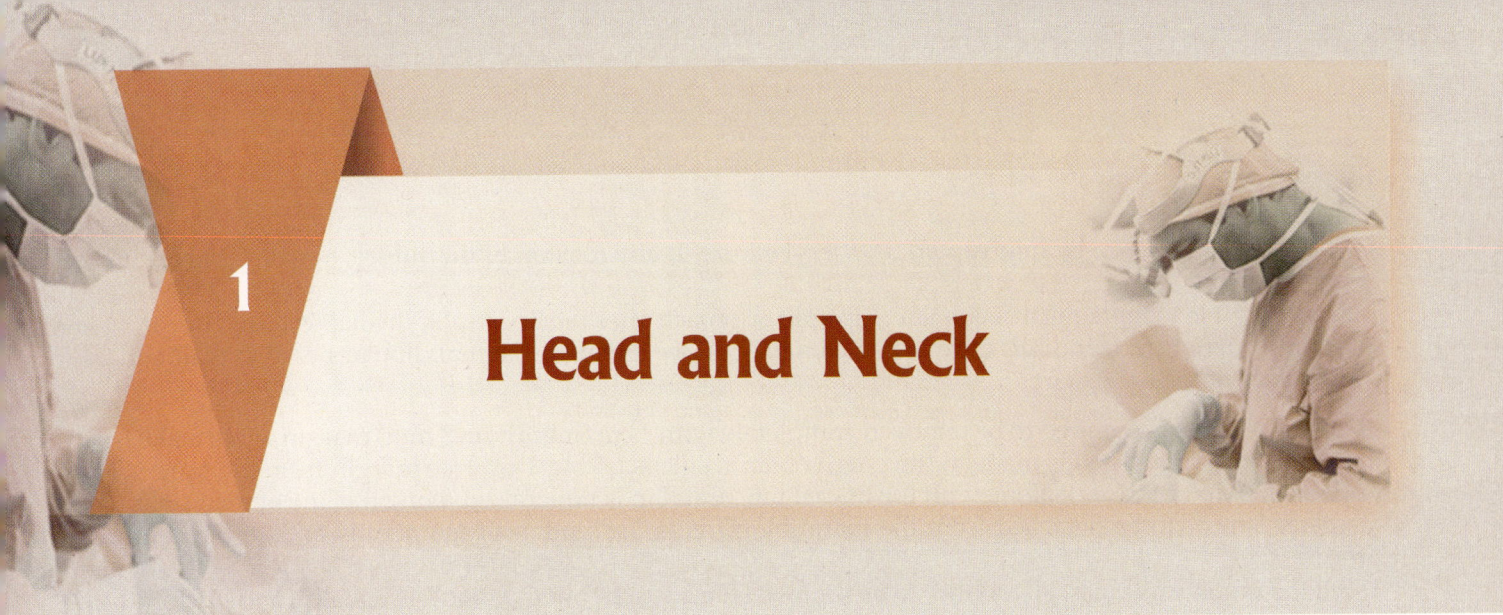

Head and Neck

1.1 COMMANDO SURGERY FOR CARCINOMA ORAL CAVITY

Commando means combined mandibular and oral surgery. Commando operation constitutes of:
1. Wide local excision of carcinoma oral cavity,
2. Mandibular resection when bone is involved or to take a clear margin, and
3. Modified radical neck dissection.

COMMANDO OPERATION

Commando means combined mandibular and oral cavity lesion (Stell and Maran). Name started during World War II and derived from the allied commando raids. Surgery continues to be the main stay in the management of carcinoma oral cavity.

I. *Wide local excision (WLE) with primary closure*

Indications

- Two centimeters size or less tumor
- Without involvement of bone.

II. *WLE for >2 cm tumor with or without bone involvement.*

Procedure

- General anesthesia with nasal intubation.
- Supine position with extended neck turned to opposite side, draping be done in three towels technique. Skin stitches to be applied to isolate the sterile arc. Cotton plug is to put into the ear.
- Ryles tube insertion and fixation.
- Mouth is opened with mouth gag which is applied opposite to the side of lesion.
- Packing of oropharynx.

Steps of Operation

1. Per oral approach
2. Excision should be in proper plane to facilitate the closure
3. Keep 1 cm of clear margin from the tumor

Life is a song, sing it. Life is a game, play it. Life is a challenge, meet it. Life is a dream, realize it. Life is a sacrifice, offer it. Life is a love, enjoy it.

4. The incision is closed by interrupted 3-0 vicryl suture. If any tension in the suture, nonabsorbable suture may be used.

It is advisable to mark the incision line. Lip split approach after the lip is split, the flap is raised beyond the inferior border of the mandible. Care to be taken to preserve the marginal mandibular nerve to maintain the competence of the oral cavity.

Step 1: The lesion is required to be removed completely with 1 cm (minimum 5 mm) margin of normal tissue, thereby; mucosal incision is made in the gingivobuccal sulcus taking 1 cm free margin from the tumor. The upper skin flap of the neck along with the buccal mucosal flap is now raised along the line of mandible. The masseter is now to be detached from the mandible. Divide the tendon of temporalis to bare the coronoid process.

- All the involved tissues, all around, to be removed, i.e. muscle, bone (mandible usually) and skin, en-bloc along with the primary tumor.
- For a larger lesion, mandibulotomy with a "mandible swing" approach or a lower cheek flap would facilitate wide local excision.

Step 2: Mandibular resection: It is indicated when the bone is involved anyway or to take clear margin of the lesion.

Every effort is to be made to keep the mandible as much as possible to give final cosmetic outcome without compromising on oncological clearance. The mandible can be divided anteriorly, the attached muscles to be divided medial to the mandible.

The different types of mandibulectomy are:
1. Marginal mandibulectomy—where the alveolus (tooth bearing area) is removed.
2. Segmental mandibulectomy—where a segment of mandible from superior to inferior margin is removed, i.e. the posterior mandibular cut is to be done.
3. Hemimandibulectomy: When one side of the mandible is completely removed in an advanced lesion, cosmetic deformity is more prominent here. Both the medial and lateral pterygoids to be divided and condyl of the mandible is to be detached from temporomandibular joint and specimen can be detached.

Step 3: Modified radical neck dissection (MRND): You can start the neck dissection first then the primary too. The basic principle is that if there is no clinically and radiologically neck node, supraomohyoid neck dissection (SOHND) is recommended. If the neck node is palpable or involved, MRND is the standard.

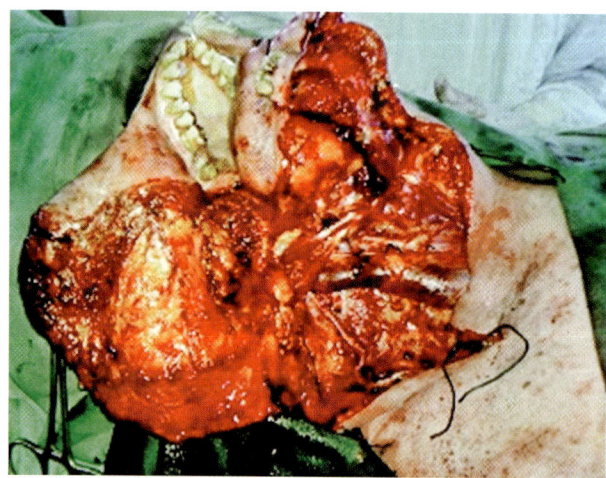

Wide local excision and neck dissection

For beautiful eyes, look for the good in others; for beautiful lips, speak only words of kindness; and for poise, walk with the knowledge that you are never alone.

Remember: Depending upon the involvement of nodes, you can offer:
1. *Type I MRND (Spare 1):* At least, spinal accessory nerve to spare, i.e. every effort to save the nerve.
2. *Type II (Spare 2):* Spinal accessory and internal jugular vein (IJV) or sternocleidomastoid, i.e. save both the structures.
3. *Type III (Spare 3):* Spinal accessory IJV and sternocleidomastoid muscle. All three structures to be saved.

When the lesion crosses the midline, at the side of origin, MRND and opposite side SOHND is recommended. Details of MRND are written in next chapter.

Step 4: Reconstruction of the defect of bone, soft tissue and the skin. % *Mandibular reconstruction:* Apart from marginal mandibulectomy, reconstruction of mandible offers immense functional and cosmetic value. The reconstruction may be either
1. By vascularized free bone grafts, or
2. By synthetic grafts.

% *Soft tissue reconstruction:*
1. Commonly used flap for a large defect is pectoralis major myocutaneous (PMMC) flap—a myocutaneous flap.
2. Deltopectoral (DP) flap—a fasciocutaneous flap. For a larger defect, both PMMC and DP flap are used.
3. Free flaps—like fabular free flap, radial forearm flap, and ribs free flap are being used by the experts.

Step 5: Hemostasis to be achieved completely both in the neck and the oral cavity (special attention to be paid, if pterygoid venous plexus is opened during the procedure).

Place a suction drain properly and close the strap muscles, platysma or all soft tissues in the oral cavity including the flap with 3-0 vicryl and wounds to be closed with 3,0 nylon.

Complications

1. Airway compromise may be obvious owing to expensive dissection and edema formation, especially in a postradiation patient. Tracheostomy may be required in such cases.
2. Reactionary hemorrhage may occur in immediate postoperative period. Re-exploration may be required.
3. Leakage of saliva from the dehiscence of mucosal closure following an infection and orocutaneous fistula (OCF) may occur.
4. Flap necrosis may occur ocassionally.

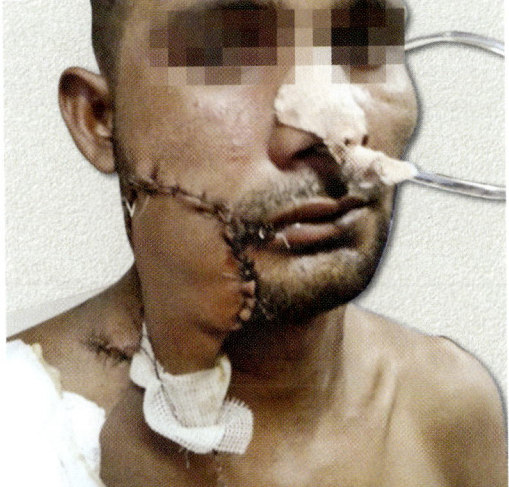

Reconstruction with pectoralis major myocutaneous (PMMC) flap and deltopectoral (DP) flap

A creative man is motivated by the desire to achieve, not by desire to beat others.

5. Problems with prolonged nasogastric feeding.

1.2 NECK DISSECTION

SURGICAL ANATOMY

The cervical lymphnodes are arranged anatomically as follows:

1. *The outer circle of superficial nodes*: These include submental, submandibular, facial, preauricular, postauricular and anterior cervical nodes.
2. *The inner circle surrounding larynx, trachea and pharynx*: These include: pretracheal, paratracheal and retropharyngeal nodes.
3. The deep cervical nodes surrounding internal jugular vein (IJV) lie between the outer and the inner circles, and drain them. These are grouped into anteroinferior, posterosuperior and posteroinferior (juguloomohyoid, supraclavicular) nodes.

The clinically useful description [originally proposed by *Memorial Sloan-Kettering Cancer Center* (MSKCC)] divides the nodes into the following groups:

  i. Submental (IA), submandibular (IB)
 ii. Upper jugular—below and medial to SAN (IIA), above and lateral to SAN (IIB)
iii. Middle jugular (III)
 iv. Lower jugular (IV)
  v. Posterior triangle (upper, middle, lower) (V)
 vi. Central compartment (VI)
vii. Superior mediastinal (VII).

Types of Neck Dissection

The terminology for describing neck dissections (NDs) was standardized by the American Academy of Otolaryngology, Head and Neck Surgery (1991, 2000). The classification is as follows:

Comprehensive Neck Dissection

- Radical neck dissection (RND)
- Modified RND
- Extended RND.

Selective Neck Dissection

- Supraomohyoid neck dissection (SOHND)
- Extended SOHND
- Lateral ND
- Posterolateral ND
- Central compartment ND.

Comprehensive Neck Dissection

Removes all lymphnode groups that would be included in a classic RND. SAN/IJV/SCM may or may not be preserved.

People say "find good people and leave bad ones". But, it should be "find the good in people and ignore the bad in them". As no one is perfect in this world, even God ownself.

RND: Lymphnode levels I to V are removed. Spinal accessory nerve (SAN), IJV, and sternocleidomastoid (SCM) are removed.

Extended RND: Extended to include one or more additional lymphnode groups, nonlymphatic structures or both. These may include parotid nodes, levels VI, VII nodes, hypoglossal nerve, digastric muscle, skin, and external carotid artery.

Modified RND: All lymphnode groups (I to V) are removed. One or more nonlymphatic structures are preserved. Some authors describe various types as follows:

- *Type I:* Preserves SAN
- *Type II:* Preserves SAN, SCM. IJV sacrificed (Jatin Shah's Cancer of Head and Neck): preserves SAN, IJV (Stell and Maran's Head and Neck Surgery; 4th Edition; Eugene M Myers' Cancer of Head and Neck, 4th Edition)
- *Type III:* Preserves SAN, SCM, IJV. In order to avoid confusion, it is desirable that the preserved structure should be named, e.g. modified RND with preservation of SAN.

Remember: Type 1, preserve 1 (SAN); type 2, preserve 2 (SAN and IJV/SCM, IJV is preferable); type 3, preserve 3 (SAN, IJV and SCM).

Selective ND: One or more lymphnode groups, which are removed in RND, are preserved. The SAN, IJV and SCM are routinely preserved. These were originally recommended for NO neck. However, they are also being advocated for N+ nodes by some surgeons.

1. *Supraomohyoid neck dissection:* Lymphnode levels I, II and III are removed.
2. *Extended SOHND:* Level IV is also removed. This is recommended for oral tongue lesions for "skip metastases" (Byers et al, 1997), but has not been accepted by others.
3. *Lateral neck dissection:* Lymphnode levels II, III and IV are removed. This is recommended for lesions of hypopharynx and larynx.
4. *Anterolateral neck dissection:* Lymphnode levels I, II, III, IV and V are removed. This is recommended for oropharyngeal lesions when surgery is used for treatment of the primary.
5. *Posterolateral neck dissection:* Lymphnode levels II, III, IV and V are removed. This is recommended for posterior scalp lesions.
6. *Central compartment neck dissection:* Lymphnode level VI is removed (lymphatics from hyoid to suprasternal notch and laterally up to carotid arteries). Recommended in differentiated carcinoma thyroid.
7. *Functional neck dissection:* Pignataro introduced the concept of conservative neck dissection in which all non-lymphatic structures are spared. Only lymphnodes are removed, interestingly in both NO and N+ neck nodes. It is claimed that this type of neck dissection is equally effective in controlling regional metastasis.

Indications

1. Clinically palpable metastatic nodes
2. Radiologically detected metastatic nodes
3. Recurrent lymph nodal mass in neck
4. Elective neck dissection for suspected micrometastases.
   - *Anesthesia:* General
   - *Position:* Supine position with extended neck. Keep a flat pillow/sand bag beneath the shoulder. Turn the face to opposite side.

Incisions

- Modified MacFee incision
- Schechter incision.

Hard work beats talent when talent does not work hard.

Procedure

Step 1: Elevation of skin flap along with platysma: Preserve the marginal mandibular nerve in the sub-mandibular area.

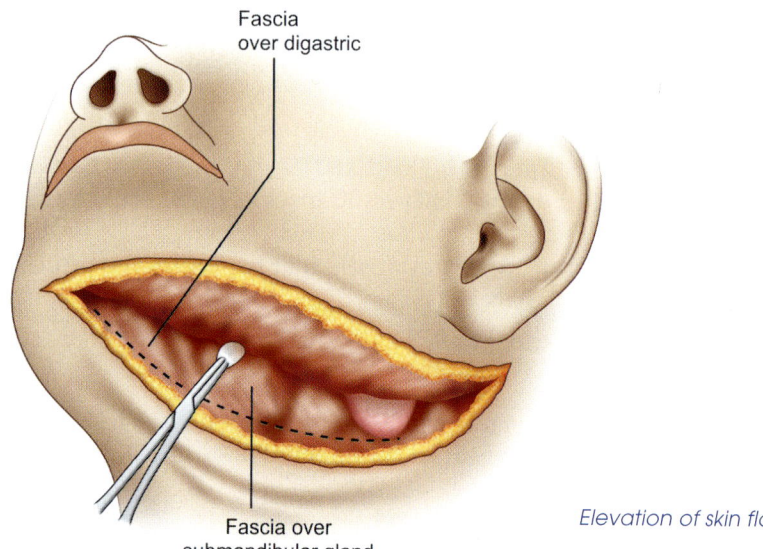

Fascia
over digastric

Fascia over
submandibular gland

Elevation of skin flap along with platysma

If nerve is not identified, make the place deeper and the plane would be on the body of the submandibular gland so that the fascia over the gland would be the part of the flap.

Step 2: Dissection may start from inferior margin: Division of both heads of sternocleidomastoid.

Remember: Divide clavicular head close (c for c) to the attachment and sternal head slightly away.

Expose carotid sheath: IJV is dissected all around and divided between ligatures. Better to put one transfixation suture on each side—vagus nerve lying between the vein and common carotid artery to be preserved.

On left side, the thoracic duct is to be divided and over sewn at this level.

Indentify and divide the inferior belly of the omohyoid muscle.

Clear the fat pad in between the vein and the muscle from underlying prevertebral fascia and overlying scalene muscles.

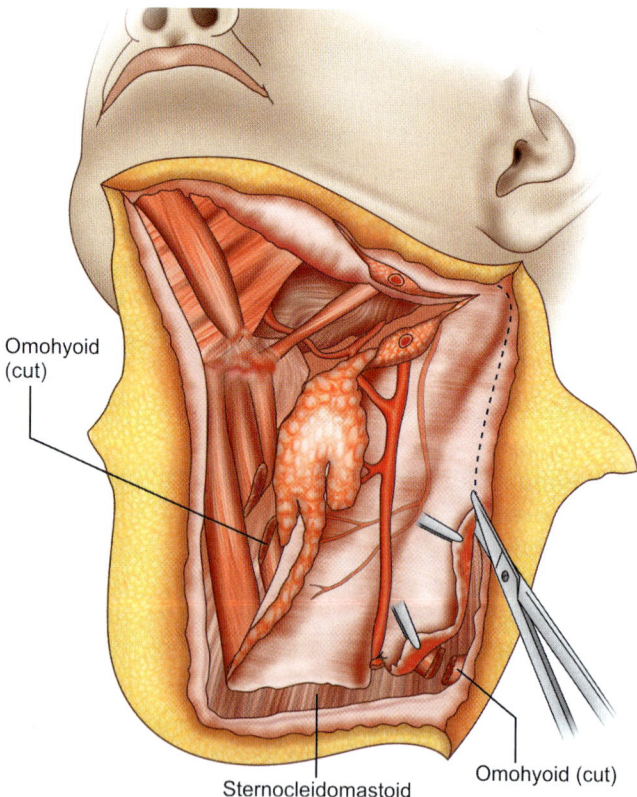

Omohyoid
(cut)

Sternocleidomastoid

Omohyoid (cut)

Division of strenocleidomastoid and below upward dissection

Man is the best judge for himself. He has to pay what he does.

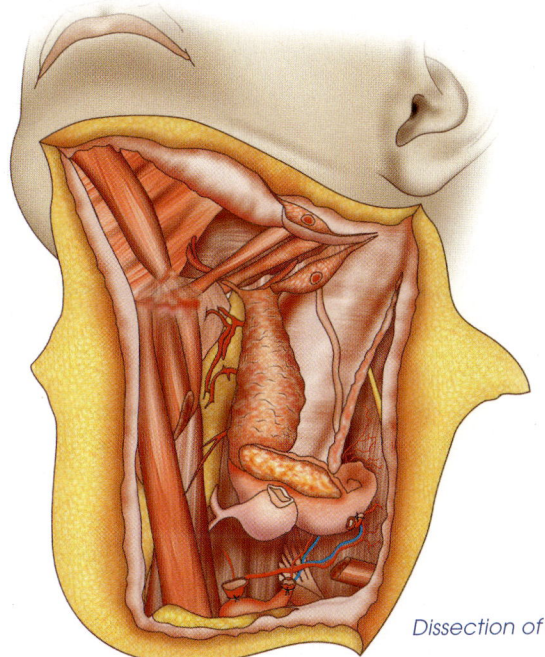

Dissection of internal jugular vein and its ligation

Phrenic nerve which runs lateral to medial and downward underneath the prevertebral fascia on the scalenus anterior is to be preserved.

Create a tunnel laterally in front of brachial plexus to the anterior border of trapezius.

External jugular vein and the transverse cervical artery are ligated during the process of dissection.

Step 3: Dissection of posterior border: Dissection of fat pad from anterior border of trapezius. Ligation and division of vertical branch of transverse cervical artery which runs up the anterior border of trapezius. Identify the accessory nerve as it enters the muscle. Try to preserve it and divide the sternomastoid at the upper part.

Step 4: Dissection of anterior margin: Superior belly of omohyoid is to be followed up to its insertion into hyoid bone and divided.

The submental fat pad is dissected off in between the anterior bellies of both digastric muscles.

Step 5: Deep dissection: The fat pad with nodes is dissected from the posterior margin of the

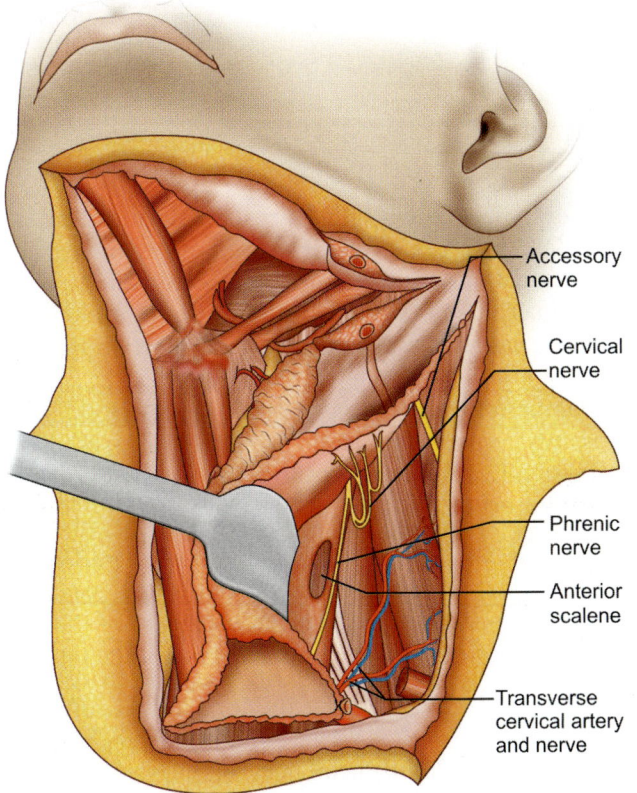

Posterior triangle dissection with identification and preservation of spinal accessory nerve

Accessory nerve

Cervical nerve

Phrenic nerve

Anterior scalene

Transverse cervical artery and nerve

_____

A perfect relationship is not ever actually perfect. It is just the thing where both people never give up.

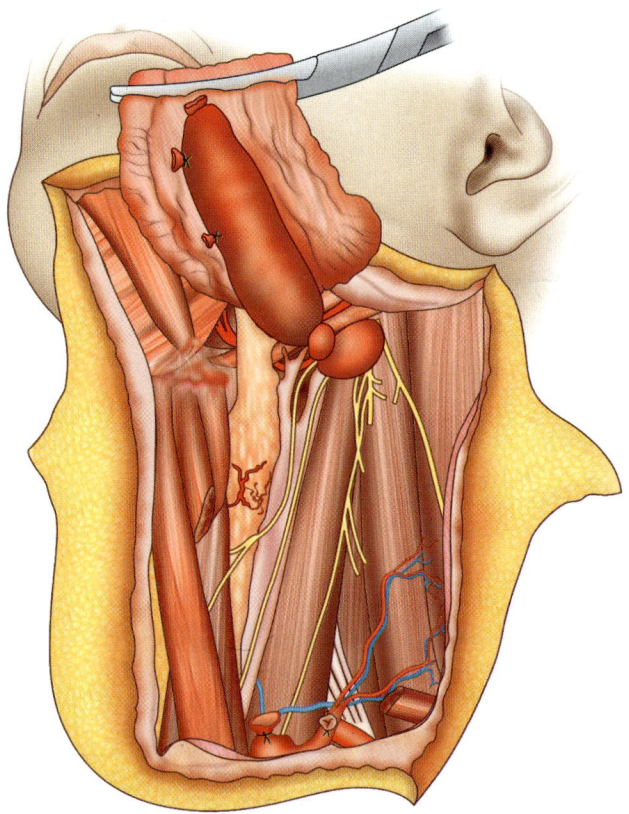

Exposure after deep dissection of neck

prevertebral fascia, levator scapulae and scalene muscles. All cutaneous branches of cervical plexus, namely the anterior cutaneous, greater auricular and lesser occipital nerves, are divided. The internal jugular vein is dissected up to jugular foramen and divided with ligation and transfixation.

Vagus nerve is to be preserved. Hypoglossal nerve crossing the external carotid artery is in turn crossed by three small veins. The veins to be divided and the nerve to be preserved.

Step 6: Superior margin: The submental pad fat, the anterior part of submandibular gland, is dissected off the lateral part of myelohyoid muscle.

Ligate and divide submental artery and facial artery.

Landmark: Just below the junction of muscular and tendinous part of diagastric, the facial artery is located. Save the lingual and facial nerves.

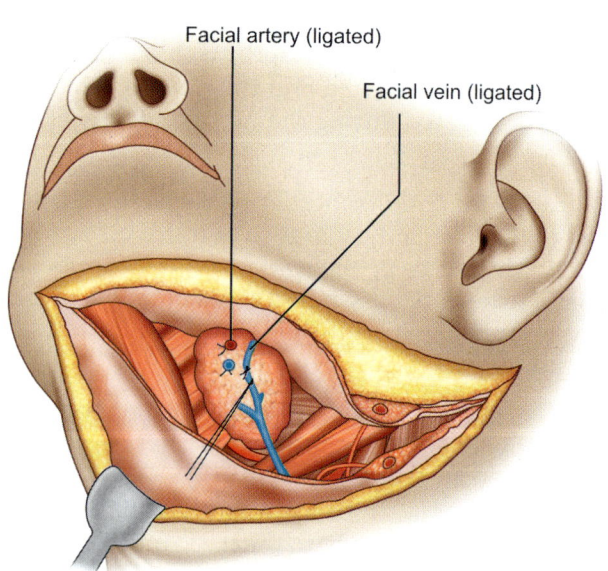

Facial artery (ligated)

Facial vein (ligated)

Exposure of facial artery and vein

Life is like making tea, boil your ego, evaporate your worries, dilute your sorrows, filter your mistakes and get taste of happiness.

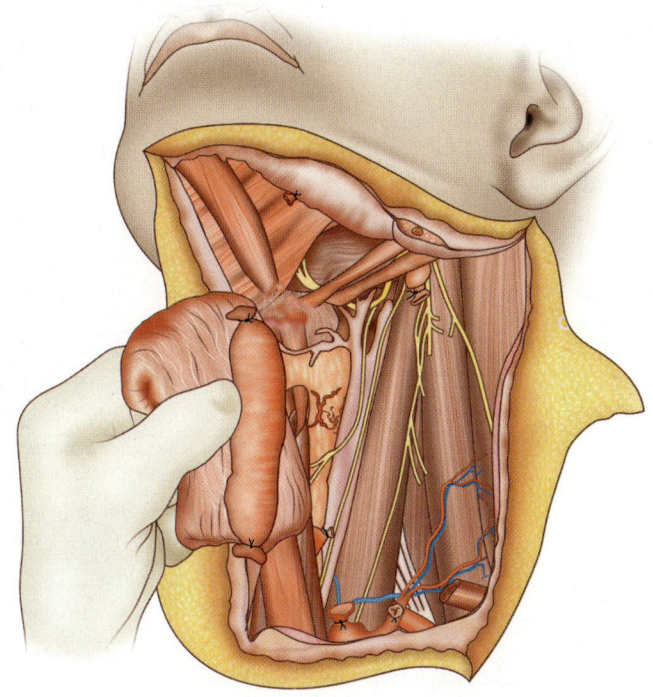

Removal of the specimen after detaching from the medial attachment

Step 7: Hemostasis to be achieved, suction drain to be placed, close the wound in two layers, platysma and skin.

Complications

Early: Hemorrhage, pneumothorax, raised intracranial tension.
Late: Skin flap necrosis, chylous fistula, carotid artery blowout, frozen shoulder, loss of accessory nerve function, keloid, etc.

1.3 OPERATIONS FOR CARCINOMA TONGUE

SURGICAL ANATOMY

Tongue is divided into two parts—anterior two-thirds and posterior one-third parts as both the parts have different biological behavior. Anterior two-thirds of the tongue is part of oral cavity but posterior one-third is in the oropharynx. Middle one-third of lateral aspect of the tongue is the most common site of malignancy.

Oral part of the tongue cancer can be treated with either surgery or radiotherapy or both, but the base of tongue lesion is treated with radiotherapy alone.

The incidence of lymphnodes involvement is high in case of carcinoma tongue. It can cross the midline, if the lesion involves median raphe of the tongue. From right and left halves, lymphnodes drain into submandibular nodes and from tip, it drains bilateral submental nodes.

Each half of the tongue is supplied by the ipsilateral lingual artery and hypoglossal nerve.

The nerve supply of the tongue is like this:
Anterior two-thirds: Taste sensation by chorda tympani branch of facial nerve.

Everything is easy, when you are crazy about it and nothing is easy, when you are lazy about it.

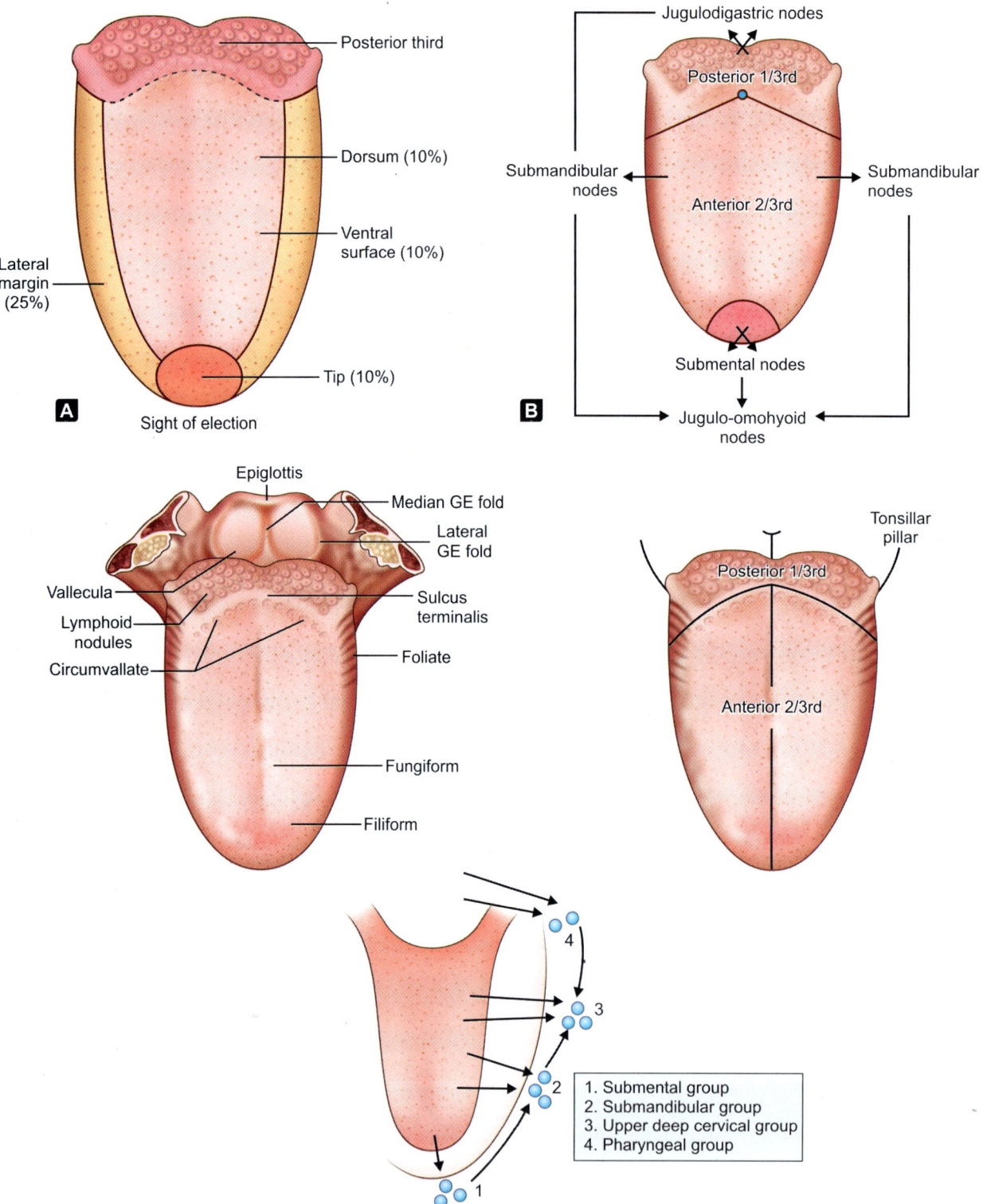

A

Posterior third

Dorsum (10%)

Ventral surface (10%)

Lateral margin (25%)

Tip (10%)

Sight of election

B

Jugulodigastric nodes

Posterior 1/3rd

Submandibular nodes

Submandibular nodes

Anterior 2/3rd

Submental nodes

Jugulo-omohyoid nodes

Epiglottis

Median GE fold

Lateral GE fold

Vallecula

Sulcus terminalis

Lymphoid nodules

Circumvallate

Foliate

Fungiform

Filiform

Tonsillar pillar

Posterior 1/3rd

Anterior 2/3rd

1. Submental group
2. Submandibular group
3. Upper deep cervical group
4. Pharyngeal group

Lymphnodes involvement in carcinoma of different parts of tongue

Weak people take revenge, strong people like to forgive, intelligent people ignore.

- General sensation by lingual nerve
- Motor supply by hypoglossal nerve to both intrinsic and extrinsic muscles except palatoglossus which is supplied by cranial accessory nerve.

Posterior one-third of tongue: Both general and taste sensation by glossopharyngeal nerve. The superior most part is supplied by the vagus nerve through internal laryngeal nerve.

To some extent, hemiglossectomy itself does not cause much more deformity and thereby, function of the tongue is more or less preserved. Like liver, compensatory hypertrophy occurs in residual part of the tongue.

Indications

1. Carcinoma anterior two-thirds of the tongue in T_1 (<2 cm), T_2 (24 cm) lesions, both wide local excision and hemiglossectomy are usually done.
2. In T_3 lesion, more extensive surgery than a formal hemiglossectomy is recommended.

Pitfalls of the Surgery

- Brisk hemorrhage from lingual artery or its branches.
- Venous bleeding or oozing may cause hematoma in the floor of mouth.
- Extensive dissection may cause severe edema leading to respiratory distress. Prophylactic tracheostomy may be required sometimes.

Procedures

- *Anesthesia*: General anesthesia with nasal endotracheal intubation.
- *Position*: Head end to be raised 10–15° to reduce venous congestion. A throat pack is placed in oropharynx, not too tight or too loose.

Incisions for hemiglossectomy: Take two stay sutures, one at each half of the tongue.

Remember: The general principles of the surgery of tongue cancer:
- Small lesion less than 2 cm (T_1 lesion) can be excised with 1 cm clear margin.
- Around 2 cm lesion, partial glossectomy with 1 cm clear margin.
- More than 2.5 cm lesion requires hemiglossectomy.

T_3 or larger lesion requires major resection with mandibulotomy via lip split incision and further reconstruction is mandatory.

The vertical incision is made on the median raphe of the dorsal aspect of the tongue extending from tip of the tongue to up to the circumvallate papilla.

On the ventral aspect, the incision from the tip is extended backward in the midline up to frenulum and from the frenulum, the incision curves and is extended on the floor of mouth up to anterior tonsillar pillar.

Step 1: On deepening the incision over the median raphe, genioglossus muscle will be visible from its origin to its insertion into the substance of the tongue. Dissect the lateral border of the muscle, reach up to its origin and divide with the cavity.

Step 2: Division of artery and nerve: After dividing the origin of the genioglossus, the tongue will be more mobile. Pull the tongue upward and to the opposite side, the hypoglossal nerve with its commitants will be visible. The lingual artery usually runs parallel to the nerve. Divide the muscle to see both the structures clearly. Ligate and divide both nerve and artery separately or together.

Step 3: The posterior transverse incision is to join with the posterior end of the dorsal incision and to the anterior pillar. Now at the side of base of tongue, the connecting muscle fibers to be separated from the diseased tongue, maintaining the plane superficial to the divided artery.

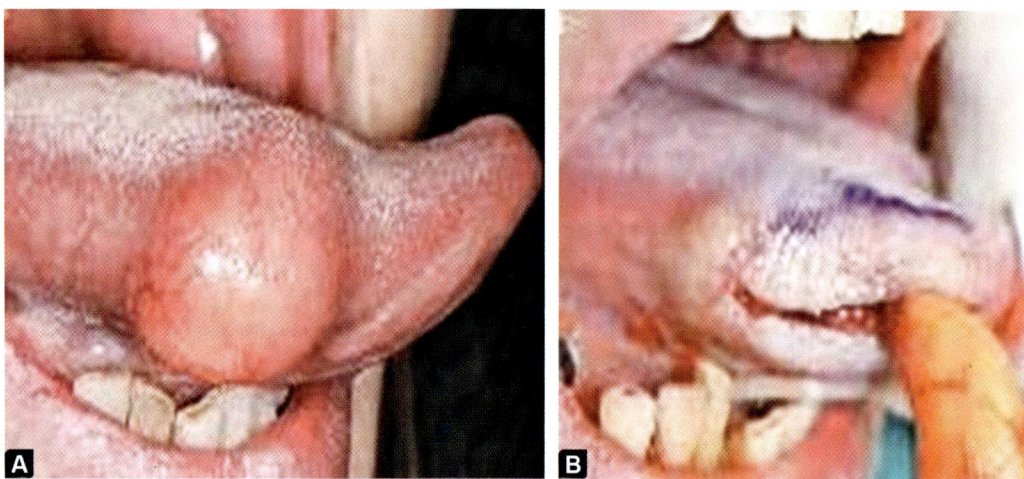

Tongue cancer typically at lateral border

Step 4: Now, the time to remove the specimen dividing the connecting muscle fibers all the sides. Check the margin and depth of the specimen carefully. Complete hemostasis to be achieved before closure.

1.4 TRACHEOSTOMY

SURGICAL ANATOMY

Indications

1. Upper airway obstruction due to growth, trauma, etc.
2. Extensive oral surgery, like central arch cancer surgery.
3. Radical oropharyngeal thyroid surgery.
4. Laryngeal obstruction, trauma, growth, surgery, etc.
5. Long-term support of ventilator.
6. Respiratory depression, like coma, head injury, spinal cord injury, etc.

Preoperative Preparation

1. *Emergency*: No preparation
2. *Elective*: Local preparation
3. Endotracheal tube insertion whenever possible.

Points to Remember (Pitfalls)

1. Injury to cricoid, first tracheal ring during surgery
2. Hemorrhage
3. Asphyxia.

Anesthesia

Local/general anesthesia.

Do or die is old fashion, do it before you die is new one.

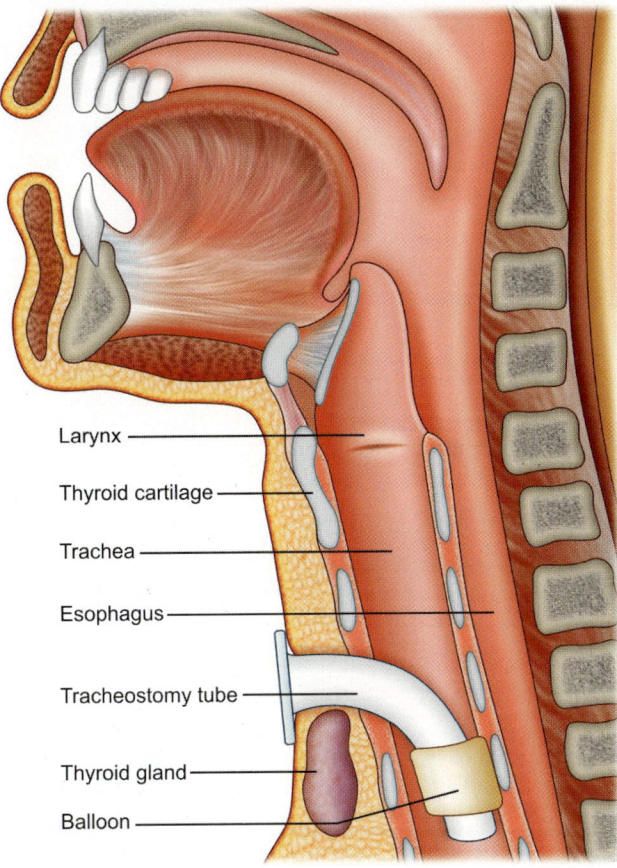

Larynx

Thyroid cartilage

Trachea

Esophagus

Tracheostomy tube

Thyroid gland

Balloon

Surgical anatomy of tracheostomy

Procedure

1. *Position*: Extended neck (keep sand bag, saline bottle or folded sheet underneath the shoulder)
2. *Incision*: Vertical preferred incision (in emergency), horizontal for better scar. Author prefers transverse incision midway between the cricoid cartilage and the suprasternal notch.

Surgical Steps

Step 1

- Incise the platysma in the same line.
- Strap muscles to be retracted on both the sides.
- Pretracheal fascia is vertically incised
- Thyroid isthmus either retracted upward or clamped, ligated and divided.

Step 2: Tackle the vessels crossing the field—inferior thyroid veins and innominate artery. Left innominate vein may cross the field. Ligate and divide all the vessels.

Don't worry about hard time because some of the most beautiful things we have in, come from mistakes and changes because of hard time.

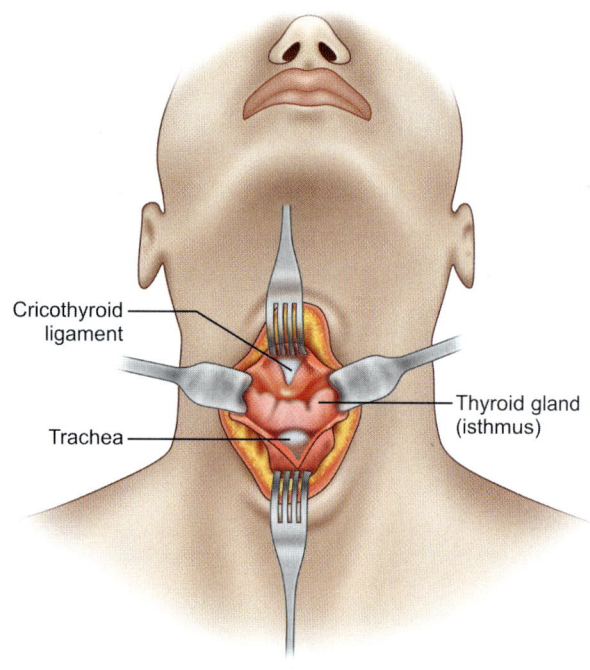

Exposure of thyroid isthmus

Step 3: An inverted "U" or a vertical incision through third, fourth tracheal ring after stabilizing the trachea (cricoid cartilage and first tracheal ring to be preserved to avoid subglottic stenosis and a failure to occlude the temporary tracheotomy).

Step 4: Remove inverted "U" shaped tracheal ring or fix it with skin at lower end of tracheostomy wound.

Step 5: Appropriate tracheostomy tube with lubricant is now inserted while anesthesiologist withdraws the endotracheal tube. Balloon of the tube is inflated.

Step 6: Aspirate blood, mucous from bronchial tree.

Step 7: Tube is fixed properly and wound is closed loosely to avoid surgical emphysema.

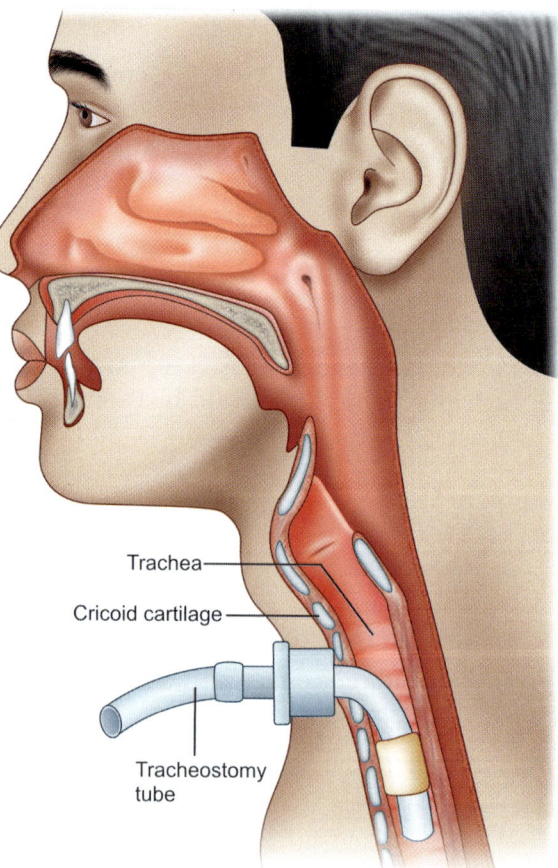

Placement of tracheostomy tube

None can destroy iron, but its own rust can. Likewise, none can destroy a person, but its own mindset can.

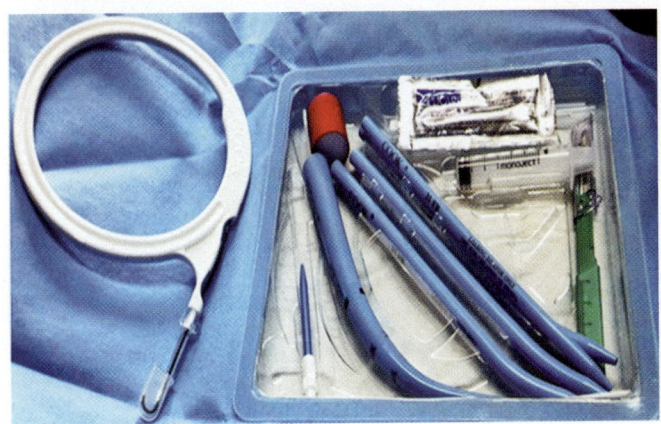 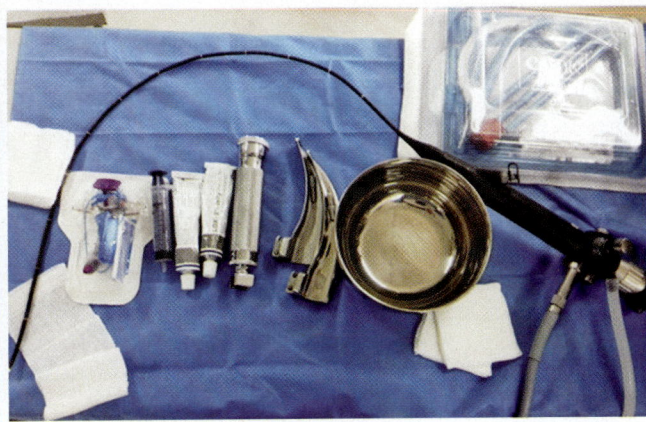

Percutaneous tracheostomy (Courtsey: Dr Sachidanand Jee Bharati, AIIMS)

Postoperative Care

1. Use light-weight swivel connector to attach tracheostomy tube to the ventilator to avoid pressure on trachea.
2. The air to pass through tracheostomy tube is to be humidified. The dry air causes crusting of secretion leading to obstruction of the tube and it may also cause damage to mucosa.
3. Tracheostomy tube must be changed between first and second postoperative weeks ensuring to have the facility of emergency endotracheal intubation or cricothyroidotomy, if difficulty is encountered to insert the metal tube. Remember the track between the skin and the tracheal stoma may not be established for a variable number of days though usually the track is established within 7–10 days. Replace the tube in proper setup with extended neck.

Complications

Early

1. Hemorrhage may occur due to tracheal erosion
2. Surgical emphysema.
3. Blockage of tracheostomy tube
4. Dysphasia
5. Difficult decannulation.

Late

Stenosis may be at the stoma or in the area of the trachea occluded by balloon cuff (a vertical incision over the trachea or an incision as small as possible).

Percutaneous Tracheostomy

Small skin incision (2–3 cm), a needle with cannula is introduced into the trachea, needle removed and a guidewire inserted through the cannula which is in turn withdrawn.

The track is to be dilated by forceps or serial plastic dilators over the guidewire.

The tracheostomy tube is now inserted and fixed.

Friendship is not just a word! Not only a relationship. It is a silent promise which says I WILL BE WITH YOU always.

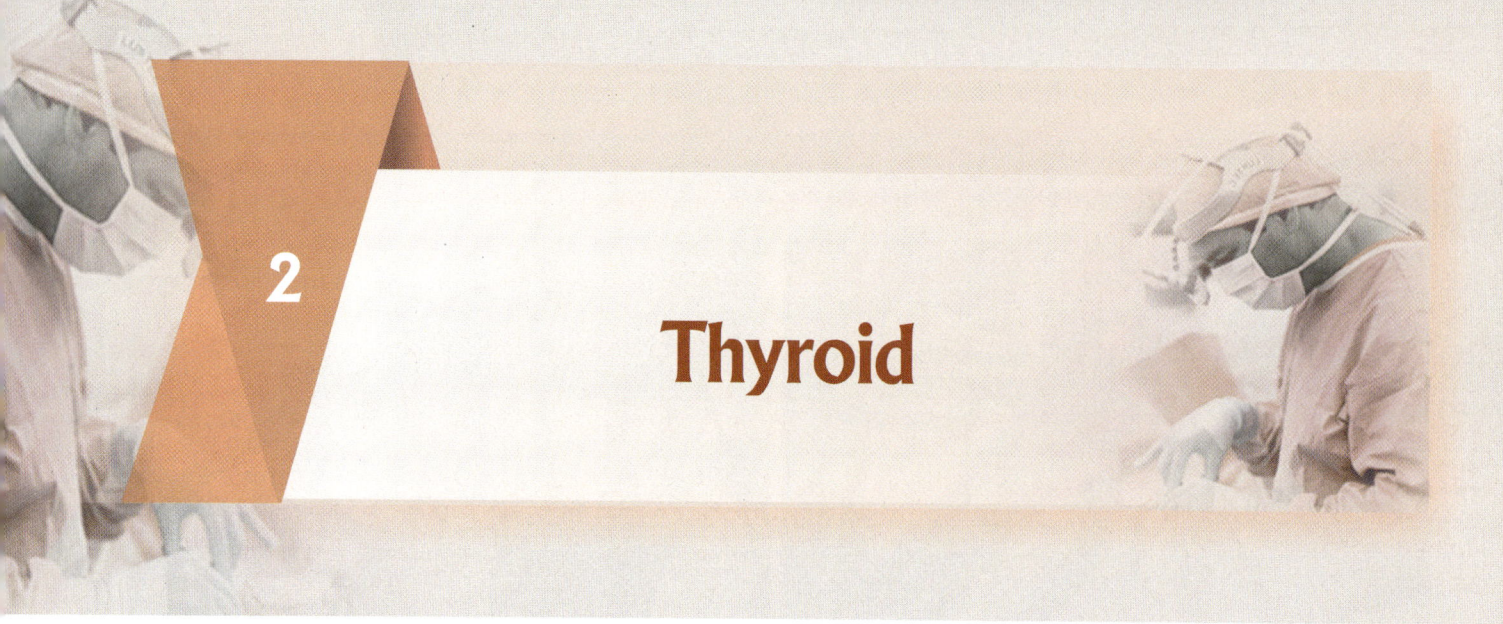

Thyroid

2

2.1 THYROIDECTOMY

Surgical Anatomy of Thyroid

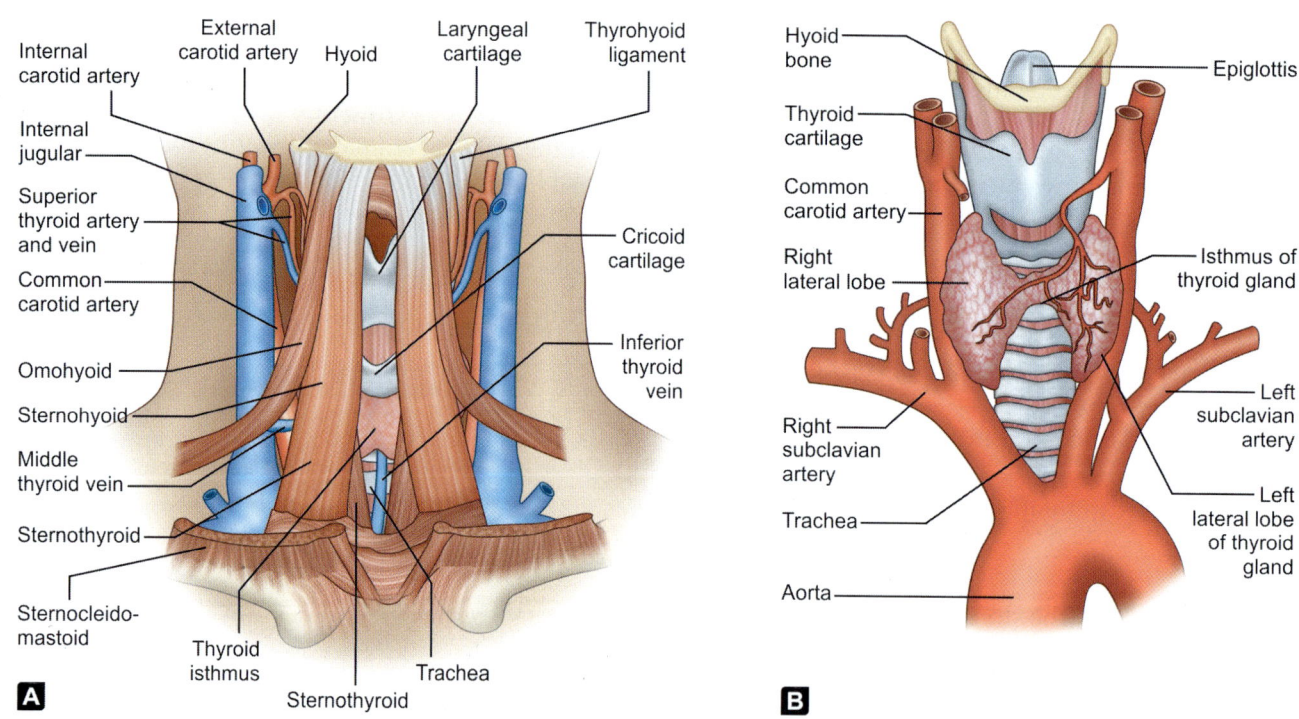

Anatomy of important structure in neck including thyroid

2.2 HEMITHYROIDECTOMY

Indications

1. Goiter and solitary nodule or multinodular
2. Hyperthyroidism at euthyroid state
3. Carcinoma thyroid (papillary carcinoma <1 cm and folicular carcinoma <4 cm)

If you want to live a happy life, tie it to a goal, not to people or objects.

Pitfalls

1. Injury or damage or inadvertent excision of parathyroid.
2. *Injury to recurrent laryngeal nerve* and superior laryngeal nerve sometimes.
3. Poor preoperative preparation of thyrotoxicosis patient may lead to thyroid storm.
4. Postoperative hypocalcemia due to damage of parathyroid glands.
5. Inadequate thyroid surgery.

Preoperative Preparation

- T_3, T_4, thyroid stimulating hormone (TSH) for all patients of thyroid disorder to exclude hypothyroid or hyperthyroid or subclinical hypothyroidism or hyperthyroidism.
- Before operation, make the patient euthyroid. For hyperthyroidism, neomercazole 10–20 mg 6 hourly 6–8 weeks and reassay.
- Propanolol 20–40 mg twice daily to relieve *cyclic vomiting syndrome* (CVS) symptoms, treatment to continue for minimum 10 days, postoperatively.
- To reduce vascularity, Lugol's iodine 10–15 drops thrice daily for 10 days prior to surgery or potassium iodide tablet 60 mg thrice daily for minimum 10 days.

Procedure

- General anesthesia (GA)
- *Position*: Supine with extended neck, sand bag or pillow to be placed beneath the shoulder and head rests on ring.
  Cleaning and draping, be sure that chin and long axis of body will be aligned at the midline.

Incision: Two to three centimeters/two fingers' breadth above the sternal notch from posterior border to opposite-sided posterior border of sternocleidomastoid (skin incision may be marked by silk thread pressure on the skin called garrote mark).

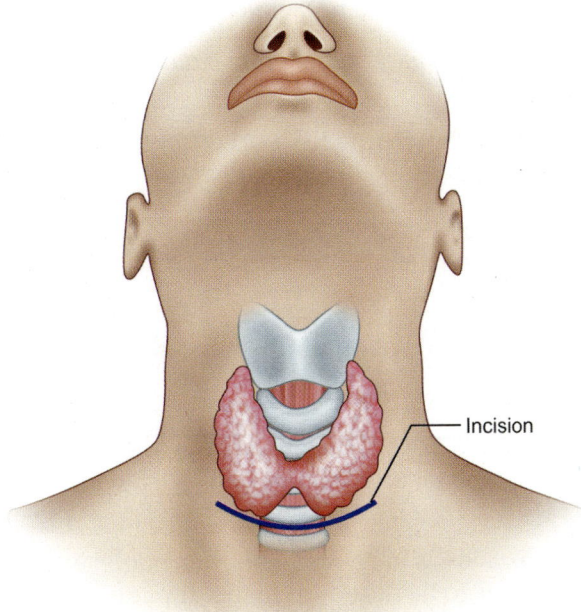

— Incision

Skin incision (Garrote mark) for thyroid surgery

Step 1: Raising of flap: Upper flap incision is to be carried out through superficial fascia and platysma. Keep at subplatysmal plane and upper flap is to be raised up to the upper border of thyroid cartilage.

Lower flap: Same way the skin, superficial fascia platysma is raised up to suprasternal notch.

Step 2: Opening of deep fascia: Longitudinal midline incision, incise the investing layer of deep fascia, anterior jugular vein to be ligated and divided on the way.

Step 3: Elevation of the strap muscles: After incising the deep fascia on the midline, the muscles are carefully lifted up from the thyroid to expose thyroid lobe with its false capsule (pretracheal fascia), the false capsule to be incised (sometime strap muscles are to be divided in case of large thyroid. Strap muscles to be divided at the upper level as the nerve enters the muscles from below).

Step 4: Exposure and mobilization of the gland: Put index finger in between the gland and the strap muscles gently to complete the separation of the gland and loose areolar tissue around the gland is also divided

Step 5: Division of veins: After dividing the loose areolar tissue, the displayed middle and inferior throid veins are to be ligated and divided. Inferior thyroid vein may be in close relation to recurrent laryngeal nerve. Be careful about it and try to identify the recurrent laryngeal nerve and save it.

Step 6: Division of superior thyroid vessels, near the superior pole of the lobe. The lobe to be exposed by retracting the muscles upward and laterally. The pedicle to be dissected close to the pole. Double ligation of proximal part of pedicle is advisable, taking care of the external laryngeal nerve.

Step 7: Division of inferior thyroid vessels: Retract the lobe medially and identify the branches of inferior thyroid artery. The branches are to be ligated and divided, sparing the branches for parathyroid glands. At this time, identify recurrent laryngeal nerve running vertically up along the tracheoesophageal groove (inferior thyroid veins to be ligated, if not ligated during ligation of middle thyroid vein).

Step 8: Division of lobe and isthmus: Dissect the lobe and isthmus from trachea. Ligate the isthmus at the junction of opposite lobe, carefully remove one lobe of thyroid along with the isthmus. Dream does not mean what you see in sleep. They are the things that do not let you sleep.

Step 9: Hemostasis to be achieved meticulously and suction drain is placed.

Step 10: Closure of the wound in layers, deep inversling layer, approximation of strap muscles, and platysma with 3-0 polyglactin then skin is closed interruptedly with 3-0 nylon or by subcuticular sutures for better cosmesis.

2.3 SUBTOTAL THYROIDECTOMY

General Anesthesia

- *Position*: Supine with extended neck, sand bag or pillow to be placed beneath the shoulder and head rests on ring.
- Cleaning and draping, be sure that chin and long axis of body will be aligned at the midline.
- *Incision*: Two to three centimeters/two fingers' breadth above the sternal notch from posterior border to opposite-sided posterior border of sternocleidomastoid (skin incision may be marked by silk thread pressure on the skin called garrote mark).

Step 1: Raising of flap: Upper flap incision is to be carried out through superficial fascia and platysma. Keep at subplatysmal plane and upper flap is to be raised up to the upper border of thyroid cartilage.

The lower flap: Same way, the skin, superficial fascia, platysma is raised up to suprasternal notch.

Good friends care for each other, close friends understand each other, but true friends stay forever beyond words, distance and time.

Step 2: Opening of deep fascia: Longitudinal midline incision. Incise the investing layer of deep fascia. The anterior jugular vein to be ligated and divided on the way.

Step 3: Elevation of the strap muscles: After incising the deep fascia on the midline, muscles are carefully lifted up from the thyroid to expose thyroid lobe with its false capsule (pretracheal fascia), the false capsule to be incised (sometime strap muscles are to be divided in case of large thyroid. Strap muscles to be divided at the upper level as the nerves enter the muscles form below).

Step 4: Exposure and mobilization of the gland: Put index finger in between the gland and the strap muscles gently to complete the separation of the gland and loose areolar tissue around the gland is also divided.

Step 5: Division of veins: After dividing the loose areolar tissue, the displayed middle and inferior thyroid veins are to be ligated and divided. Inferior thyroid vein may be in close relation to recurrent laryngeal nerve. Be careful about it. Try to identify the recurrent laryngeal nerve and save it.

Step 6: Division of superior thyroid vessels at superior pole of the lobe: The lobe to be exposed by retracting the muscles upward and laterally. The pedicle to be dissected close to the pole. Double ligation of proximal part of pedicle is advisable taking care of the external laryngeal nerve.

Step 7: Division of inferior thyroid vessels: Retract the lobe medially and identify the branches of inferior thyroid artery. The branches are to be ligated and divided, sparing the branches for parathyroid glands. At this time, identify recurrent laryngeal nerve running vertically up along the tracheoesophageal groove (inferior thyroid veins to be ligated, if not ligated during ligation of middle thyroid vein).

Now apply multiple hemostatic artery forceps and transect the lobe leaving behind a cuff of posterior thyroid tissue of either side of the trachea. Continuous hemostatic suture may be applied in each side of the remnant of thyroid tissue (it is usually 8 g; 4 g each side, measured by equal part of distal phalanx of the patient's thumb). Every attempt is to make to preserve recurrent laryngeal nerve and the parathyroid glands.

Step 8: Hemostasis to be achieved meticulously and suction drain is placed.

Step 9: Closure of the wound in layers: Deep investing layer, approximation of strap muscles, platysma with 3-0 polyglactin then skin is closed interruptedly with 3-0 nylon or by subcuticular sutures for better cosmesis.

2.4 TOTAL THYROIDECTOMY

It is same as bilateral hemithyroidectomy but risks are more in total thyroidectomy in term of recurrent laryngeal nerve and parathyroid's injury. Unilateral nerve damage causes deeper voice with less strength and cough. Bilateral damage may create emergency as paralyzed vocal cords obstruct airway. Tracheotomy may be required. Damage of external laryngeal nerve alters the voice significantly. Bilateral parathyroid damage for inadvertent excision or ligation of supplying artery (especially in singers as the nerve supplying to cricothyroid muscle which is a tensor of the vocal cord, may produce symptomatic hypothyroidism usually it manifests after 48 hours of surgery).

Lymphnode dissection in carcinoma thyroid: There are therapeutic values of prophylactic dissection in clinically negative node.
1. Well differentiated cancer
2. Medullary cancer:
   - Prophylactive level VI (central). Lymph node dissection in N0 nodes
   - MND-III in N1 nodes

How to find parathyroid glands during thyroid surgery: The best anatomical landmark khaki or brown in color but frequently covered with fat making them difficult to recognize.

Be sincere and absolute in your consecration to the divine and your life will become harmonious and beautiful.

The superior glands are more constant and lie on the posterior surface of the middle third of the posterior border of thyroid gland. If enlarged, they may descend into posterior mediastinum. The two inferior parathyroid glands usually lie close to the posterior surface of the interior poles of the thyroid gland within 1 cm below the pole. They lie on more anterior plane than the upper glands. The parathyroid gland is located within the surgical false capsule of the thyroid. The gland may be also embedded in the thyroid gland.

The strategy for finding of abnormally located parathyroid glands:

- Explore the superior surface of the thyroid gland, middle thyroid veins to be ligated and the lobe to be retracted medially and anteriorly and the recurrent laryngeal nerve will be exposed.
- Dissect anterosuperior mediastinum, see the thymus and its remnant behind the manubrium.
- Dissect above the upper pole of thyroid gland as far as the hyoid bone.
- Retroesophageal and retropharyngeal spaces may be explored.
- Subtotal thyroidectomy may be performed to find out the parathyroids.
- In near total thyroidectomy, a rim of thyroid tissue to be kept to prevent recurrent laryngeal nerve injury and to save the parathyroid glands. Practically total thyroidectomy is very difficult to perform. Almost every cases, it is recommended total or near total thyroidectomy performed, even in a very expert hand.
- In case of total thyroidectomy, particularly in carcinoma thyroid, better you divide the sternothyroid muscle as high as possible. So that you can ligate and divide the superior thyroid pedicle far away from the pole. Otherwise you definitely leave some thyroid tissue along the pedicle inadvertently.

Remember: Sternothyroid lies below the sternohyoid.

- Recently, most inferior approach is becoming popular to identify the recurrent laryngeal nerve. You know right recurrent laryngeal nerve is more difficult to identify than the left.
- The IMA approach is the dissection along the common carotid artery and division of the most lateral tributory of inferior thyroid vein.
- The nerve will be identified at the same level, especially at the bottom of the triangle of recurrent *laryngeal nerve* (RLN). [The RLN triangle is bounded by trachea/esophagus, carotid artery/IJV and inferior thyroid pole.]
- It is an easy, quick and safe approach for identifying the RLN.

2.5 PARATHYROIDECTOMY

SURGICAL ANATOMY

Indications

1. Primary hyperparathyroidism with the following:
   - Hypercalcemia more than 14.5 mg% (3.62 mmol/L)
   - Renal stone
   - Bone pain
   - Urinary excretion of calcium more than 400 mg/day
   - Age less than 50 years, etc.
2. Secondary hyperparathyroidism: As a result of chronic renal failure (CRF), malabsorption with the following:
   - Bone pain and spontaneous bone fracture
   - Serum calcium more than 12 mg%
   - Vascular calcification
   - Psychoneurologic symptoms, etc.
3. Parathyroid adenoma
4. Parathyroid carcinoma.

Always do your best and the Lord will take care of the result.

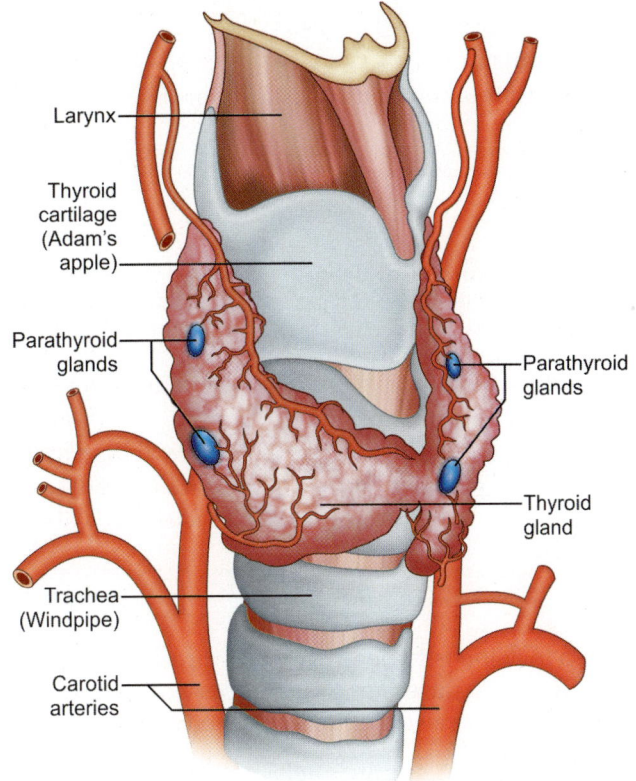

Larynx

Thyroid cartilage (Adam's apple)

Parathyroid glands

Parathyroid glands

Thyroid gland

Trachea (Windpipe)

Carotid arteries

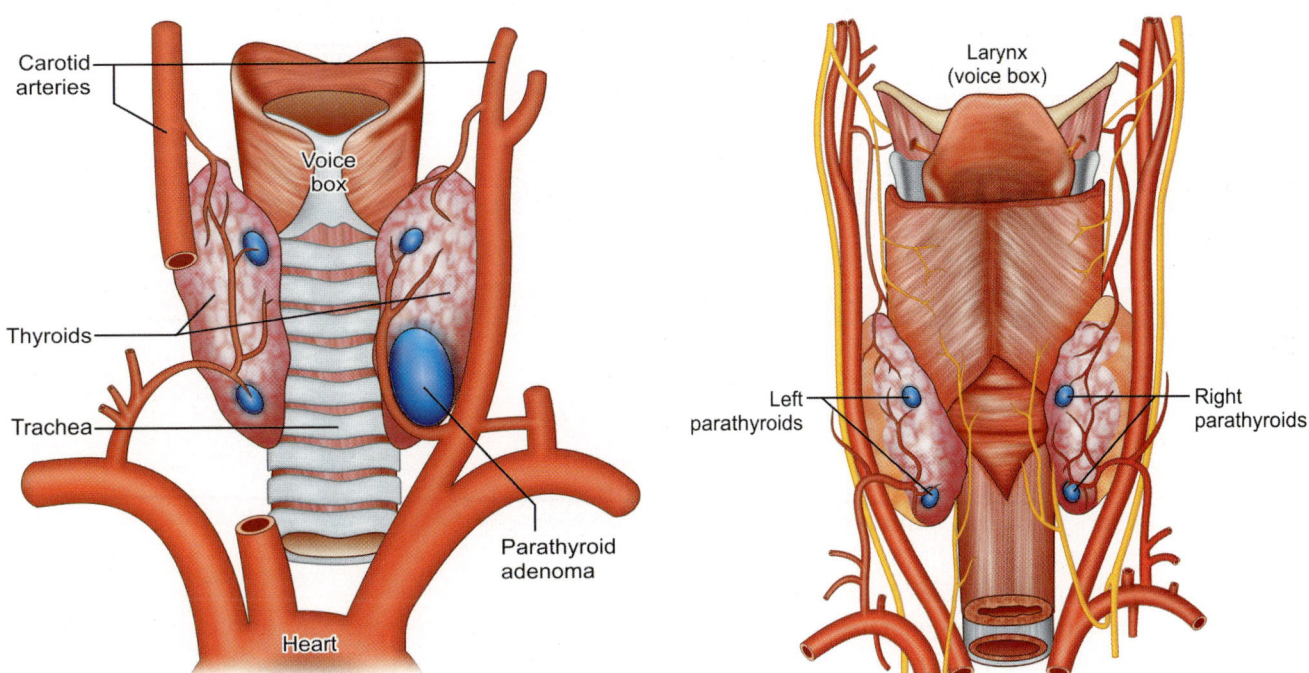

Carotid arteries

Voice box

Thyroids

Trachea

Parathyroid adenoma

Heart

Larynx (voice box)

Left parathyroids

Right parathyroids

Anatomy of parathyroid glands

Don't you feel bad if people remember you only when they need you. Feel privileged that you are like a candle that comes to their minds, when there is darkness in their lives.

Pitfalls

1. Failure to find out the offending adenoma
2. Failure to cure the disease owing to missing of multiglandular disease
3. Recurrent laryngeal nerve injury.

Preoperative Preparation

- Laryngoscopy
- Serum calcium and potassium day before operation.

Procedure

1. Position supine with extended neck, sand bag or pillow to be placed beneath the shoulder and head rests on ring.
2. Cleaning and draping, be sure that chin and long axis of body will be aligned at the midline.
3. *Incision:* Two to three centimeters/two fingers' breadth above the sternal notch from posterior border to opposite-sided posterior border of sternocleidomastoid (skin incision may be marked by silk thread pressure on the skin called garrote mark).

Steps of Operation

Step 1: Raising of flap: Upper flap incision is to be carried out through superficial fascia and platysma. Keep at subplatysmal plane and upper flap is to raised up to the upper border of thyroid cartilage, lower flap same way the skin superficial fascia platysma is raised up to suprasternal notch.

Step 2: Opening of deep fascia: Longitudinal midline incision will incise anterior jugular veins, the investing layer of deep fascia veins to be ligated and divided on the way.

Step 3: Elevation of the strap muscles: Incised deep fascia along with strap muscles is carefully lifted up from the thyroid to expose lateral lobe with its false capsule (pretracheal fascia), the false capsule to be incised (sometime strap muscles are to be divided in case of large thyroid. Strap muscles to be divided at the upper level as the nerves enter the muscles from below).

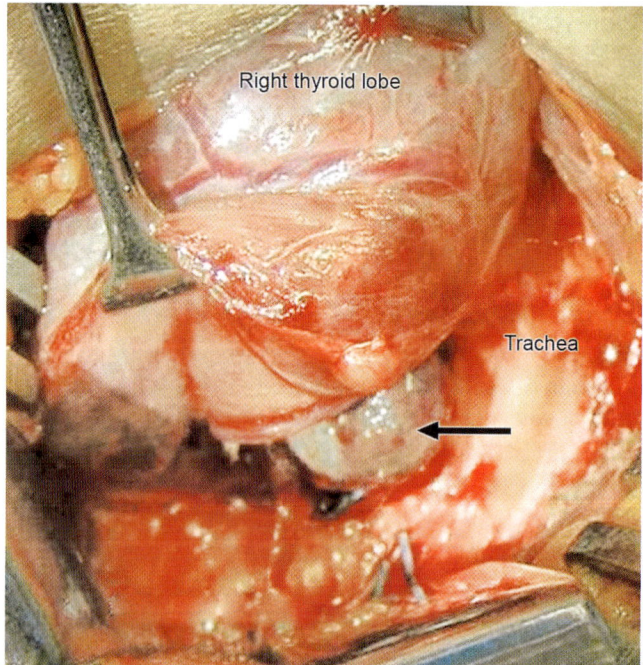

Parathyroid adenoma

Step 4: Exposure and mobilization of the gland: Put index finger in between the gland and the strap muscles gently to complete separation of the gland and loose areolar tissue around the gland is also divided.

Step 5: Strategy for finding parathyroid gland:

1. Exposure to superior surface of thyroid gland
2. Ligate middle thyroid vein
3. Retract the thyroid lobe anteriorly and medially
4. Identify the recurrent laryngeal nerve and save it
5. Dissect toward anterosuperior mediastinum as far as possible. Thymus or its remnant may be identified.

If you want to keep long relationship, follow a simple rule – never lie.

6. Above dissect the upper pole of the gland close to hyoid bone
7. Find the parathyroid like this way:
   - Superior parathyroid glands are more constant in position usually lies at the middle of the posterior border of the lobe of thyroid.

And it is usually dorsal to recurrent laryngeal nerve.
- Inferior parathyroid glands are more variable in position may be:
  - Within the thyroid capsule below inferior thyroid artery and near the lower pole of thyroid.
  - Behind and outside of thyroid capsule, just above the inferior thyroid artery.
  - Within the substance of the lobe near its posterior border.
  It is usually ventral to the recurrent laryngeal nerve.

Step 6: Excision of the adenoma:
- Mobilize it from the surrounding structure.
- Preserve the recurrent laryngeal nerve.
- Tackle the hilar blood supply to the adenoma (the terms subtotal parathyroidectomy that means three and half glands to be removed is usually not done).
  In case of carcinoma parathyroid along with the tumor, additional hemithyroidectomy to be done.
  Remove all four parathyroid glands, one by one, mobilizing from the surrounding tissues and tackling the vascular supply. And then, a small piece of one of the parathyroids is implanted into the muscle.

Step 7: Auto-transplantation: Fragments of the glands to be implanted in brachioradialis muscle of the forearm or in sternocleidomastoid muscle in the neck. Marker stitch is to be placed at the site of implantation.

Procedure

1. A longitudinal incision to be made in the volar aspect of the non-dominant forearm.
2. Divide subcoutaneous tissue, down to the forearm muscles, especially brachioradialis.
3. Create 10–12 pockets in the muscle along the direction of its fibers.
4. Place the piece of parathyroid $1 \times 1 \times 1$ mm³ in the small pocket. 1–2 mm pieces of parathyroid tissue to be transplanted. Minimum one-third of total volume [200 mg (as each parathyroid weighs approximately 50 mg) × one-third = 66.67 mg] to be implanted.

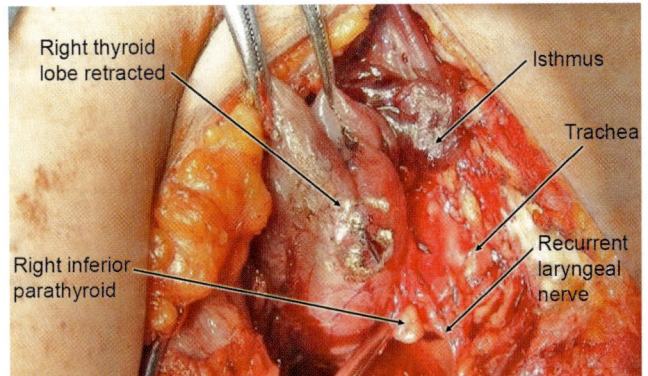

Relations of thyroid, parathyroids and recurrent laryngeal nerve

If you want to live a happy life, tie it to a goal, not to a people or object.

5. Close it over after putting a mark suture or with clips.
6. Close the subcutaneous tissue and skin.

Step 8: Closure of the wound in layers: Deep investing layer, approximation of strap muscles, platysma by 3-0 polyglactin then skin are opposed interruptedly or by subcuticular sutures.

Suppose adenoma (enlarged parathyroid) not found, what to do then?

- Once again search the usual locations of parathyroids.
- Next follow the branches of inferior thyroid artery. Look for any enlarged branch, trace it. It may lead to suspected adenoma.
- Otherwise, incise thyroid capsule over any area of discoloration that might be due to devascularization of intrathyroid and parathyroid glands.
- If still not found, trace thymothymic ligament and search for intrathymic adenoma.
- Otherwise inspect and palpable behind the pharynx and esophagus.
- Next open the carotid sheath, look along the vagus nerve. Otherwise look for its embryonic course from hyoid to aortic arch.
- Other techniques are:
  - Thyroid lobectomy at the missing side
  - A cervical thymectomy may be another way.

Complications

Immediate

- Bleeding
- Upper airway obstruction
- Laryngospasm
- Recurrent laryngeal nerve injury
- Tracheomalacia with upper airway obstruction
- Superior laryngeal nerve palsy—though it is rare
- Hypocalcemia usually manifests after 48 hours as circumoral paresthesia and twitching, carpopedal spasm (twiching and weakness of tongue muscles, forearm muscles, hand, foot and digits). Hypocalcemia is usually temporary. It lasts for 46 weeks.
- Additional thyroidectomy may be required
- Postoperative hungry bone syndrome may be developed where suddenly—calcium absorption is increased by the bone.

Late

- Permanent hypoparathyroidism.
- One percent chance of recurrent laryngeal nerve palsy.
- Five percent chance of persistent hyperparathyroidism.

Management of Hypoparathyroidism and Hypocalcemia

Send blood for serum ionized calcium on second postoperative day, i.e. after 48 hours.

↓

If it is normal, i.e. 9–11 mg%, nothing to be done just observe for the symptoms

↓

If patient is symptomatic and serum calcium is between 6 mg% and 8 mg%, start oral calcium 500 mg to 1 g QDS.

Dose is 3 g elemental calcium orally per day.

↓

If it is less than 6 mg%.
- Start injection calcium gluconate 10% (10 mL) intravenous (IV) 6–8 hourly, depends upon the severity of symptoms. One amp calcium gluconate (10 mL of 10% calcium gluconate contains 1 g calcium gluconate) in 500 mL of 5% dextrose over 5–6 hours.

Recheck calcium after an hour, check magnesium and correct it, if necessary, 10 mL of 10% magnesium. Intravenous (IV) OD

↓

Then switch over to oral elemental calcium 1 g with vitamin D (1–2 µg daily).

↓

When consecutive, two values of calcium are stable or increasing, the patient can be given oral. Calcium in tapering dose as follows:
- One gram elemental calcium TID for 1 week
- One gram elemental calcium BID for 1 week
- One gram elemental calcium OD.

Remember: 2.5 g of calcium carbonate is equivalent to 1 g of elemental calcium.

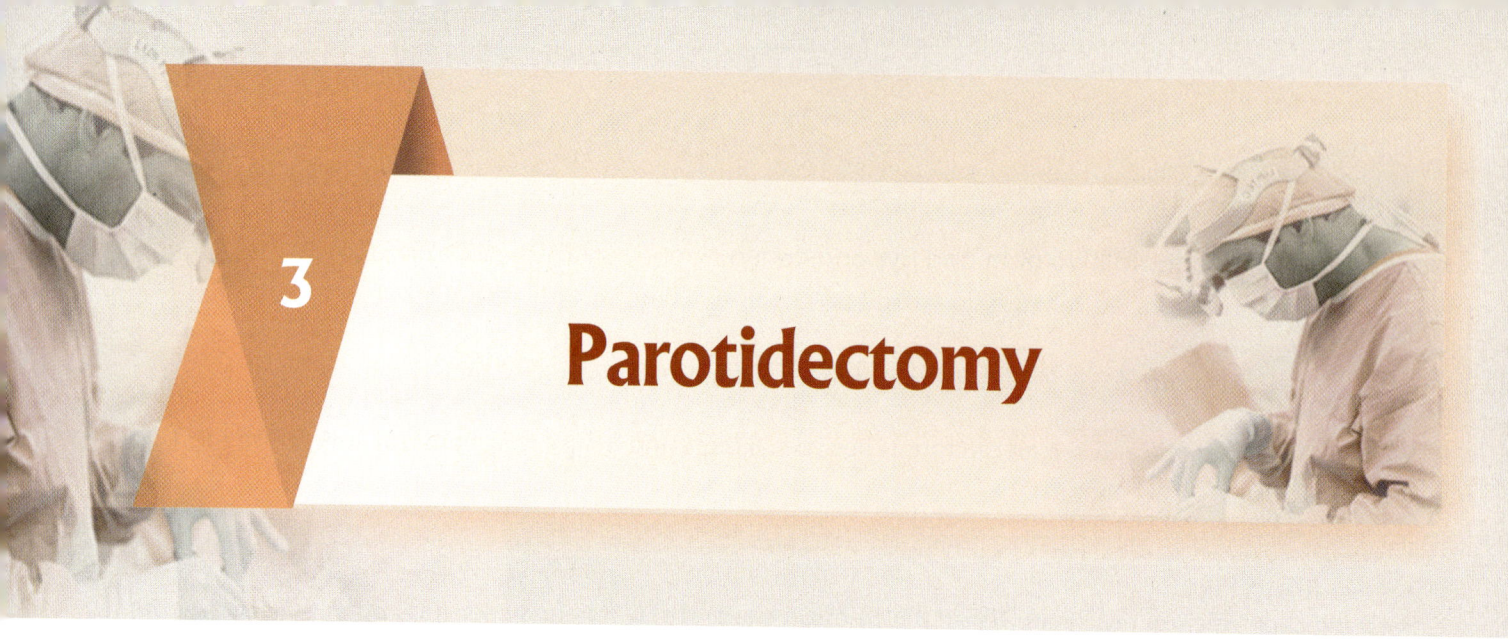

SURGICAL ANATOMY

Surgical anatomy and relations of parotid gland.

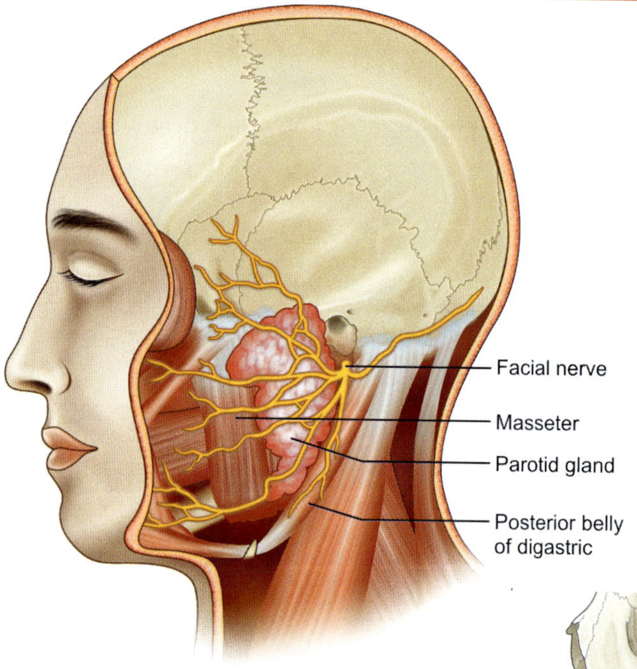

- Facial nerve
- Masseter
- Parotid gland
- Posterior belly of digastric

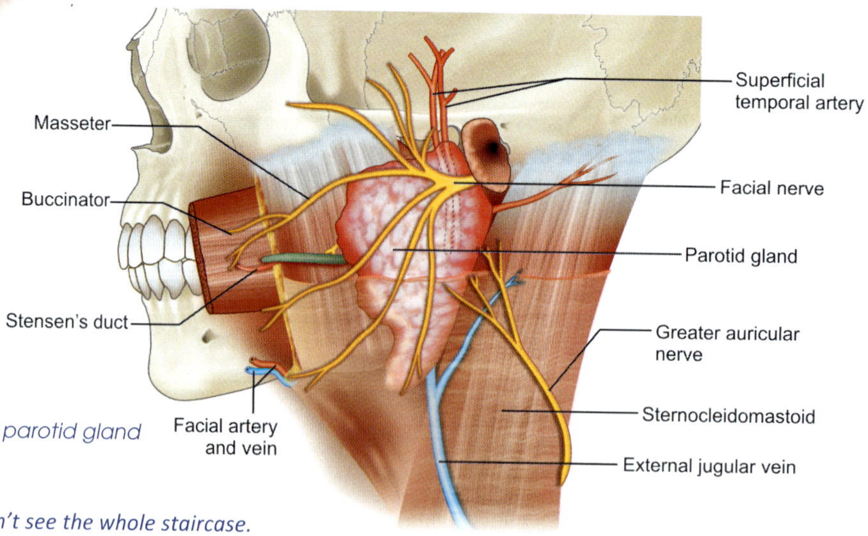

- Masseter
- Buccinator
- Stensen's duct
- Facial artery and vein

- Superficial temporal artery
- Facial nerve
- Parotid gland
- Greater auricular nerve
- Sternocleidomastoid
- External jugular vein

Surgical anatomy and relations of parotid gland

Faith is taking the first step even when you can't see the whole staircase.

3.1 SUPERFICIAL PAROTIDECTOMY

Indications

- Parotid tumors benign or malignant (most common)
- Chronic sialadenitis
- Parotid duct calculus.

Pitfalls

- Facial nerve injury or injury to its branch or branches.
- Inadequate margin for mixed protid tumor there by high chance of local recurrence.
- Frey's syndrome 25–50% of patients.

Procedure

1. General anesthesia
2. *Position*: Extended neck with face turned to opposite side. Uncover the outer canthus of the eye and the angle of mouth. Clean the external auditory canal (to see the facial nerve stimulation during dissection, so that we can avoid inadvertent injury to the nerve or its branches).
3. *Incision*: Lazy "S", inverted "T" or modified "Y".

   Lazy "S": Make an incision just below the zygomatic process 3 mm in front of the tragus, it curves backward around the ear lobule, it extends close to mastoid process then descends downward along the anterior border of upper third of sternomastoid muscle.

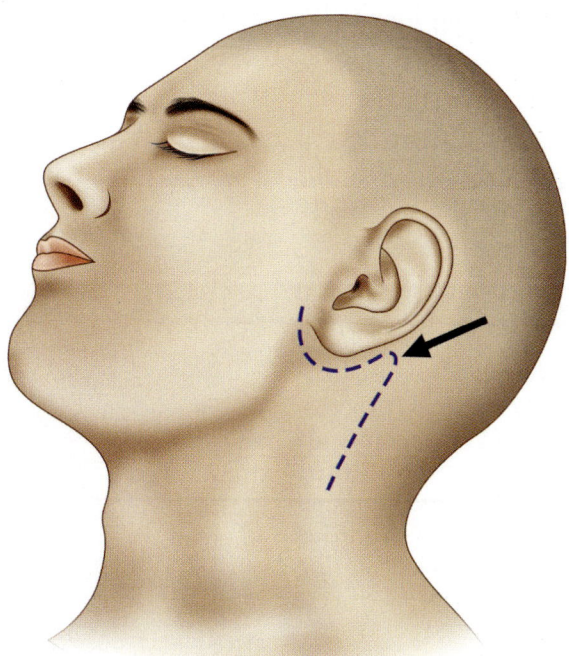

Lazy "S" incision: Most commonly used incision for parotidectomy

---

Maturity is not when we start speaking big things. It is when we start understanding small things.

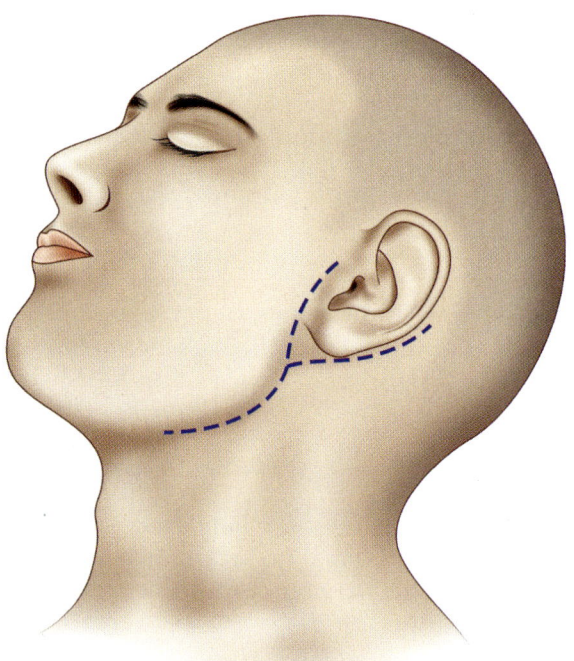

Modified "Y"

Inverted "T" incision: Some surgeons prefer inverted "T" incision about 3–4 mm in front of the tragus with downward-curved extension at the posterior angle of the mandible. Make a transverse-curved incision 3 cm below the mandible with posterior extension close to the mastoid.

Modified "Y" incision: Vertical preauricular or postauricular incisions which join at the angle of the mandible form a Y-shape which meets a transverse incision 3 cm below the mandible.

Step 1: Deepening the incision deep into superficial fascia fat, platysma anteriorly and fat posteriorly.

Step 2: Formation of flaps: Elevate the flap at subplatysmal plane, upward up to zygomatic process, laterally toward the external auditory canal, below up to posterior belly of diagastric and posteriorly toward the mastoid process with proper traction and counter-traction (in the vicinity of lower flap and lower border of parotid, the greater auricular nerve and posterior facial vein are very close so they are usually sacrificed during the raising of lower flap).

Step 3: Identification of facial nerve

1. Place the distal phalanx of the index finger over the mastoid process pointing toward the eye of the patient. The direction of the facial nerve in this direction.

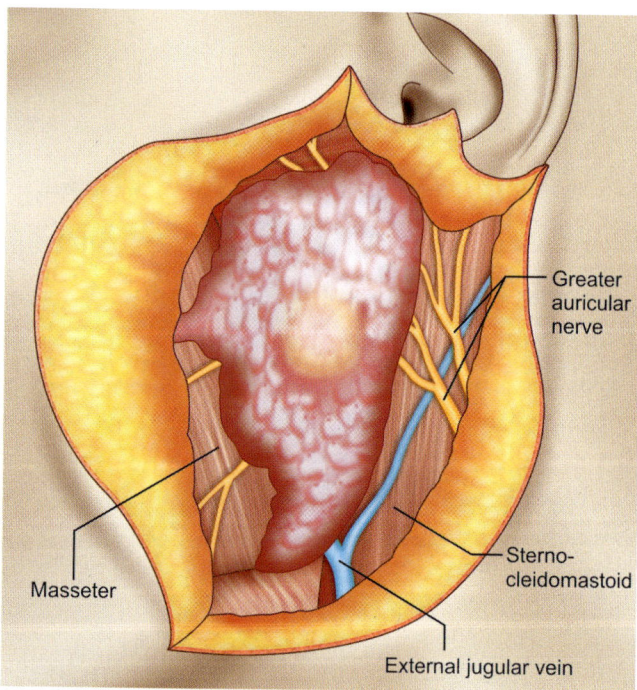

Skin flaps are raised and the surrounding structures related with parotid are exposed

The inner peace begins the moment you choose—not to allow another person or event to control your emotion.

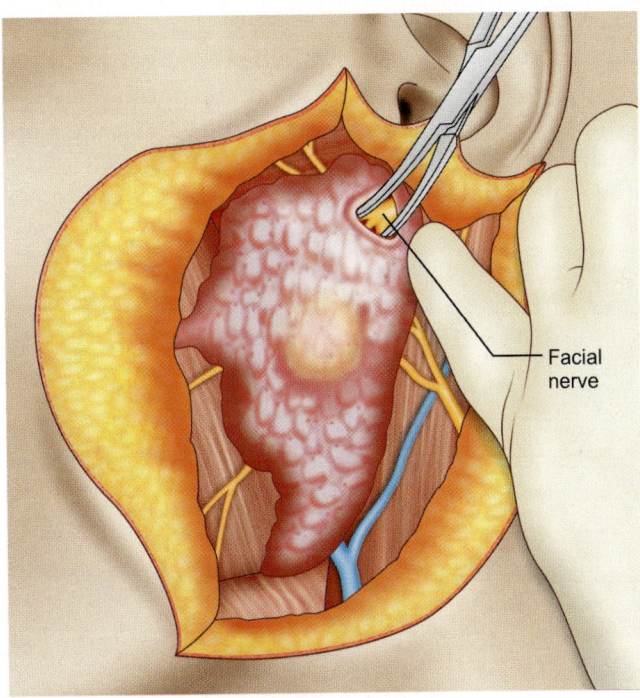

Exposure of facial nerve trunk

2. The end of tragal cartilage is termed as Conley's pointer. The facial nerve lies 1 cm deep and inferior to this pointer.

3. The nerve lies at the junction of bony and cartilaginous part of external auditory canal.

4. There is a groove between mastoid process and bony external auditory canal. The nerve lies deep to this groove.

5. Near the insertion of posterior belly of digastric muscle into the mastoid process, look the nerve at medial border of the muscle close to its insertion. Author prefers this technique.

6. The nerve emerges from stylomastoid foramen. The facial nerve can be identified just lateral to the styloid process.

Author prefers to identify the nerve in this way: After incising the deep fascia at the lower part of parotid, it is to be lifted up. Digastric muscle to be mobilized up to its origin. At this time, junction of bony and cartilaginous part may be exposed where the nerve can be identified otherwise palpate the styloid process and just lateral to the foramen identify the nerve or trace the nerve at the medial border of digastric attachment (practically, the nerve lies in deeper plane than expected). If there is any doubt about the nerve, electric stimulation can be used.

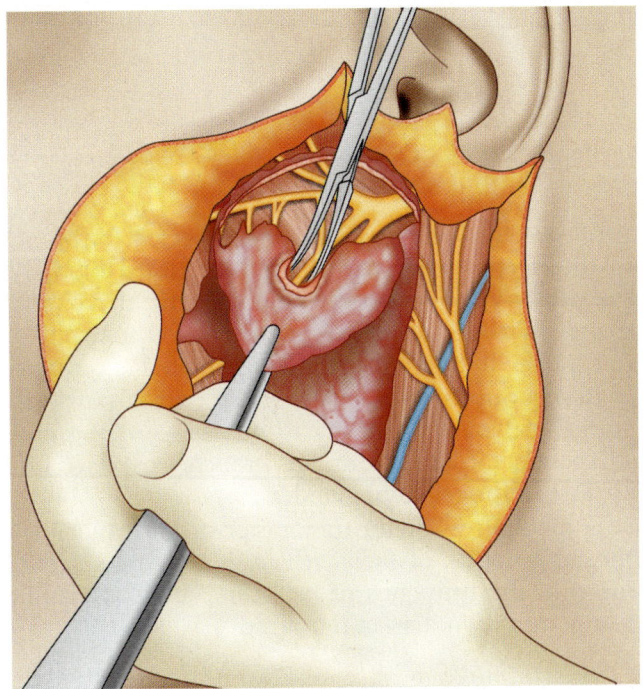

Exposure of individual branches of facial nerve

It is a long journey between human being and being a human. Let us walk at least one step daily to cover the distance.

Another way to identify the facial nerve

- Place the distal phalanx of index finger over the mastoid pointing toward the eye of the patient.
- Incise the parotid facia and mobilize the superficial pat of the parotid.
- Dissect carefully between mastoid process and the gland and retract the gland medially stem of the nerve is found at the depth of centimeter.
- Give traction upward on the superficial lobe and start dissecting over the nerve.

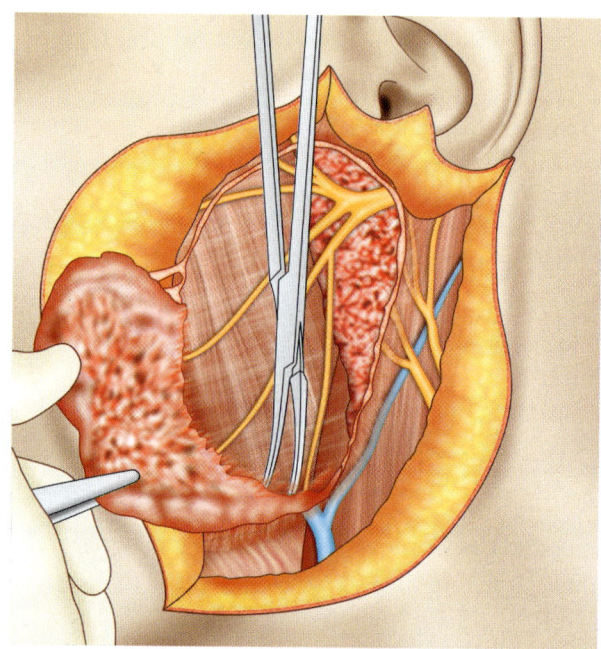

Exposure of facial nerve branches after superficial parotidectomy

Step 4: Removal of superficial lobe of parotid: Put a gentle traction over the gland and dissect all the branches of the nerve along with their directions toward the periphery. Mobilize the whole superficial part of the gland. During the process of dissection, parotid duct (Stensen's duct) will be dissected, ligated and divided.

Resect out the whole superficial part of parotid, i.e. superficial parotidectomy to be done. At the end of dissection, facial nerve and its branches exposed on the surface of the residual gland.

Sometimes when the tumor is posteriorly placed near the main trunk of facial nerve, it may be simpler to identify the branches of facial nerve away from the tumor and then dissect retrograde.

Step 5: Drainage and closure: Place a closed suction drain through a puncture wound posterior to the incision.

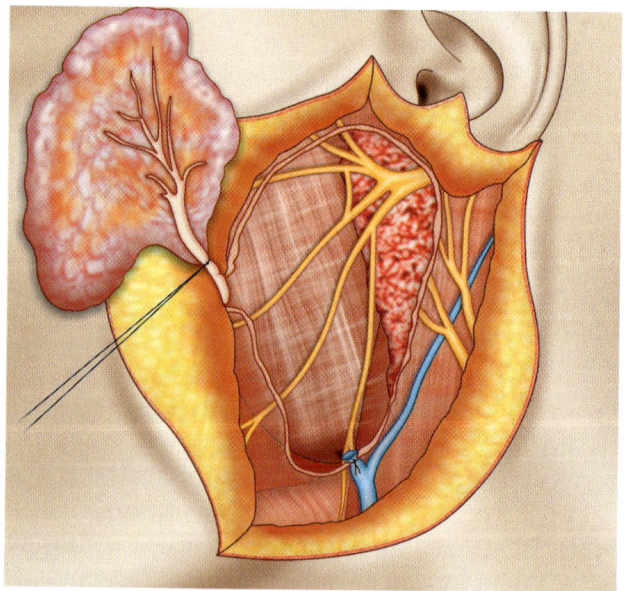

Identification and ligation of parotid duct before removal of superficial lobe

---

A strong and positive attitude creates more miracles than any other things, because life is 10% how you make it and 90% how you take it.

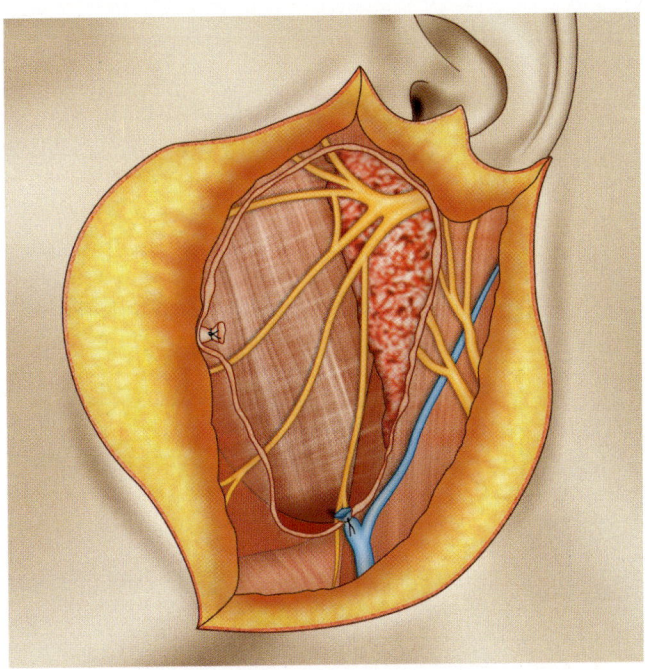

Before closing, the parotid bed should be looked like this

Incised wound is closed in layers, initially platysma and subcutaneous fat with 3-0 vicryl and skin is closed with 4-0 nylon (keep the drain for 3, 4 days till the drainage is less than 30 mL).

Complications

1. Facial weakness can be either temporary (due to neuropraxia) or permanent (due to injury to the facial nerve or as a result of radical parotidectomy).
2. Hemorrhage, hematoma (primary, reactionary, secondary)
3. Infection
4. Frey's syndrome gustatory sweating and flushing over the skin of parotid region after parotidectomy. As a result of injury of the innervations of the salivary gland during dissection, there is in appropriate regeneration of parasympathetic autonomic nerve fibers which stimulate the sweat gland of the overlying skin during chewing of food.
5. Facial numbness
6. Sialocele
7. Numbness over the ear lobule due to injury to greater auricular nerve.

3.2 TOTAL PAROTIDECTOMY

Step 1: Deepening the incision deep into superficial fascia fat, platysma anteriorly and posteriorly fat only. If you never taste bad apple, you would never appreciate a good apple. Sometimes, we need to experience bitterness of life to understand the value of sweetness.

Step 2: Formation of flaps: Elevate the flap at subplatysmal place upward up to zygomatic process laterally toward the external auditory canal below up to posterior belly of digastric and posteriorly toward the mastoid process with proper traction and counter-traction. (In the vicinity of lower flap and lower border of parotid,

Someone who knows how to smile in all circumstances is very close to true equality of soul.

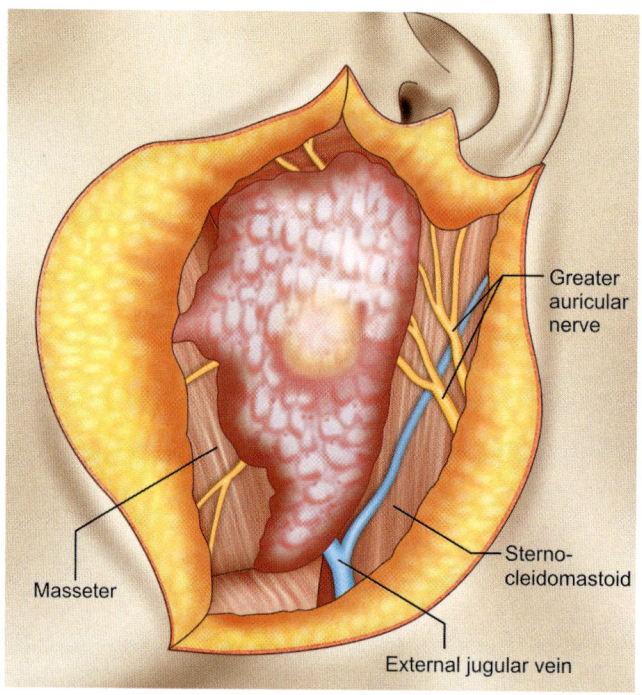

Skin flaps are raised and the surrounding structures related with parotid are exposed

the greater auricular nerve and posterior facial vein are very close so they are usually sacrificed during the raising of lower flap.)

Step 3: Identification of facial nerve

1. Place the distal phalanx of the index finger over the mastoid process pointing toward the eye of the patient.
2. The end of tragal cartilage is termed as Conley's pointer. The facial nerve lies 1 cm deep and inferior to this pointer.
3. The nerve lies at the junction of bony and cartilaginous part of external auditory canal.
4. There is a groove between mastoid process and bony external auditory canal. The nerve lies deep to this groove.
5. Near the insertion of posterior belly of digastric muscle into the mastoid process, look the nerve at medial border of the muscle close to its insertion.
6. The nerve emerges from stylomastoid foramen. The facial nerve can be identified just lateral to the styloid process.

   After incising the deep fascia at the lower part of parotid, it is to be lifted up. Digastric muscle to be mobilized up to its origin. At this time, junction of bony and cartilaginous part may be exposed where

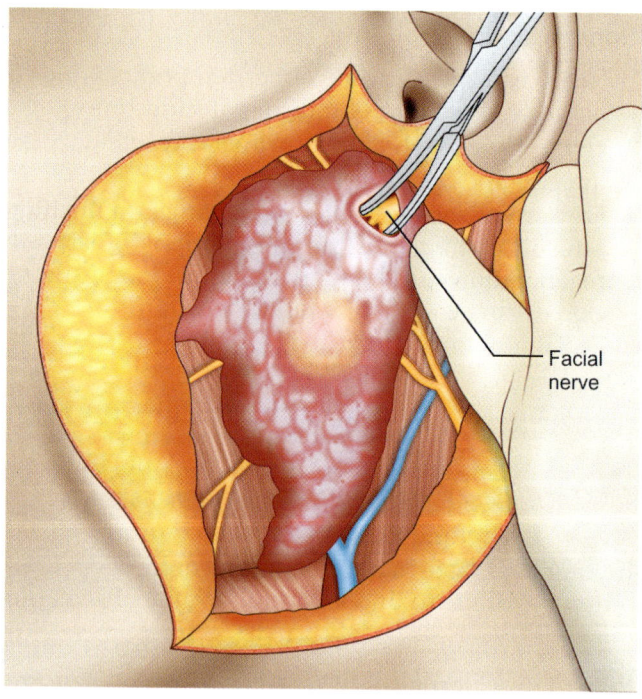

Exposure of facial nerve trunk

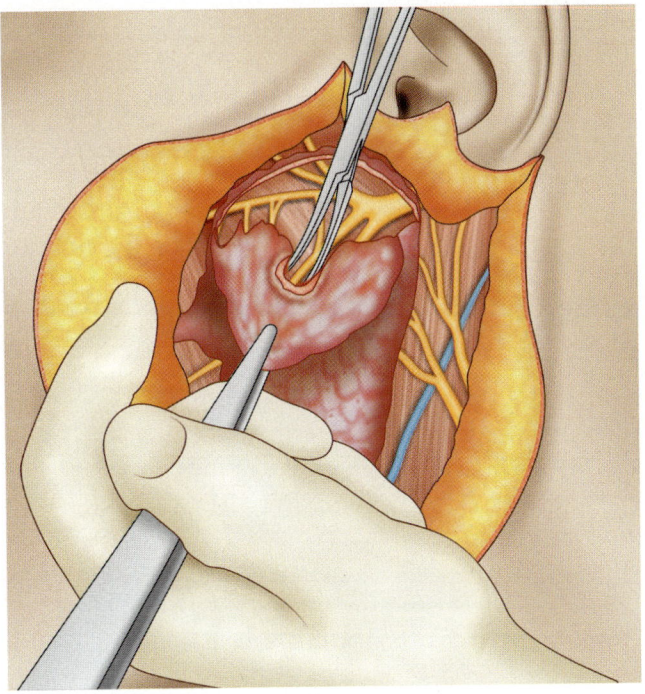

Exposure of individual branches of facial nerve

the nerve can be identified otherwise palpate the styloid process and just lateral to it identify the nerve (practically, the nerve lies in deeper plane than expected). If there is any doubt about the nerve, electric stimulation can be used.

Another Way to Identify the Facial Nerve

- Place the distal phalanx of index finger over the mastoid pointing toward the eye of the patient.
- Incise the parotid facia and mobilize the superficial part of the parotid.
- Dissect carefully between mastoid process and the gland and retract the gland medially, stem of the nerve is found at the depth of half centimeter.
- Give traction upward on the superficial lobe and start dissecting over the nerve.

Step 4: Removal of superficial parotid lobe: Put a gentle traction over the gland and dissect all the branches of the nerve along with their directions toward the periphery. Mobilize the whole superficial part of the gland. During the process of dissection, parotid duct (Stensen's duct) will be dissected, ligated and divided.

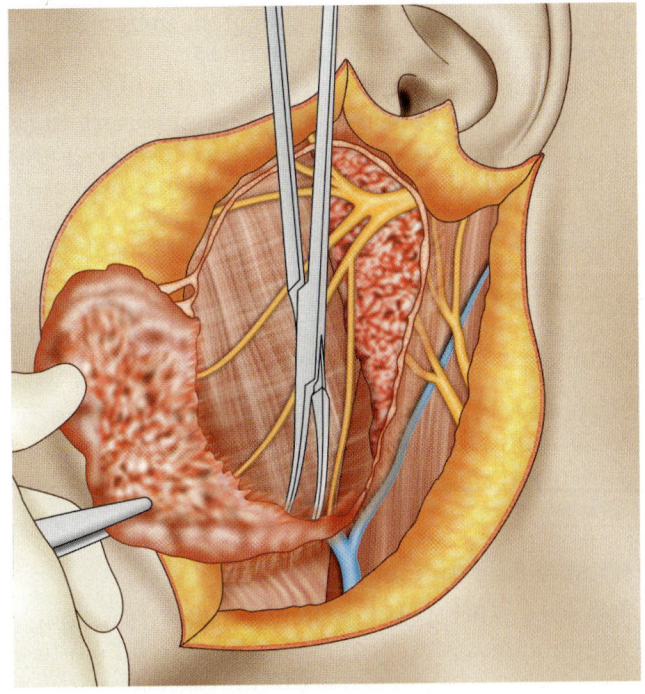

Exposure of facial nerve branches after superficial parotidectomy

Time decides whom you met in life, your heart decides whom you want in life and your behavior decides who will stay in your life.

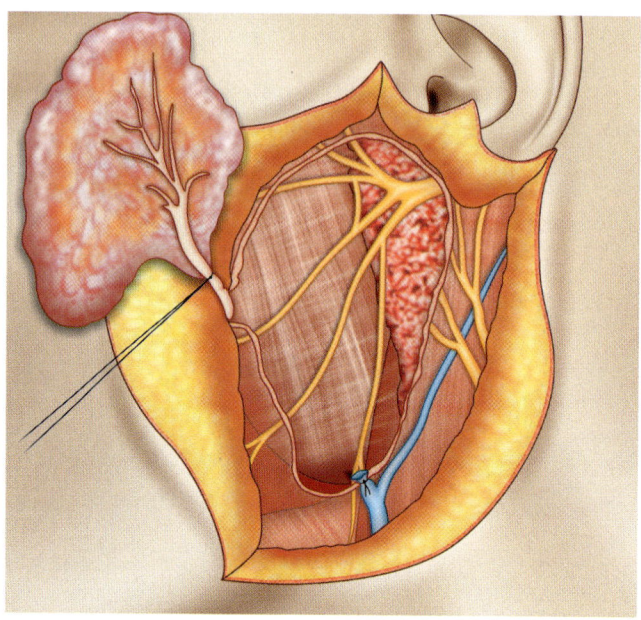

Identification and ligation of parotid duct before removal of superficial lobe

Resect out the whole superficial part of parotid, i.e. superficial parotidectomy to be done. At the end of dissection, facial nerve and its branches exposed on the surface of the residual gland.

Step 5: Resection of deep lobe: Mobilization of deep part of parotid gland begins with separation of facial nerve and its branches form underlying residual tissue. Posterior facial vein to be dissected, ligated and divided after careful separation of the marginal mandible nerve. Now, superficial temporal artery and vein to be encountered, ligated and divided.

Maxillary and superficial temporal arteries to be encountered. Elevate the lower border of the gland and now the branches from external carotid artery to be ligated and divided. At the anterior border of the gland, internal, maxillary and transverse facial arteries are to be ligated and divided. Sometimes, the external carotid artery is to be ligated and divided to mobilize the lobe. The deep part may now be removed (bleeding from pterygoid venous plexus may be stopped by compression for 5 minutes). Working under facial nerve piecemeal, dissection technique may be used. Obtain complete homeostasis.

Step 6: Drainage and closure: Place a closed suction drain through a puncture wound posterior to the incision. Incised wound is closed in layers, initially platysma and subcutaneous fat is closed with 4-0 nylon (keep the drain for 3, 4 days till the drainage is less than 30 mL).

Remember: Complete removal of parotid gland reveals the following structures. The pneumonic is *video-assisted neck surgery* (VANS), i.e. (1) vein: internal jugular; (2) artery: external crotid artery; (3) nerves: glossopharyngeal, vagus, spinal, accessory and hypoglossal and (4) "S" for styloid process and styloglossus, stylopharyngeus and stylohyoid muscles.

Radical Parotidectomy

The term radical parotidectomy is used when along with excision of parotid gland into the facial never regional lymphnodes are to be removed. Ipsilateral modified neck dissection may be necessary sometimes. Even in locally aggressive malignant tumor, excision of the temporomandibular joint, the mastoid process, the external auditory meatus and overlying soft tissue to be removed. Such radical surgery is being done rarely as the result is not satisfactory and gross disfigurement is obvious.

Management of Complications

1. *Parotid fistula* may be glandular or duct fistula. Glandular fistula usually regresses spontaneously within two to three weeks. Anticholinergic, like propanthaline bromide 50 mg QDS or hyoscine bromide 15 mg twice in divided doses for 10–15 days may be given in case of duct fistula. If there is stenosis at the terminal part of the duct, surgical intervention (papillotomy) may allow good drainage and fistula may heal automatically.

   If the fistula is related to main duct and stenosis, other site than terminal part resection and reconstruction is the option. If it fails, total parotidectomy is the curative option.

2. *Frey's syndrome:* Management

   a. *Preventive:*
      i. Following parotidectomy, sternomastoid muscle flap may be placed on parotid bed.
      ii. Alternative is temporalis fascial flap.
      iii. Artificial membrane is placed between the parotid bed and the overlying skin.

   b. *Established case:*
      i. Surgical intervention is not satisfactory so patient is to be counseled to adjust mentally with this syndrome that is the best way.
      ii. Local antiperspirants may relieve the symptoms to some extent.
      iii. Some time injection botulinum toxin into the affected skin may give relief.
      iv. Tympanic neurectomy has got some role to play in selective cases.

3.3 SUBMANDIBULAR SALIVARY GLAND EXCISION

Indications

- Chronic inflammation and pain of the gland
- Repeated stone formation
- Pleomorphic adenoma of the gland
- Submandibular gland tumors—mostly malignant.

Procedures

1. General anesthesia
2. Extended neck with turning to opposite site
3. Cleaning and draping.

Incision: A transverse incision is made 3 cm (two finger breadths) below the ramus and lower border of the mandible.

Step 1: Raising of superficial flap: The incision is deepened down to body of the gland. The superficial flap, consisting of skin, platysma and investing layer of the gland is raised up to the ramus and lower border of mandible.

   Incise the superficial fascia from the anterior border of the sternocleidomastoid muscle to 3 cm short of midline.

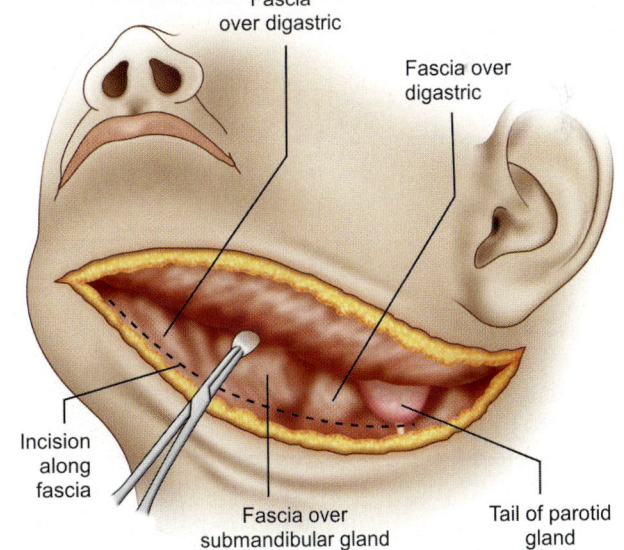

Upper flap is raised to see the submandibular salivary gland and its surrounding structures

Labels: Fascia over digastric; Fascia over digastric; Incision along fascia; Fascia over submandibular gland; Tail of parotid gland

---

A person is happy not because everything is right in his life. He is happy only because his attitude toward everything is almost right.

Carefully, preserve marginal mandibular nerve and cervical branch of facial nerve which lies between platysma and deep fascia and usually 2 cm below the inferior border of the mandible.

Remember: The marginal mandibular nerve is easily injured if the raised upper flap is more superficial).

Step 2: Raising the inferior, medial and lateral flap:
The flap is already raised:
- Superiorly, up to inferior border of the mandible
- Inferiorly, up to digastrics and stylohyoid muscles
- Laterally, up to sternocleidomastoid muscle
- Medially, up to mylohyoid muscle
- The facial vein crosses superficial to the gland which is to be ligated and divided. But, facial artery can be dissected out of the gland and to be ligated, if required above and below the gland.

Now, raise the inferior, medial and lateral flap to expose the area completely.

(Remember: During the dissection of facial vessels, try to prevent marginal mandibular nerve injury as it, lies superficial to these vessels.)

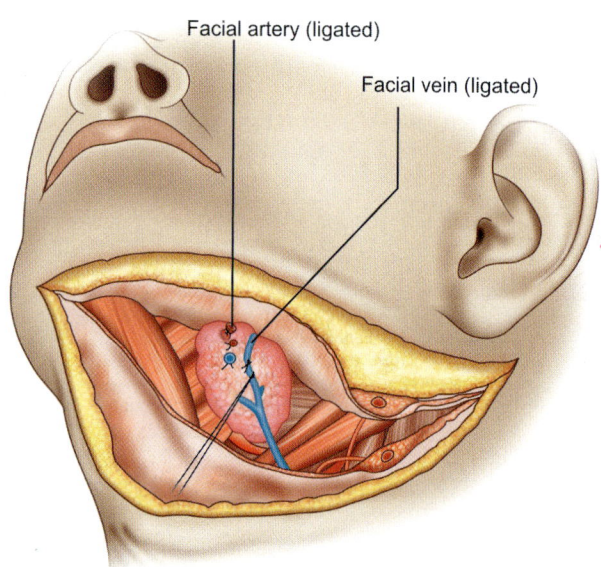

Exposure of facial vessels and their ligations

Step 3: Mobilization of the gland: The gland is now to be mobilized all around. The gland is dissected off the ramus of mandible and then the anterior part of the gland to be dissected off anterior belly of digastric and mylohyoid muscles. The hypoglossal nerve is located very close to digastric tendon and accompanied by lingual vein and in deep external maxillary artery. Both vessels to be ligated and divided.

Now retract the posterior border of mylohyoid to expose the deep part of submandibular gland which is to be dissected slowly, as cephalad to it, lingual nerve,

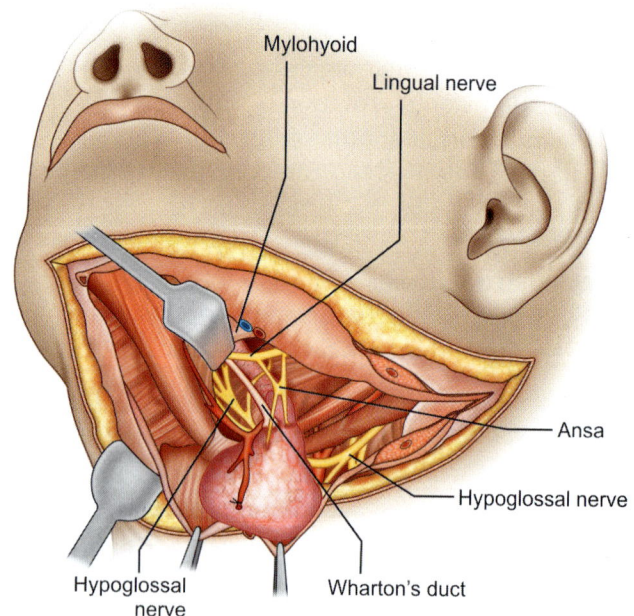

Exposure of lingual, hypoglossal, ansa cervicalis and Wharton's duct

---

Live the life you want to live. Never be ashamed of anything. Make decisions, make mistakes. If you fall, at least you fell because you tried. No regrets, its life.

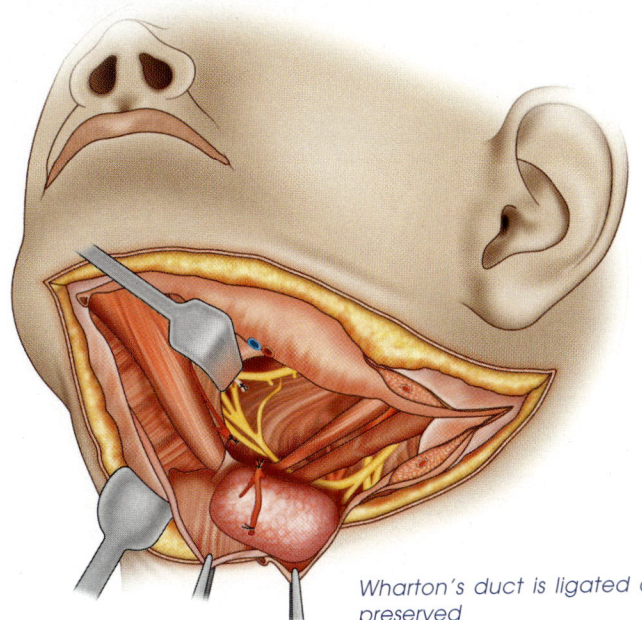

Wharton's duct is ligated and hypoglossal nerve which passes under digastrics muscle is preserved

chorda tympani nerve, Wharton's duct and deep to it, hypoglossal nerve.

Step 4: Ligation of Wharton's duct: Dissect the Wharton's duct, ligate with absorbable suture (2-0 vicryl) and divide as far anteriorly as possible (to ensure removal of any small calculi lodged into the duct).

Wharton's duct is ligated and hypoglossal nerve which passes under digastrics muscle is preserved.

Step 5: Remove the gland: Hemostasis is to be achieved completely. Place a small suction drain in the bed of the gland and brought out posteriorly.

Wound to be closed in layers and the skin is closed with 3-0/4-0 nylon or subcuticular closure may be done for better cosmetic results.

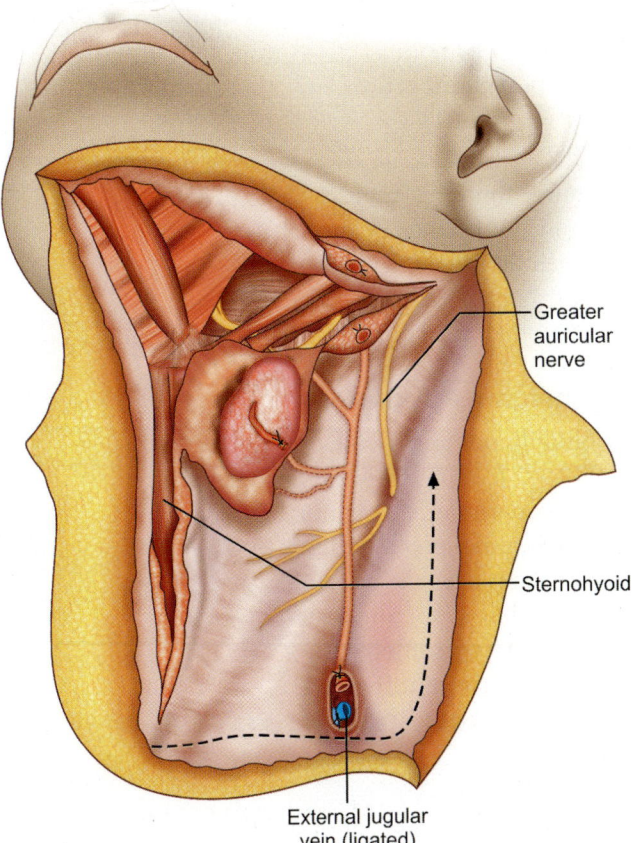

Greater auricular nerve

Sternohyoid

External jugular vein (ligated)

After completion of submandibular salivary gland dissection

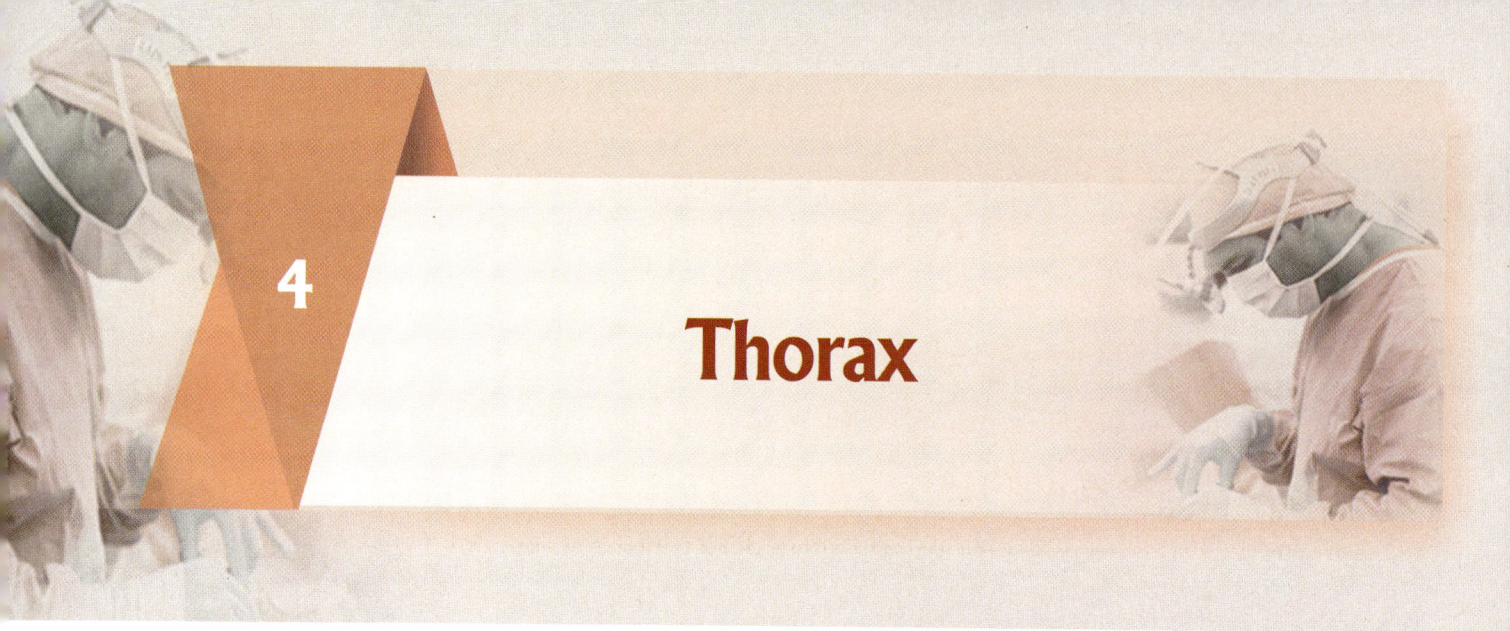

4

Thorax

4.1 TRANSTHORACIC ESOPHAGECTOMY (TTE)

Indications

1. Carcinoma esophagus: Middle or distal part with lymphadenopathy.
2. When extra-esophageal spread suspected in locally advanced tumor.
3. When transhiatal esophagectomy (THE) is not possible, i.e. tumor is fixed to mediastinum.

Remember: A group of surgeons prefer TTE in middle one-third tumor where chance of bronchus involvement is more and for field dissection of lymphnodes and THE is reserved for lower one-third tumor without lymphnodes dissection.

Pitfalls

1. Injury to vital structures, like great vessels
2. Injury of trachea or bronchus
3. Anastomotic leak and stenosis
4. Necrosis of gastric conduit
5. Higher chance of postoperative pulmonary complication because of thoracic component.

Preoperative Preparation

- Nutritional improvement
- Forced feeding through nasogastric (NG)
- Total parenteral nutrition (TPN)
- High intake protein diet
- Maintain hygiene
- Pulmonary function tests
- Incentive spirometry
- Preoperative antibiotic
- Stomach wash.

Procedure

1. General anesthesia with double lumen intubation.

Steps to a happy life: 1. Do not stress yourself with useless people who do not even deserve to be an issue in your life. 2. Never invest too much emotion at one thing, because if you do, you will end up hurting yourself. 3. Learn to live life without worries because God will take care of everything, trust and just have FAITH.

2. Position: Put a sand bag to elevate patient's right side approximately 30°. Right arm to be abducted and kept rest. Head is turned to the right. (For Iver-Lewis two stage operation position to be altered. First for thoracic part, the position to be in the left lateral position and abdominal part on supine position.)

3. Cleaning and draping of neck, chest and abdomen.

Thoracic Part—at Right-sided Thorax

Incision: Two fingers' breadth below the tip of the scapula. The incision is made from the angle between the spine and the medial edge of the scapula through 5th/6th intercostal space up to inframammary fold.

Step 1: The skin incision is deepened through latissimus dorsi which is at about 90° to the incision line. The incision is extended upward under the scapula. Explore the chest (as described in posterolateral thoracotomy) and rule out metastatic lesion, if any.

Step 2: Superior dissection: During superior dissection, see the vagus nerve running over the trachea and save the recurrent laryngeal nerve.

Ligate and divide the thoracic duct immediately above the diaphragm on the right lateral part of descending aorta.

[*Remember:* Knowledge of the course of thoracic duct is very important to prevent the complications.]

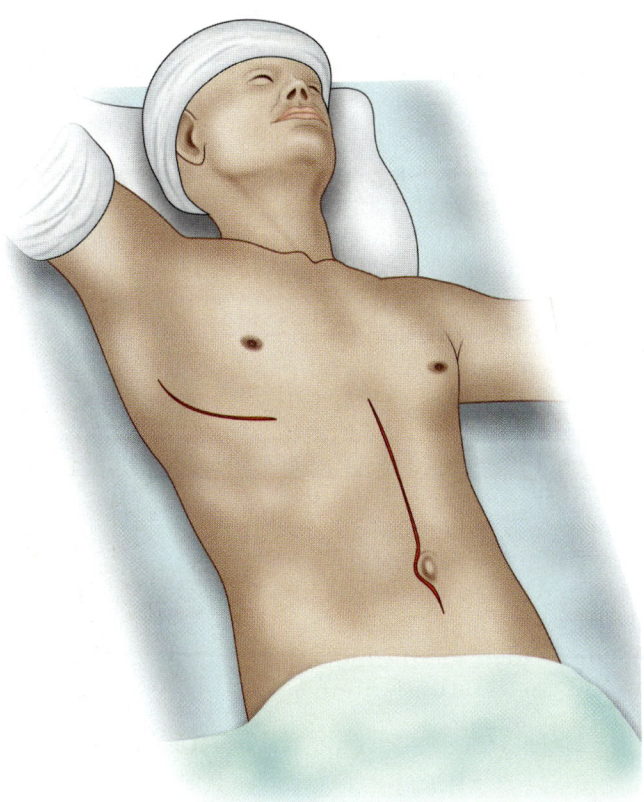

Thoracic and abdominal incision for esophagectomy

Being honest may not get you a lot of friends around, but it will make sure you will have right ones always around you.

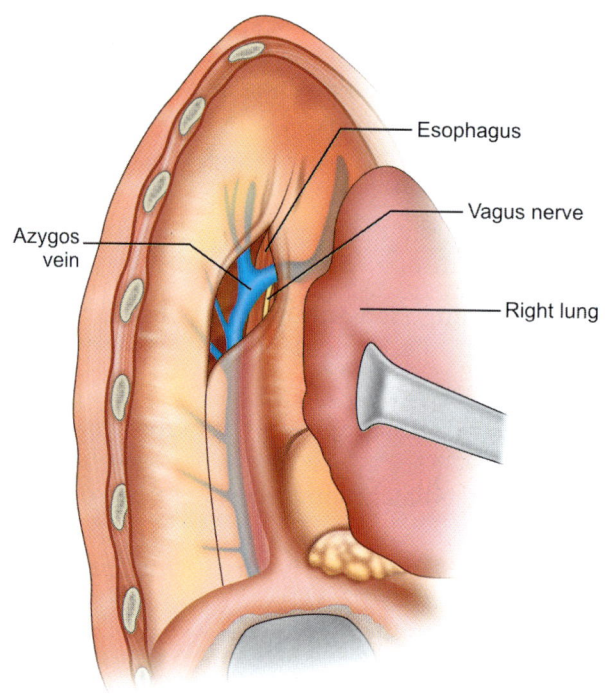

Incision of parietal pleura at the level of azygos vein to mobilize the thoracic esophagus and for the lymphnode dissection

Step 3: Lymphnodes dissection: The first field lymphnode dissection involves intra-abdominal part of paraeso-phageal lymphnodes and lymphnodes of proximal part of the stomach (like D2 lymphadenectomy for proximal gastric cancer).

- The two-field lymphadenectomy includes the additional clearance of intrathoracic nodes, i.e. subcarinal, right paratracheal nodes, pulmonary hilar nodes.
- The three-field lymphadenectomy includes, in addition to above two fields, brachiocephalic, deep internal and external cervical nodes. (Most of the surgeons recommend the two-field lymphadenectomy and others believe that positive nodes do not mean incurable disease, chemotherapy—neoadjuvant or adjuvant will take care of the lymphnodes, so they prefer THE). The inferior pulmonary ligament is divided and the lung is gently retracted. Open the mediastinal pleura longitudinally overlying the esophagus.
- Azygos vein is divided by ligating double. Dissection to continue to free the esophagus. All esophageal branches of arteries are to be ligated or clipped and divided.

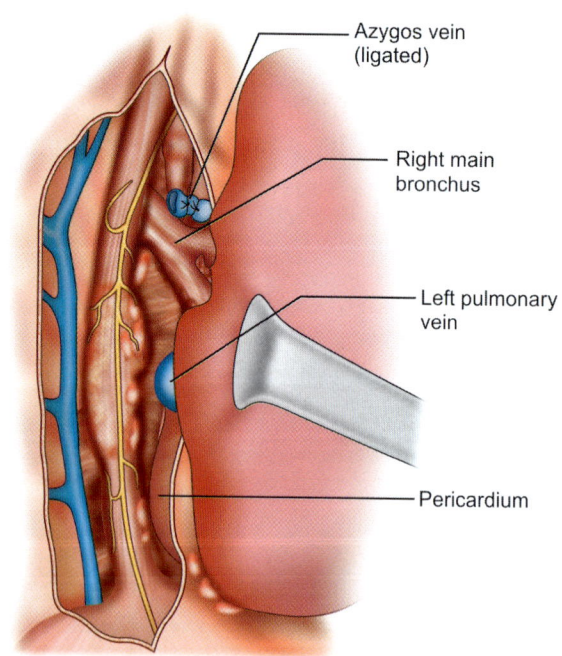

Ligation and division of azygos vein and the lymphnode dissection

Step 4: When the intrathoracic esophagus has been mobilized sufficiently, the gastroesophageal junction is to be mobilized at the level of hiatus and the distal limit is identified.

Abdominal Part

Incision: The operation table is rotated toward the right and the abdominal incision is made in the midline from xiphoid to umbilicus.

Step 1: Perform restaging once: Apply self-retaining retractor for better exposure. Divide the left triangular and left coronary ligaments of the liver. Retract the left lobe of the liver.

Now, detach the greater omentum from the stomach, preserving the right gastroepiploic vessels. Preserve the right gastric artery too.

Step 2: Vessels ligation: Doubly ligate and divide left gastric vessels, short gastric vessels too. Ligate and divide the left gastroepiploic close to its origin from splenic artery, to give additional vascularity to the stomach conduit. Excise all nodal tissues around the vessels with the specimen.

Step 3: Divide the phrenicoesophageal ligament, encircle the esophagus at the hiatus with a feeding tube, bilateral truncal vagotomy to be done.

Step 4: Mobilization of duodenum: Mobilize the duodenum, i.e. Kocher's maneuver is to be performed to add additional length of the stomach tube. Next pylorotomy or pyloroplasty or finger fracture of pylorus to be done.

Step 5: Make stomach tube: By using linear cutter stapler (GIA/NTLC) 75 mm, make the stomach tube, i.e. remove the portion of lesser curvature of the stomach and LNs along with. The max 3 fingers' breadth stomach

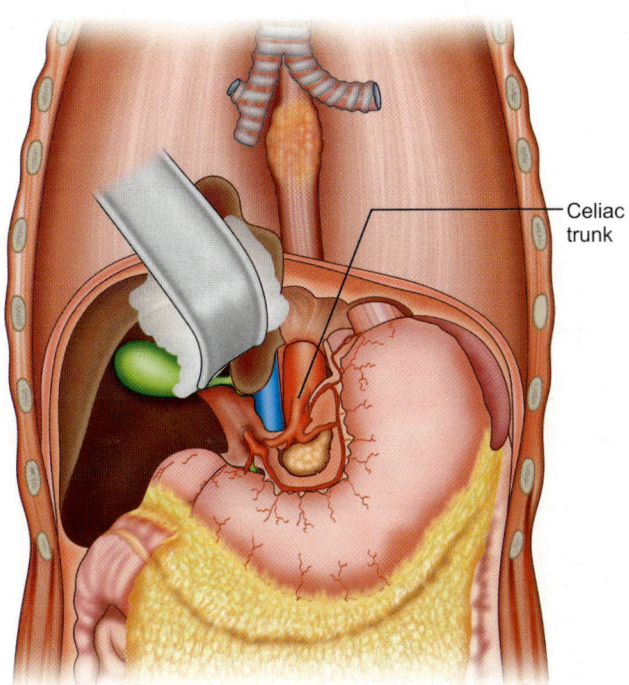

Celiac trunk

Ligation of left gastric, gastroepiploic, short gastric vessels

Golden rules for success—be honest when in poverty, simple when in wealth, polite when in authority, silent when in anger.

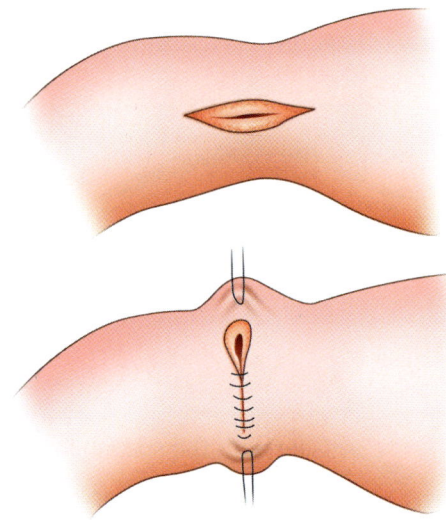

Pyloroplasty: incise the pylorus longitudinally and close it transversely

tube is made, keeping greater curvature along with its vascular arcade. It is better to oversew the staple lines with 3,0 silk either interrupted or continuous.

Step 6: Dilate the hiatus with three fingers so that stomach tube is passed easily.

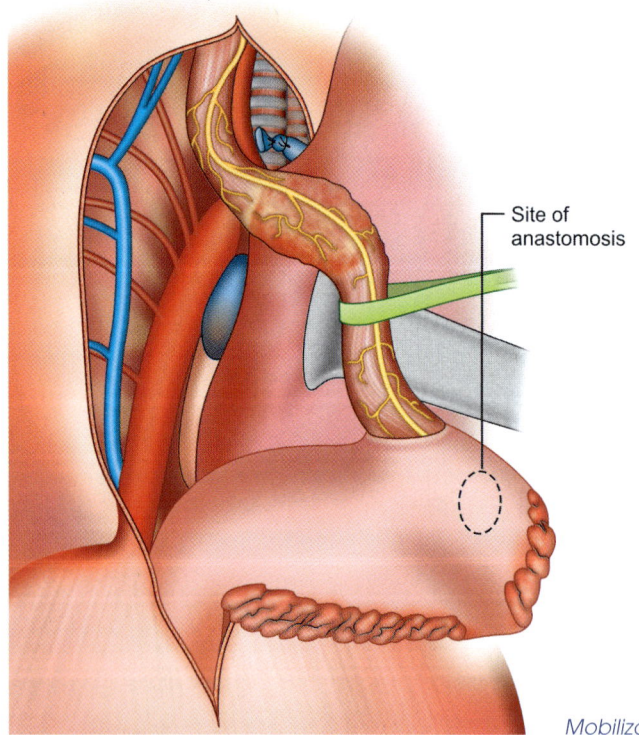

Site of anastomosis

Mobilization of esophagus and entry of stomach tube through the chest

Life is flowing like a river with unexpected turns. May be good, may be bad. Learn to enjoy each turn because these turns will never RETURN.

Neck Portion

Incision: Make an oblique left cervical incision along the medial border of sternocleidomastoid from the sternal notch to three fingers breadth below the mandible.

Step 1: Retract the sternocleidomastoid laterally: Omohyoid and sternothyroid muscles may be divided into two: (1) inferior thyroid artery, (2) middle thyroid vein. Now, retract the carotid sheath laterally.

Step 2: Mobilization of cervical esophagus: Identify left recurrent laryngeal nerve and save it. Retract the thyroid gland and trachea medially. Enter the retroesophageal space medial to carotid and jugular vessels. Mobilize and clear all around the esophagus and put a feeding tube.

Step 3: Division of cervical esophagus: Cervical esophagus to be divided 5 cm distal to cricopharyngeal muscle after withdrawing the Ryle's tube. A feeding tube or Ryle's tube to be fixed at the distant end of the esophagus. Now pull the stomach downward, the esophagus will be reached into the abdomen via hiatus.

Step 4: Specimen resection: Now, specimen to be resected out and the same tube is fixed to the healthy fundus of stomach and pull it from neck side, the fundus along with stomach tube will reach to neck.

Step 5: Esophagogastric anastomosis: Before anastomosis look for vascularity at both the end and the anastomose, and if vascularity is not good, cut that end slightly more and construct one layer anastomosis with 3-0 silk or polydioxanone (PDS). Stapled anastomosis can be done instead of hand sewn.

Step 6 Feeding jejunostomy (Witzel)

1. Select a loop of proximal jejunum approximately 15 cm from the ligament of Treitz (distal to one peristaltic segment of jejunum).
2. Make a stab wound in the abdominal wall and insert the catheter.
3. Take a purse string suture with 3-0 mars silk or vicryl and make a small incision on the jejunal wall inside the purse string and insert the catheter (12/14 F Foley's) and tighten the purse string suture around the catheter.

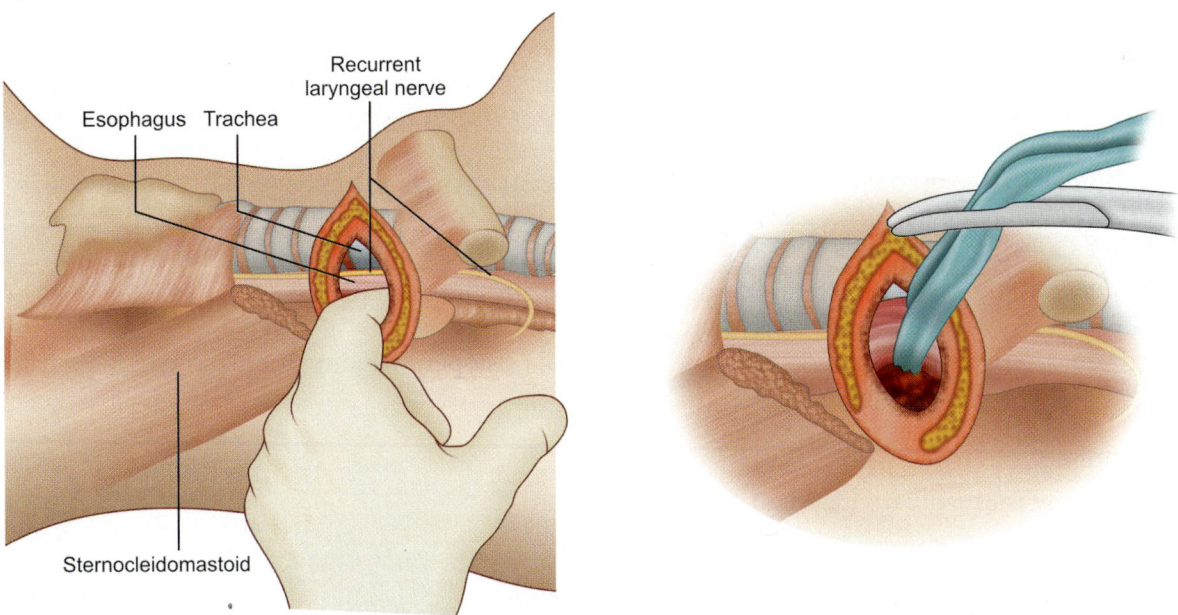

Mobilization of cervical esophagus

A relation is not a business where you give only when you get, but it is a beautiful feeling for someone where you like to give everything, even if you do not have or get anything.

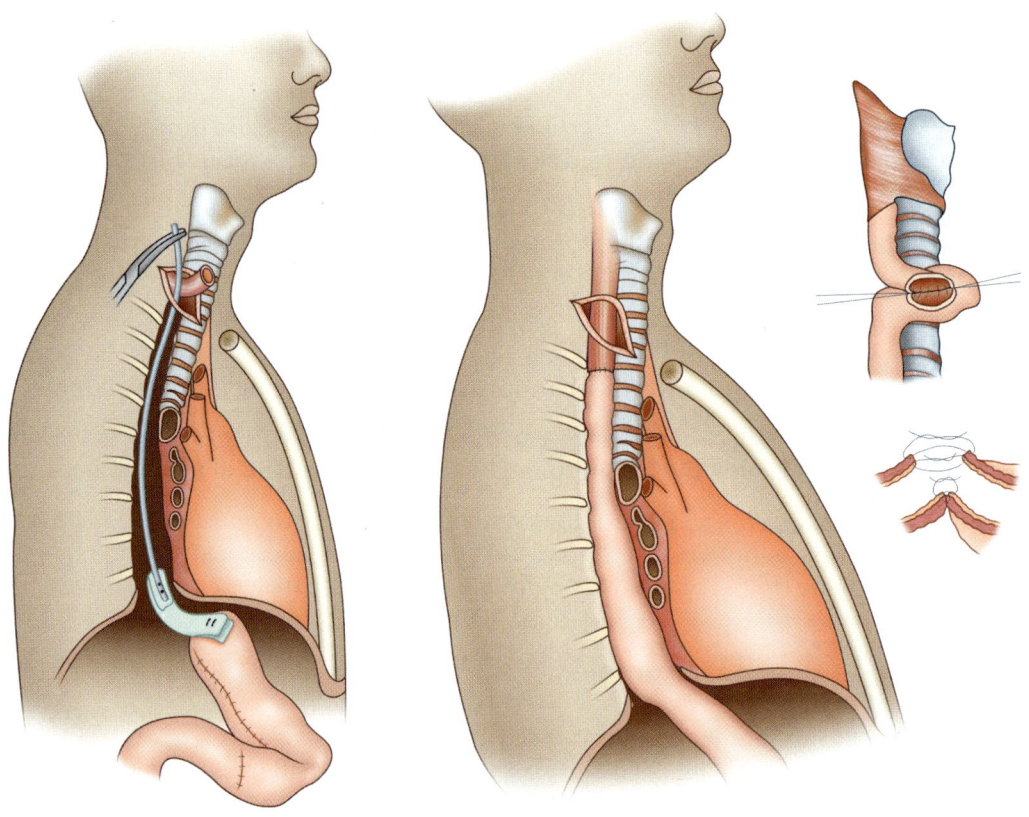

Residual omentum may be loosely placed over the anastomosis. Put a corrugated rubber drain and close it

4. Create a seromuscular tunnel 5–6 cm in length and fix the catheter using interrupted 2-0 silk suture.
5. Fix the tunnel to the parietal wall too, at least three points keeping the direction of the catheter tip downward.
6. Fix the catheter to the skin properly.
   Now, abdomen to be closed with or without putting a drain after complete hemotasis.

Postoperative Care

1. Keep NG tube till the bowel function returns (usually on 4th/5th postoperative day)
2. Chest tube to be kept till the drain is less than 100 mL.
3. Gastrografin contrast swallow study is performed on 8th postoperative day. If no leakage or obstruction, the diet is advanced from soft to solid.

Types of Esophagectomy

A. Esophagectomy is broadly divided into two types:
   a. THE (Orringer)
   b. TTE.
   TTE is divided into (1) three-stage procedure (McKown), (2) Two-stage procedure (Ivor-Lewis). Ivor-Lewis esophagectomy may be either en bloc esophagectomy or esophagectomy and fields lymphadenectomy. Lymphadenectomy may be standard or extended two fields or three fields. Lymphnodes to be dissected from

mediastinal pleura, crus of diaphragm, pericardial tissue along with lower paraesophageal lymphnodes and continuously upward till the carina en-bloc.

Esophagectomy may be classified as follows:

1. TTE (Akiyama)

Indication: For mid one-third of esophageal carcinoma where there is a fair chance of adherence to tracheobronchial tree, even to aorta.

Step I: Right thoracotomy to be done and mobilization of thoracic esophagus and separation from tracheobronchial tree and/or aorta.

Step II: Laparotomy and preparation of gastric conduit.

Step III: Cervical exploration and gastroesophageal anastomosis to be done.

2. TTE

- Via right thoracotomy (Ivor-Lewis)
- Via left thoracotomy (Sweet-Garlock).

Indication: Gastroesophageal (GE) junction tumor specially adenocarcinoma, spreading toward stomach and large part of stomach to be resected.

Abdominal approach to surgically stage the disease and mobilize the stomach. Resection of involved stomach with 5 cm distal clear margin.

Right thoracotomy to resect the involved esophagus and to reestablish gastrointestinal continuity with an esophagogastric anastomosis in the chest (as a result of resection of stomach, the smaller gastric conduit which may not reach the neck for a cervical anastomosis).

3. THE (Orringer)

Indications
1. Carcinoma lower third esophagus
2. Carcinoma GE junction
3. Many surgeons routinely do THE even in carcinoma middle third.

Advantage: Chest is not opened. So, it is considered as less morbid procedure.

Disadvantage: Lymphnode dissection is not possible so survival benefit is compromised to some extent.

All steps are more or less same as TTE but here thorax is not opened. So, blind mobilization of thoracic esophagus is to be done through the hiatus.

Remember: Mobilization through cervical and hiatal approach using right and left index finger. Both fingers will meet each other close to or just above carina in the THE.

Here, chest drain is as per the requirement not mandatory always.

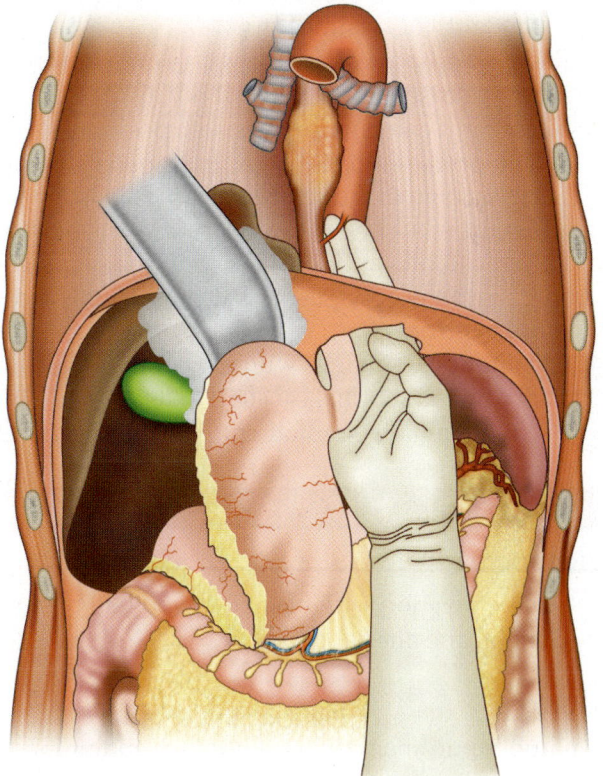

Transhiatal esophagectomy

Life is like a FLUTE. It may have many holes and emptiness in it. But, if you work on it carefully, it can play magical melodies.

4. *Radical En Bloc Esophagectomy*

Like TTE, thoracotomy, laparotomy and cervical exploration to be done. But, the procedure is more radical including thoracic esophagus, mediastinal nodes, stomach, spleen, celiac nodes, etc. And to be replaced by colonic conduit. Not routinely done as radical resection performed in this operation and it is a highly morbid procedure and no significant survival benefit as compared to other procedures. The plane of the dissection is different in contrast to parietal pleura. Azygos vein, thoracic duct, pericardium and aortic nodes will be en bloc along with the specimen.

5. *Total Laryngopharyngoesophagectomy with Gastric Pull Up*

Indications

- Carcinoma cervical esophagus involving hypopharynx or the posterior membranous trachea. In the procedure, the gastric conduit is anastomosed to the pharynx.
- The trachea is brought out as tracheostomy.
- In some cases, free jejunal inter-position graft may be used to replace the resected esophagus provided the resection does not extend beyond the thoracic inlet. This procedure requires specialized microvascular technique.

In Special Problems in Esophageal Surgery

1. An identification of unresectable disease during dissection—sometime after mobilization of esophagus and preparation of gastric conduit, some gross disease is discovered.
   a. In such cases, we should proceed with resection of the esophagus and gastroesophageal anastomosis and mark the gross disease with clips for postoperative radiotherapy, chemoradiotherapy is a good modality of treatment too.
2. Resected gastric carcinoma with development of carcinoma esophagus.
   a. In this case, gastric conduit not available.
   b. So, right colon in isoperistaltic position.
   c. Transverse colon is placed in isoperistaltic position. Both right and left colon can be used. Advantage of right colon is the segment would be isoperistaltic but the length issue is there, but in case of left colon length would be sufficient but the segment will be antiperistaltic.
   d. Left colon in antiperistaltic position.
3. In Barrett's esophagus, it is a premalignant condition. Presence of severe dysplasia is an indication for esophagectomy.
4. Carcinoma esophagus with tracheoesophageal fistula
   a. A covered esophageal stent to tamponade the fistula region is desirable.
   b. Next, palliative radiotherapy is the treatment of choice.

4.2 TRANSHIATAL ESOPHAGECTOMY (THE—DESCRIBED BY ORRINGER)

Procedure

- Supine position with placing a sand bag behind the hiatus
- General anesthesia

Incisions

An upper midline incision is used for abdominal exploration from xiphisternum to below umbilicus.

If you never taste bad apple, you would never appreciate a good apple. Sometimes, we need to experience bitterness of life to understand the value of sweetness.

In the neck, an oblique incision is made along the anterior border of left lower sternocleidomastoid muscle extending from the left side of suprasternal notch to the level of thyroid cartilage.

Abdominal Dissection

Step 1: The abdomen is opened and carefully examined for the presence of liver metastasis or ascites. The resectability of the tumor is assessed. The stomach to be used as a conduit for esophageal replacement is also examined. It should be long enough to reach the neck for a tension free cervical anastomosis. A self-retaining retractor is very useful for exposure and retraction of the left liver lobe. The left triangular ligament is divided and the left lobe of liver is retracted to the right.

Step 2: Gastric mobilization

The lesser sac is entered by serially ligating vessels in the greater omentum about 2–3 cm from the greater curvature of the stomach, **preserving the right gastroepiploic vessels** which will be the main supply of the gastric conduit. The greater omentum is divided up to the pylorus and the posterior aspect of stomach is separated from the stomach bed.

The greater curvature of the stomach is then freed by serially ligating the left gastroepiploic vessels and the short gastric vessels. These vessels should be ligated well away from the greater curvature to prevent ischemia to the stomach.

The gastrophrenic ligament is similarly divided, and the entire greater curve from the pylorus to the gastroesophageal junction is freed. The posterior aspect of stomach is lifted up and dissected free from the retroperitoneum by dividing few avascular adhesions.

The peritoneum over the lower esophagus is incised, and the esophagogastric junction is encircled and separated from the retroperitoneum. The lesser curve of the stomach is then similarly freed by entering an avascular part of the gastrohepatic omentum well away from the right gastric vessels. While dividing the gastrohepatic omentum, carefully look for an **aberrant left hepatic artery arising from the left gastric artery.**

The greater curve of the stomach is retracted upward and to the right. The left gastric vein and artery are identified and doubly ligated and divided one by one. Dissection then proceeds upward toward the high lesser curvature and esophageal hiatus.

All the lymphnodes and soft tissue along the lesser curve are sequentially dissected and reflected toward the stomach, taking as much margin as is possible. In this way, the entire lesser curvature and greater curvature of the stomach is mobilized up to the esophageal hiatus.

The peritoneum overlying the diaphragmatic hiatus is incised, and the phrenoesophageal ligaments are divided, separating the lower esophagus circumferentially from the hiatus. If the tumor adheres to the hiatus, a rim of diaphragm at the hiatus may be excised.

Step 3: Mediastinal dissection and esophageal mobilization

Larger arterial supply, to the esophagus, branches into small capillaries approximately 1 cm away from the esophageal wall. Dissection within this immediate paraesophageal space disrupts only these small capillaries, which rapidly spasm and subsequently, thrombosis occurs. Dissection of the esophagus should be carried out in this safe paraesophageal plane. Dissection outside this safe paraesophageal plane may cause injury to the larger vessels, resulting in more blood loss.

Most of the esophageal dissection is performed under vision from below, through the esophageal hiatus. The hiatus is, therefore, widened adequately by incising the hiatus anteriorly. This usually requires ligation of phrenic vein.

Step 4: Widening of hiatus and transhiatal mobilization of esophagus

A Devers or Harrington retractor is placed in the hiatus to improve exposure. An infant feeding tube is used to encircle the lower end of esophagus and keep it taut. It also helps to retract the esophagus on either side to facilitate dissection.

Life is flowing like a river with unexpected turns. May be good, may be bad. Learn to enjoy each turn because these turns will never RETURN.

Gentle dissection of the esophagus is performed with fingers through the hiatus. This dissection is carried out circumferentially. This way, by sequentially dividing small bits of paraesophageal tissue on both sides and by dividing branches of vagal trunk entering the esophagus, the whole of the esophagus is gradually mobilized and completely freed up to the level of carina. Care is taken to not to breach the pleura during this portion of the dissection.

(If the pleural cavity is entered, a chest tube should be inserted on that side and **while** retraction and dissection is performed near the left atrium, the anesthetist should be watchful for hypotension.) Once esophageal mobilization is complete, a pack is placed in the mediastinum through the hiatus, and preparation is done for the cervical part of operation. By this time, cervical esophagus would have already been looped.

A similar paraesophageal dissection is performed in the upper mediastinum through the neck. Both hiatal and cervical dissection should meet in the mediastinum.

Step 5: Esophagogastric anastomosis at neck: As described in TTE. Rest everything like TTE except those extrathoracic complications.

4.3 POSTEROLATERAL THORACOTOMY

Indications

- Elective surgery for any lung pathology, like metastasectomy, lobectomy, etc.
- Right posterolateral thoracotomy for the access of thoracic esophagus.

Pitfalls

- Hemorrhage
- Injury to lung, trachea
- Injury to recurrent laryngeal, vagus or phrenic nerve
- Apnea, cardiac arrhythmia.

Procedures

Position: Right lateral position with slightly prone. Right arm to be kept on the arm board. (For left—left lateral position)

Incision: Two fingers' breadth below the tip of the scapula. The incision is made from the angle between the spine and the medial edge of the scapula through 5th/6th intercostal space up to inframammary fold or minimum up to anterior axillary line.

Incision for Posterolateral Thoracotomy

Step 1: The skin incision is deepened through latissimus dorsi which is at about 90° to the incision. The incision is extended upwards under the scapula.

Step 2: The ribs and intercostal muscles are now exposed. Plan the level of thoracotomy. The edge of second rib can be felt under the scapula and count the space as per the requirement. Now, lower border of serratus anterior is divided as low as

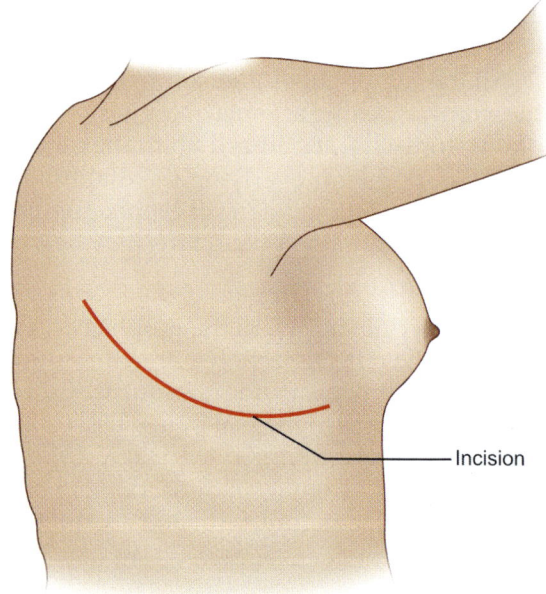

Incision

Incision for posterolateral thoracotomy

possible to preserve the innervation (if more space is required, trapezius can be divided).

Life is the art of drawing without eraser. So, be careful while taking your decision about any valuable page of your life. Be a good artist of your own life.

Step 3: Enter into the chest through intercostal muscles particularly along the upper border of the rib to save neurovascular bundle or through the bed of the rib. If through bed of the rib, incise the periosteum and stripped off its upper border with diathermy or periosteum elevator. And stripping should be from back to front along the fibers of the muscle. Dissect at the upper border of the rib.

Step 4: Now, through posterior peritoneum, enter the pleural cavity. Divide costotransverse ligament posteriorly to allow extra mobility of upper rib (rib resection is better to be avoided). Now, self-retaining retractor is introduced.

Step 5: The pleura is incised with double lumen tube in place and ask the anesthetist to collapse the lung. Now, do the dissections, like mobilization of the esophagus, mediastinal mass, etc.

Step 6: Cosure: Place one-sided chest drain or both sides (deepend on the extensive dissection and opposite pleura is opened). Ribs apposition is to be done by 1, 0 ethibond. Approximate the divided upper leaf periosteum to the fascia over the intercostal muscles. The chest wall muscles are repaired with absorable sutures.

Muscles Sparing Posterolateral Thoracotomy

Conventional posterolateral thoracotomy with a division of latissimus dorsi (LD) and serratus muscles provides a good exposure to any intrathoracic structures. But with this muscle cutting approach, there are so many disadvantages like severe postoperative pain, reduced shoulder girdle movement and respiratory difficulty. So, the muscle sparing posterolateral thoracotomy has come up in a great way to avoid the significant complications.

Technique

1. General anesthesia
2. Position: Lateral decubitus position

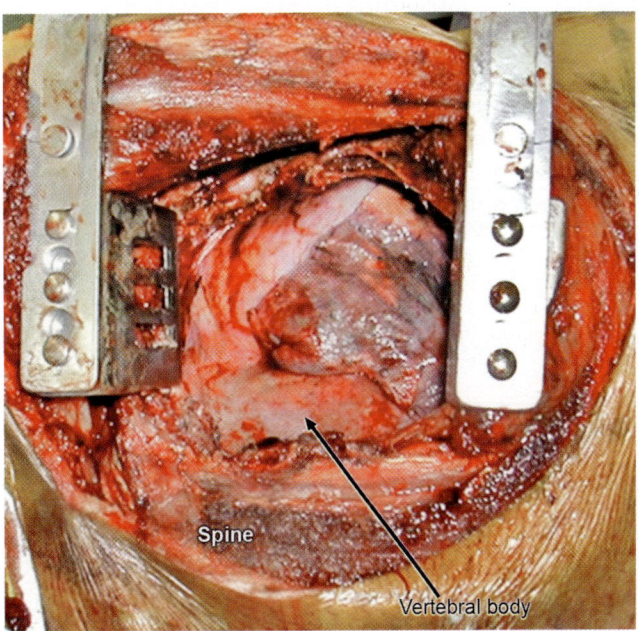

Thoracic cavity is entered with retraction of ribs

Be slow in choosing friend, slower in loosing them because friendship is not an opportunity, but it is a sweet responsibility.

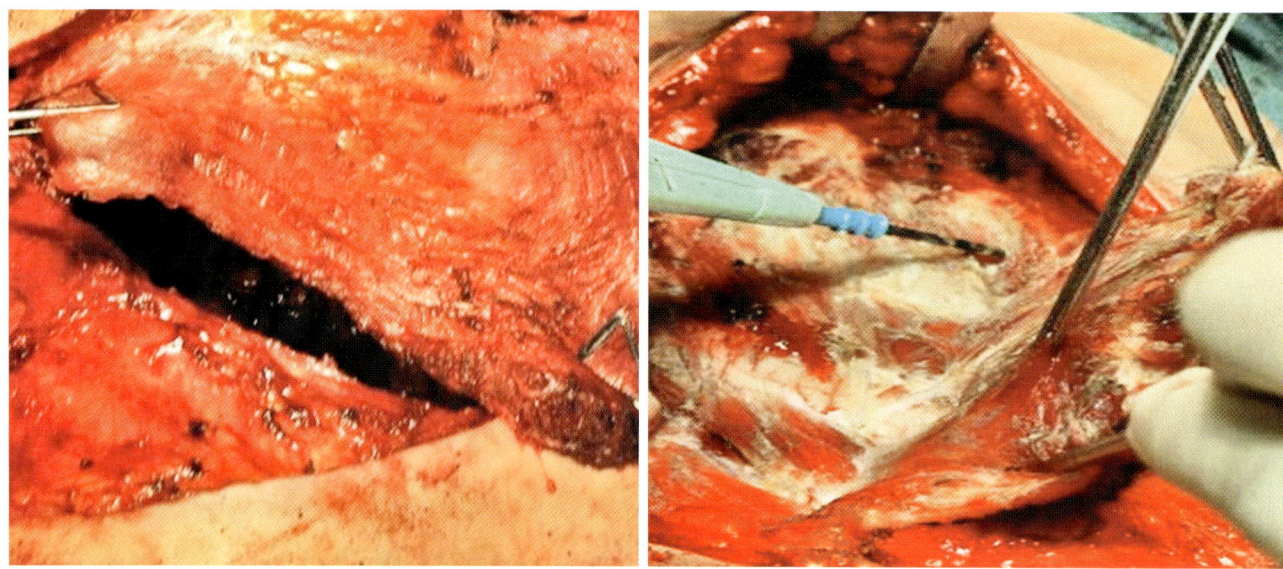

Muscles sparing thoracotomy

3. Incision: Two fingers' breadth below the tip of the scapula. The incision is made from the angle between the spine and medial edge of the scapula through 5th/6th intercostal space up to inframammary fold or up to anterior axillary line minimum.

Step 1: The incision is carried down through the subcutaneous and superficial layers of LD as much as close to its insertion and exposed it. The anterior attachment of LD is defined and a plane is made between the muscle and chest wall and the LD is retracted posteriorly in this plane and flap is raised behind the muscle. The muscle is elevated from the chest wall. (Some surgeons detach it from the iliac crest to avoid dividing the muscle fiber. This procedure is similar to latissimus dorsi myoplasty.)

Step 2: Now, the serratus is retracted anteriorly and a few fibers are detached from the ribs of its insertion. And the posterior border of the muscle is exposed.

Step 3: Both muscles are dissected and freed but their fibers to be kept intact.

Rest of the steps are like the posterolateral thoracotomy, but at the end of the operation both the muscles to be fixed to the chest wall. (If you detached from the origin you should reattach with origin and place suction drain in the subcutaneous layer.)

It is only when we are not disturbed that we can always do the right thing at the right time in the right way.

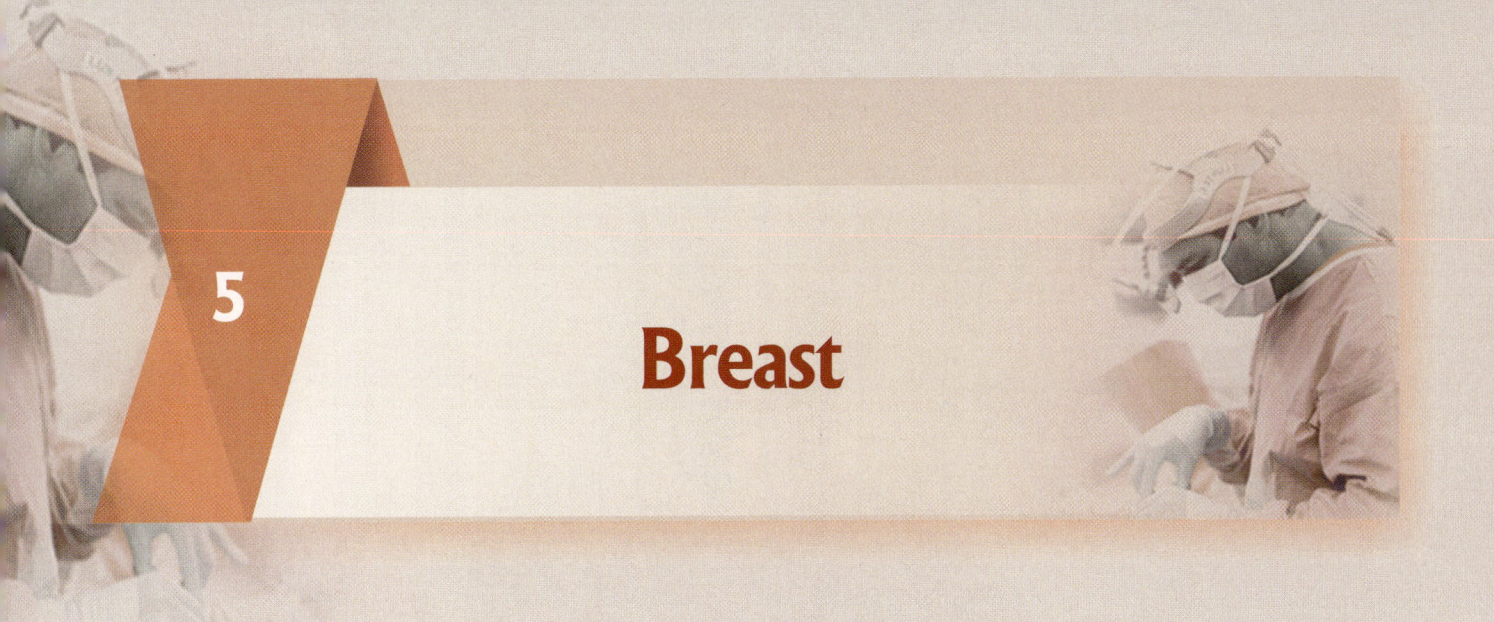

5

Breast

5.1 MODIFIED RADICAL MASTECTOMY (MRM)

SURGICAL ANATOMY FOR MASTECTOMY

- Anatomy of triangular bed in MRM.
- Boundary of the triangular bed is:
  - Medially: The lateral margin of pectoralis major
  - Laterally: Medial border of latissimus dorsi muscle
  - Superiorly: Axillary vein and floor is formed by serratus anterior and subscapularis muscles.
- After the breast and underlying fascia is removed, good dissection consists of:
  - Removing the fascia of pectoralis major at its axillary border
  - Incising the axillary fascia, enter into the axilla
  - Striping the fascia of pectoralis minor
  - Exposing the axillary vein, preserving the fascia over axillary vein—to prevent lymphedema.
  - Dissection of axillary fat and lymphnodes downward, ligation of the tributaries of axillary vein
  - Removing the fascia partially of serratus anterior, subscapularis and medial border of LD muscles.
- Identification of:
  - The thoracodorsal nerve: It lies on subscapularis muscle and innervates the LD muscle.
  - The pedicle is usually found close to the medial border of LD about 5 cm above the plane at the level of 3rd sternochondral junction. (If the nerve is cut, abduction and internal rotation of the shoulder will be weakened without any deformity.)
  - The long thoracic nerve (nerve of Bell): It lies on serratus anterior and innervates it.
- The landmark of location of the pedicle is the point at which axillary vein passes over the 2nd rib. The nerves usually descend on the 2nd rib, posterior to axillary vein.
- The injury of this nerve causing winging of scapula.
- The medial and lateral anterior thoracic nerves.
  - The medial anterior thoracic nerve is superficial to axillary vein and lateral to pectoralis minor.
  - The lateral is also superficial to axillary vein and lies at the medial edge of the pectoralis minor.
  - Injury of one or both nerves causes atrophy of pectoralis major and minor muscles.
- Intercostal brachial nerve: The second intercostal nerve is joined to the medial cutaneous nerve of the arm by a branch, called intercostals brachial nerve, that is similar to the lateral cutaneous branch of other nerves. Usually, these nerves are cut during the dissection of breast and axilla. But, it is always better to try to preserve it.

Strength grows when we dare, unity grows when we pair, love grows when we share and relationships grow when we care.

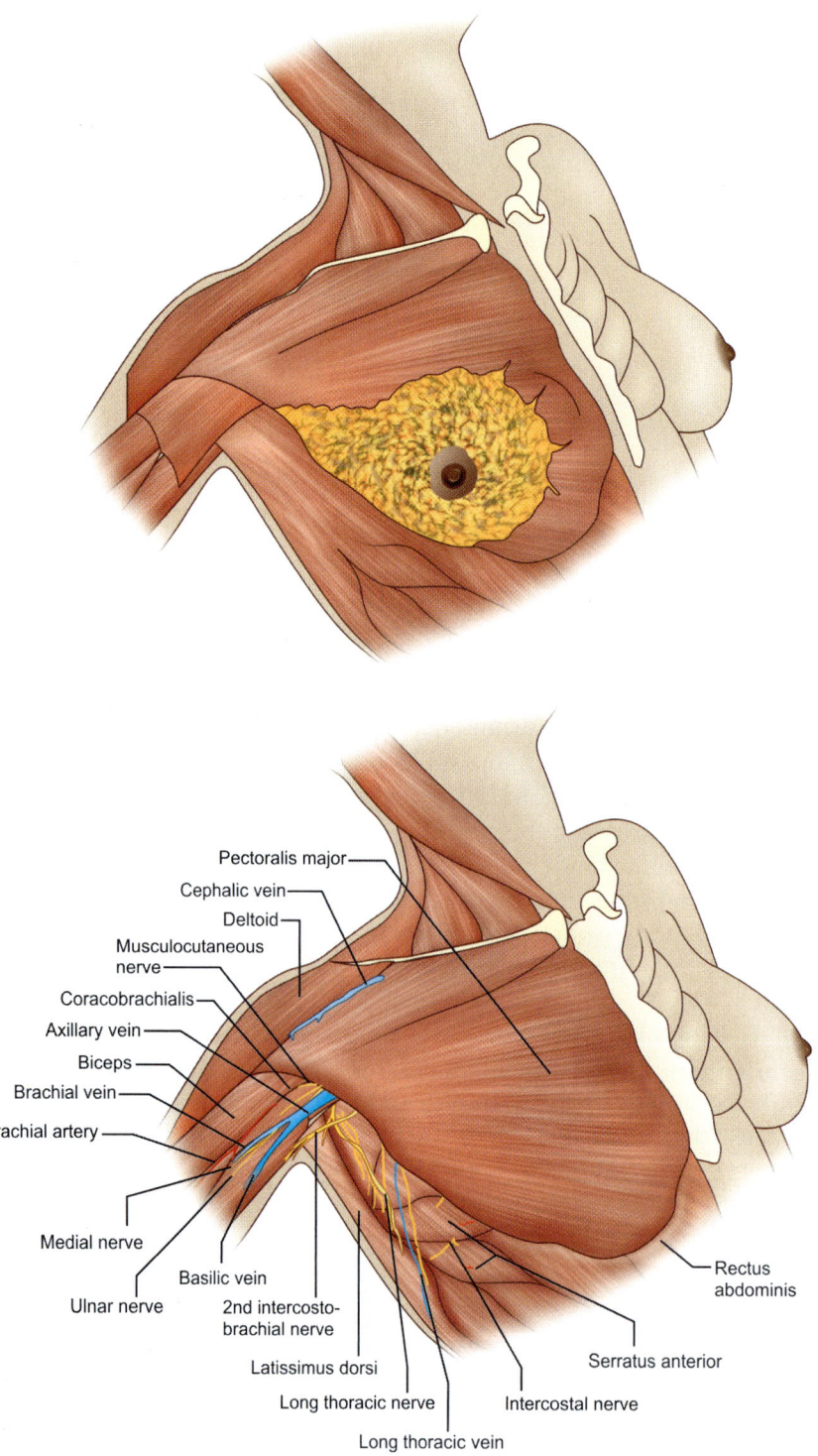

Pectoralis major
Cephalic vein
Deltoid
Musculocutaneous nerve
Coracobrachialis
Axillary vein
Biceps
Brachial vein
Brachial artery
Medial nerve
Basilic vein
Ulnar nerve
2nd intercosto-brachial nerve
Latissimus dorsi
Long thoracic nerve
Intercostal nerve
Long thoracic vein
Rectus abdominis
Serratus anterior

Surgical anatomy of breast and its surrounding structures

To be kind is more important than to be right. Many times what people need is not a brilliant mind that speaks but special heart that listens.

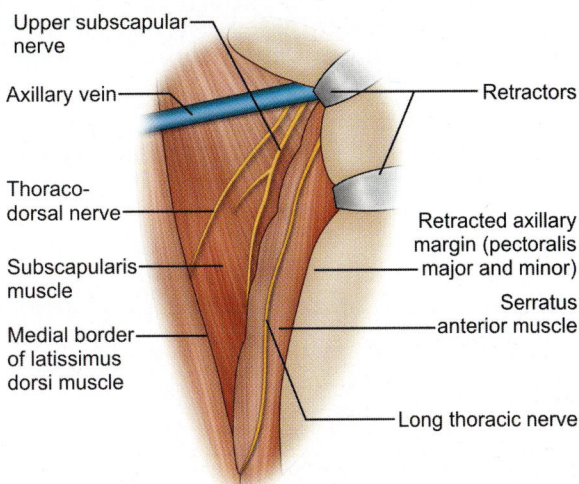

The triangular bed of modified radical mastectomy

- Axillary nodes:
  - Level I: Below and lateral to pectoralis minor. Anterior (pectoral), lateral and posterior (subscapular)
  - Level II: Behind the pectoralis minor, central group of nodes
  - Level III: Above and medial to pectoralis minor—apical nodes

  Minimum 10 nodes to be removed for staging of the cancer and for the prognosis. Level I and II must be removed.

  Removal of level III is not required unless they are enlarged. Involvement of level III denotes worst prognosis.

Procedures

1. General anesthesia
2. *Supine position:* Arm of the affected side to be kept straight on arm rest or arm to be abducted up to 90° and kept on arm rest. Antiseptic cleaning draping to be done.
3. *Incision:* The skin ellipse is marked a transverse elliptical incision (FT Stewart) 4–5 cm around the lump.

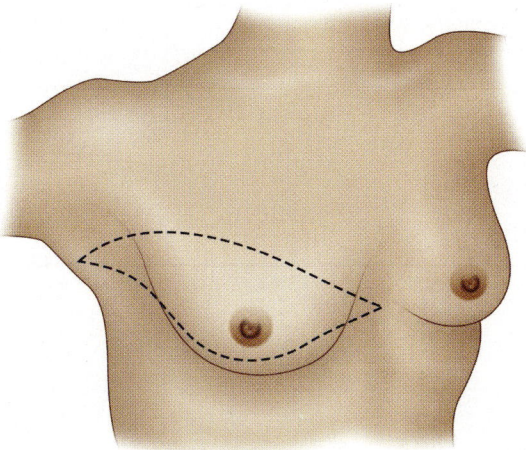

FT Stewart incision for MRM

Step 1: Raising of flaps: Upper flap to be raised first up to the edge of the breast or where you see the subclavius muscle. The plane of dissection between subcutaneous fat and breast fat (Remember: "B for B", i.e. breast fat is bigger than subcutaneous fat).

Lower flap to be raised up to 2–3 cm below inframammary fold, i.e. when you see the upper rectus sheath. Medially up to midline and laterally till the medial border of LD (flap thickness should be 8–10 mm). In each steps, bleeding points to be coagulated with diathermy.

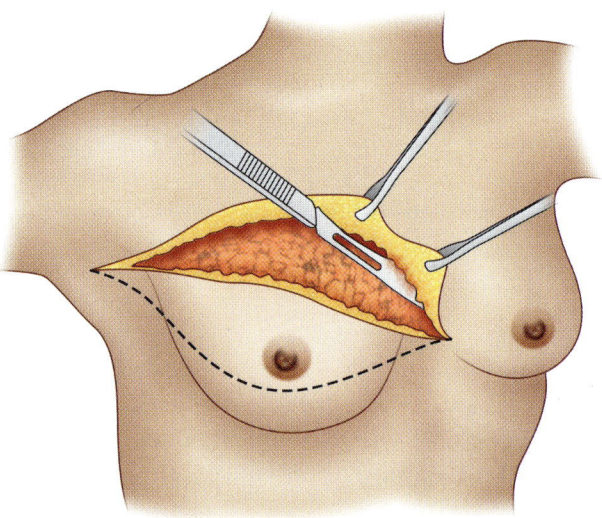

Raising of upper flap

Step 2: Raising of breast: Start form medial side, whole breast to be taken off from pectoralis major fascia from all sides, perforators are to be controlled either by diathermy or by ligation. Now, the whole breast is allowed to hang laterally with axillary tail in continuity with axilla. Elevate the lateral border of pectoralis

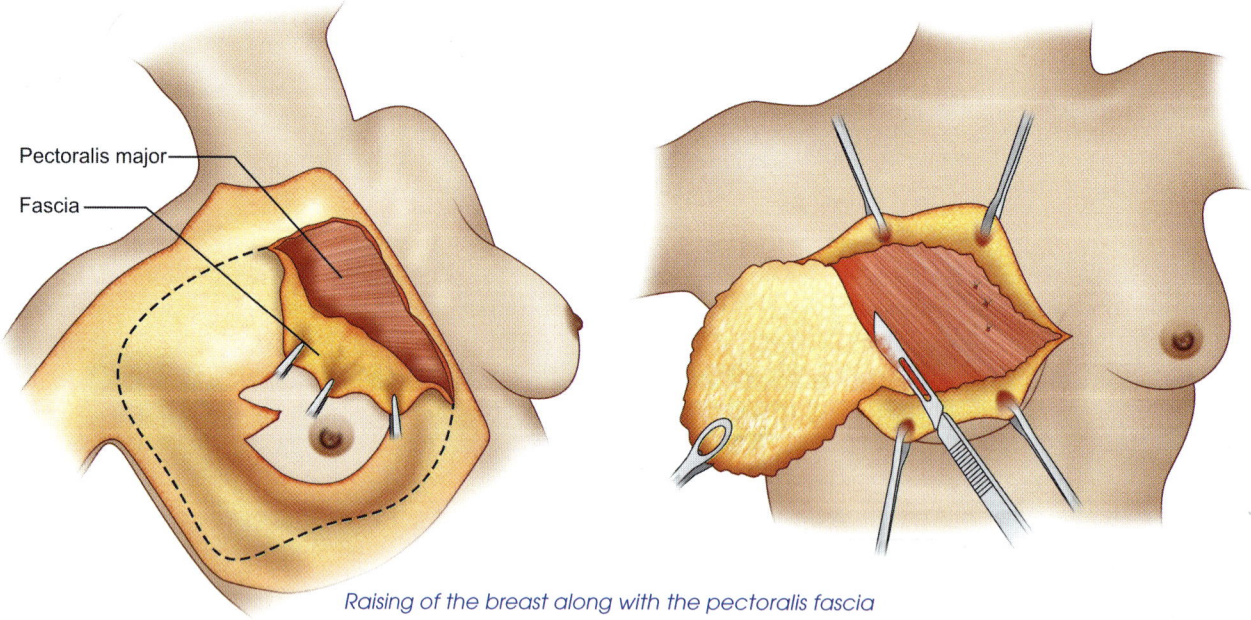

Pectoralis major

Fascia

Raising of the breast along with the pectoralis fascia

We are shaped by our thoughts. We become what we think. When the mind is pure, joy follows like a shadow that never leaves.

major with two Allis forceps and clear loose areolar tissue and fally tissue along with interpectoral nodes, if any. Retract pectoralis minor and clear the loose areolar tissue, fatty tissue behind the muscle.

Step 3: Axillary dissection: Axilla is now widely opened the boundary of axillary dissection is above axillary vein, laterally LD and medially the pectoralis major. Along with the clearance of lateral border of pectoralis major, level I lymphnodes are cleared to clear level II and III, pectoralis minor muscle may be removed from coracoid process (Patey's procedure), the muscle may be divided (scanlon) or it may be retracted (auchinclos), the lymphatics and loose areolar tissue to be cleared up to axillary vein, from below upward few tibuteries of axillary vein to be tied in the dissected field of axilla. The nerve to serratus anterior (long thoracic nerve) to be identified under the fascia along the lateral chest wall and to be preserved, nerve to LD (thoracodorsal nerve) close to anterior border of latissimus dorsi along with subscapular vessls to be preserved. The intercost brachial nerve may or may not be preserved.

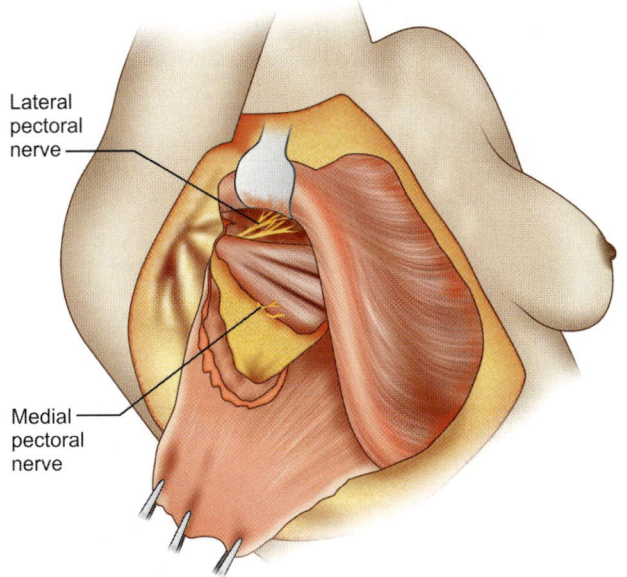

Lateral pectoral nerve

Medial pectoral nerve

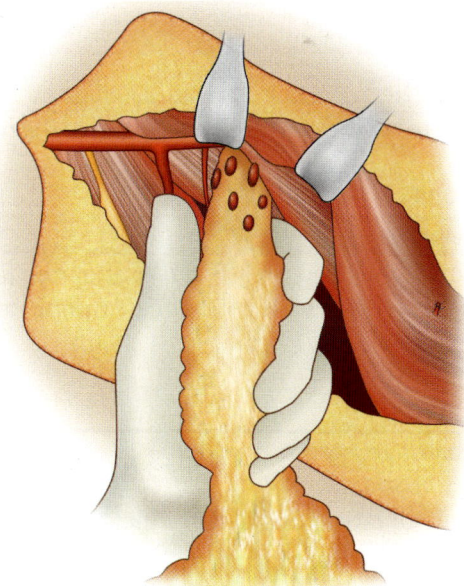

Axillary dissection

Smile will be complete when it begins with your heart, reflects in your eyes and ends with a glow on your face.

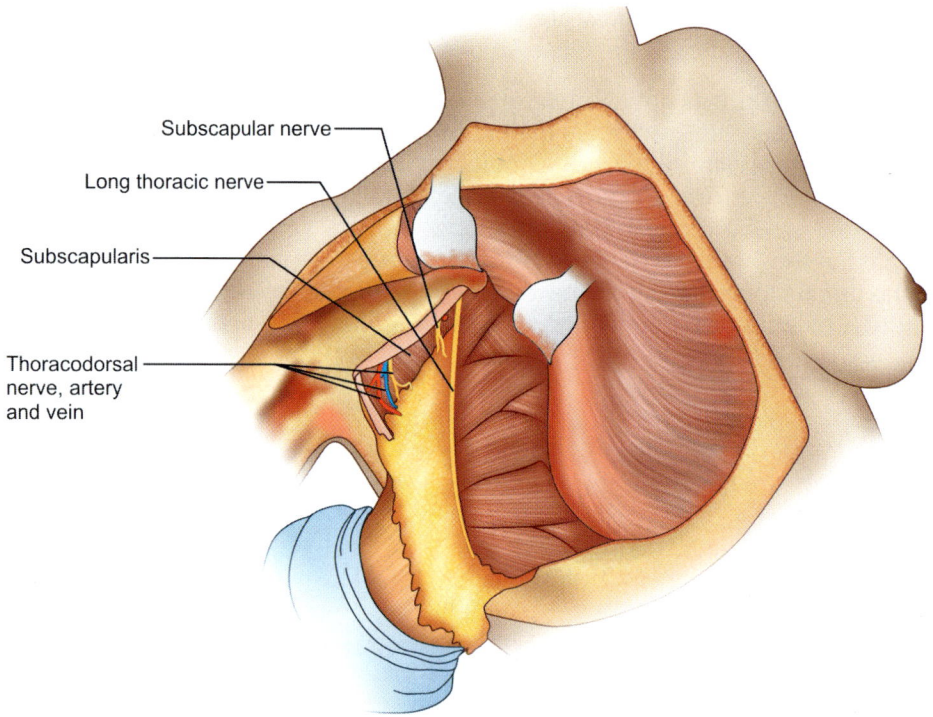

Subscapular nerve

Long thoracic nerve

Subscapularis

Thoracodorsal
nerve, artery
and vein

Pedicle of latissimus dorsi along with thoracodorsal nerve and nerve to serratus anterior preserved

Step 4: Closure: Hemostasis is secured. Suction drain is placed at axilla (another drain may be placed below the flap). Skin may be closed with subcuticular suture or interrupted nylon/silk/stapler.

5.2 BREAST CONSERVATION SURGERY (BCS)

SURGICAL ANATOMY

BCS includes wide local excision (WLE) of the tumor with 1 cm clear margin plus a complete axillary dissection.

Indications

- Early breast cancer T1, T2 lesion
- Locally adveanced breast cancer after neoadjuvant therapy
- Even T3 lesion with a good breast tumor ratio.

Pitfalls

Same as MRM.
- Hemorrhage, seroma
- Flap necrosis
- Damage of latissimus dorsi pedicle, nerve to serratus anterior and thoracodorsal nerve.

Procedure

- Supine position, ipsilateral arm is abducted at 90° position

---

Watch your thoughts; they become words. Watch your words; they become actions. Watch your actions; they become habits. Watch your habits; it becomes your destiny.

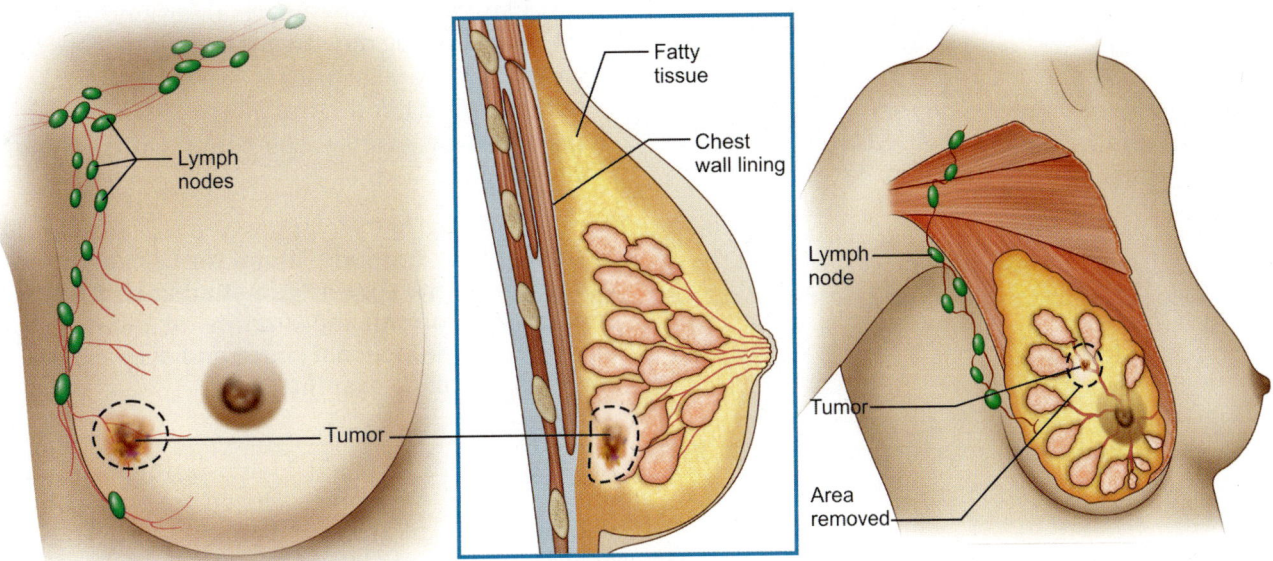

Anatomy of breast conservation surgery

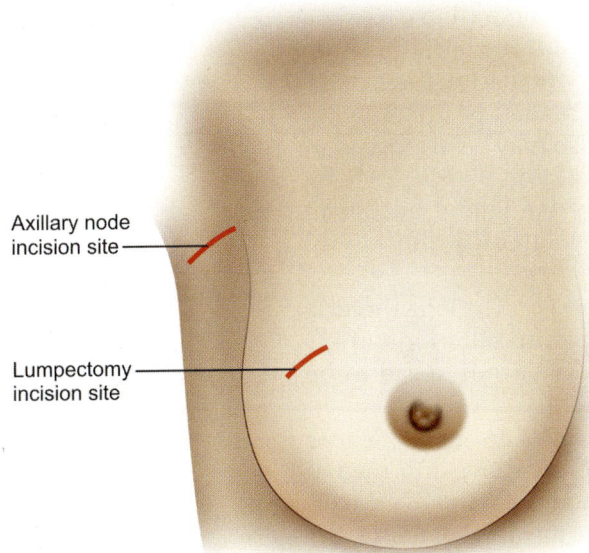

Incision on the tumor

- General anesthesia
- Incision: It is to be made over the lump. For upper half circumferential incision and for lower half radical incision are preferred for better cosmesis.

Step 1: Excision of the lump
- Flap elevation or tunneling is not advisable.

Be more eager for truth than for success.

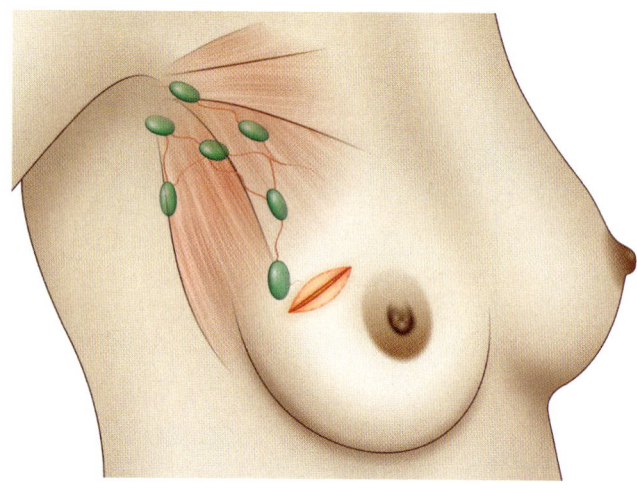

Wide local excision of the tumor with 1 cm clear margin

- Place your index finger all around the tumor and keep dissecting downward to the pectoralis major.
- Fascia of pectoralis major is also to be excised along with the tumor and normal breast tissue.
- Like this way, excise whole tumor with minimum 1 cm margin.

Step 2: Mark the lumpectomy specimen by silk suture: Short superior and long lateral for the identification of margin by the concerned pathologist. Take tissue separately, from all the margins of the defect, i.e. superior, inferior, medial lateral and deep margin too, for histopathology examination.

Step 3: Closure of the breast wound: Breast tissue is not to be reapproximated. Hemostasis to be achieved meticulously. Wound is closed in a single layer without placing a drain as seroma formation inside the cavity will give rise the shape of the breast. This concept has recently been questioned; cavity is being managed by various oncoplasty techniques (volume displacement) to achieve better cosmetic outcome. Now, the concept is not to keep seroma cavity by different oncoplastic techniques.

Step 4: Axillary clearances: A separate transverse or curvilinear incision is made just below the lower axillary hairline, starting from the lateral pectoral fold up to the fold of lateral border of LD.

- The clavipectoral fascia over the axillary vein is incised parallel to the vein and all fat, fibrofatty tissue and level I and level II axillary nodes are dissected.
- Downward off the vein: The medial pectoral nerve, and the clavipectoral nerve also may be preserved, if possible. The limit of the dissection is superiorly by axillary vein, anteromedially the lateral border of pectoralis major and posterolaterally the lateral border of latissimus dorsi.
- Preservation of pedicles and nerves: The long thoracic nerve (the nerve of Bell) to serratus anterior and LD pedicle along with thoracodorsal nerve are to be preserved.
- The level III, i.e. the apical nodes are to be cleared separately which are located just above and medial to the pectoralis minor. The nodes are removed with lying bare of axillary vein. At the apex of axilla, the limit of dissection is costoclavicular ligament of Halsted.
- At the same time, excise all the interpectoral fatty tissue clearly. Care to be taken that there should no communication between the primary tumor cavity and the axillary cavity.

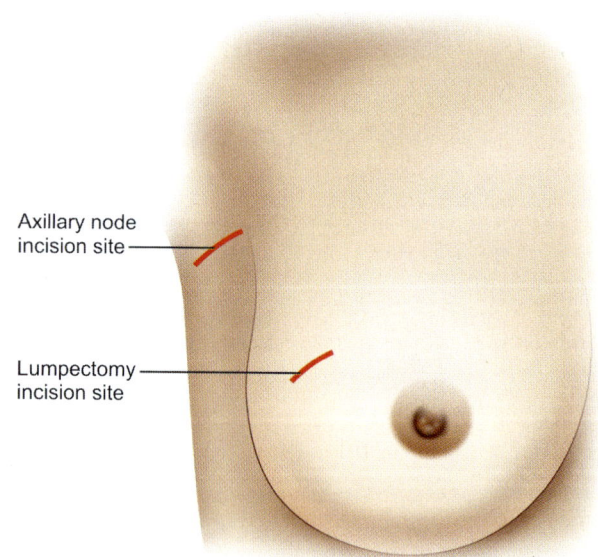

Axillary node incision site —

Lumpectomy — incision site

Axillary incision just below lower axillary hairline

Hemostasis to be achieved. Irrigate the wound thoroughly. Place a closed suction drain which is to be brought out close to the lower end of axillary incision.

Everything that shocks me in others means a work I have to do in myself.

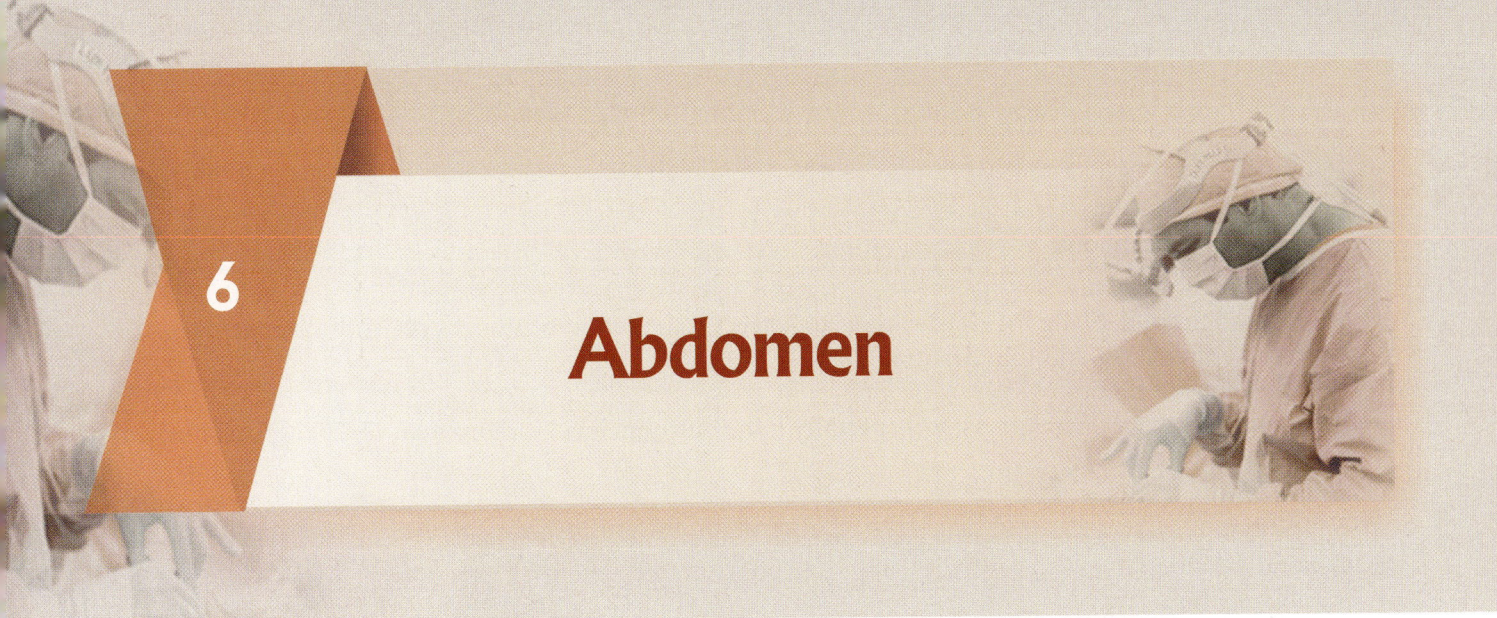

6

Abdomen

6.1.1 WHIPPLE'S PANCREATICODUODENECTOMY

History

Allen Oldfather Whipple was an American surgeon who performed the first two-stage pancreatico-duodenectomy in 1935.

In first stage, cholecystogastrostomy and gastrojejunostomy was performed to reduce the clinical jaundice. After reducing jaundice and improvement of nutrition, he performed 2nd stage procedure.

In second stage, he used to resect en bloc, duodenum and wedge of pancreas. Pancreatic stump was closed without pancreaticoenterostomy.

The mortality rate was too high (>45%) in that procedure. For that in 1941, Trimber performed one-stage pancreaticoduodenectomy.

Ultimately in 1946, Whipple's described pancreaticoduodenectomy in proper way and since then the procedure bears his name.

Till 1960, the perioperative mortality rate was 25%. In present days, mortality rate in specialized centers should be under 5%.

Indications

1. *Malignant carcinoma:*
   - Head of pancreas
   - Ampulla
   - Distal common bile duct (CBD)
   - Duodenum (D_2)
2. *Possibly benign:* Chronic pancreatitis with head mass

Pitfalls

1. Intraoperative bleeding
2. Injury to superior mesenteric artery, vein, aberrant hepatic artery, portal vein or ligation inadvertently.
3. Leakage of pancreaticojejunostomy or hepaticojejunostomy
4. Postoperative bleeding, like hemosuccus pancreaticus.
5. Postoperative pancreatitis.

If in work you meet with some difficulties, look sincerely into yourself and there you will discover their origin.

Preoperative Preparations

- Correct nutrition status
- Injection vitamin K 10 mg IM OD 3–5 days to correct coagulation profile, hypoprothrombinemia.
- Correct hypovolemia and rehydration
- Prophylactic antibiotics
- Preoperative biliary decompression, especially if the bilirubin level is more than 15–20 mg% (controversial and institution based).

Procedure

- General anesthesia
- Supine position
- Cleaning and draping
- Incision: Bilateral subcostal incision also called "Roof Top" or Chevron's incision or long midline incision.

Assessment of the disease: Abdomen is explored.

- Exclude peritoneal and hepatic metastases which would be the contraindication for the surgery.
- Invasion of tumor to infracolic part of transverse mesocolon.
- Involvement of superior mesenteric artery (SMA) is a contraindication to the procedure, while a limited involvement of SMV/portal vein (PV) can be dealt with venous resection and reconstruction.
- An extended Kocher's maneuver is performed, i.e. to see the left-sided renal vein clearly, to confirm that pancreas is not adherent to the inferior vena cava (IVC).
- Open lesser sac and mobilize the whole pancreas before committing to resection. It is to exclude that pancreas is not adherent to the PV.

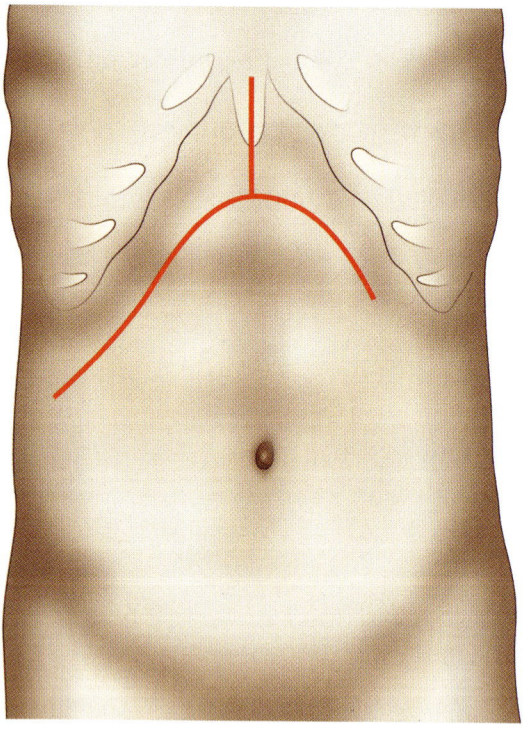

Roof top or Chevron's incision

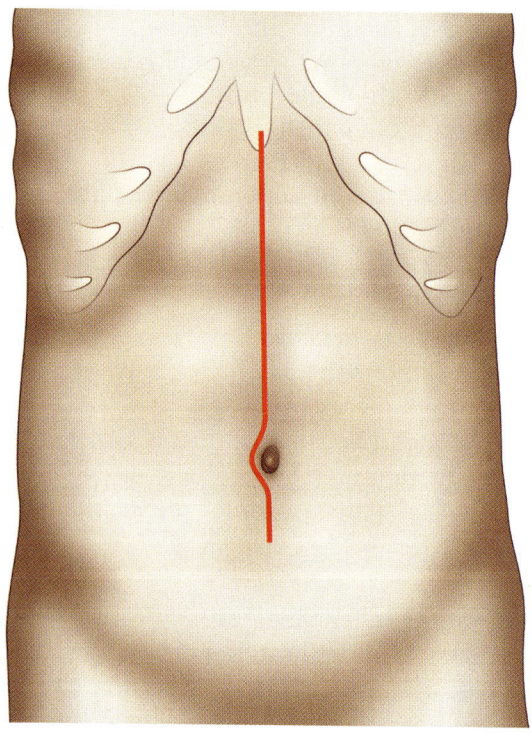

Long midline incision—particularly when the costal angle is narrow

Life's most deepest feelings are often expressed in silence and the one who can read volumes from your silence is your true friend.

If the tumor is resectable, the following dissection and resection to be performed in the clockwise manner as follows:

Step 1: Cattell-Braasch maneuver exposing SMV: Mobilizing the right colon, hepatic flexure and incise the peritoneum to the ligament of Treitz. Now, retract the right colon and pack the small intestine, 3rd and 4th parts of duodenum will be exposed.

The middle colic vein is identified, ligated and followed to its junction with SMV. Involvement of SMA is a contraindication to the procedure, while a limited involvement of SMV/PV can be dealt with by venous resection and reconstruction.

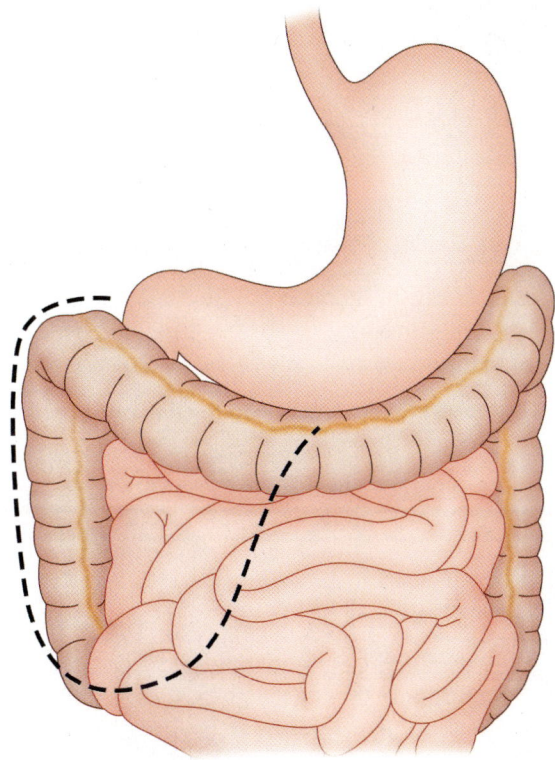

Cattell-Braasch maneuver

Step 2: Extended kocherization of duodenum: Kocherization of duodenum starts at the junction of right gonadal vein and ureter. The right gonadal vein may be ligated and divided. The Kocher maneuver is to continue to the left lateral edge of aorta and identify the left renal vein.

Now, the relationship between SMA and the tumor is assessed by palpation of the tumor. The lesser sac is entered through the mid-part of greater omentum by ligating epiploic vessels which also facilitates the dissection of greater omentum from transverse colon. Lesser sac dissection is continued toward the head of pancreas. Dissection of colon from second and third parts of duodenum across the anterior surface of the pancreas exposes the SMV and SMA.

The SMV passes over the uncinate process and receives number of fragile veins on its anterior surface. Tackle this vein very carefully, i.e. we should take time during the dissection of uncinate process in order to prevent troublesome bleeding.

Love is self-giving without asking anything in return.

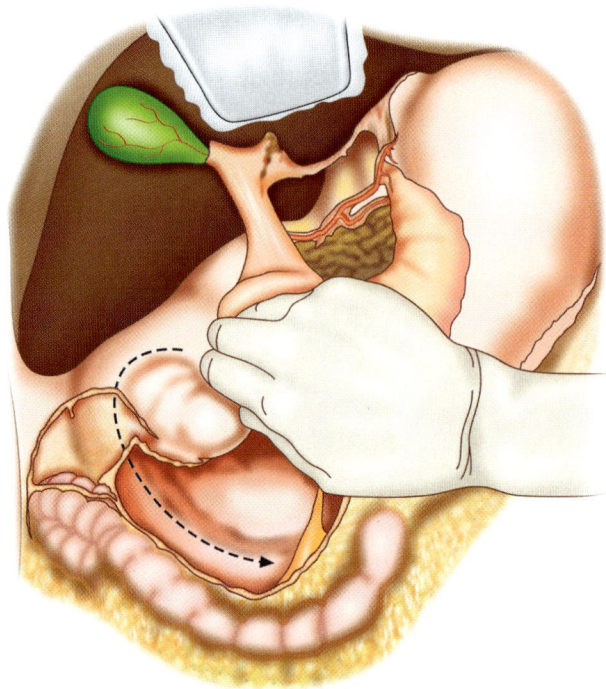

Division of mesentery between hepatic flexure and the liver and kocherization of duodenum

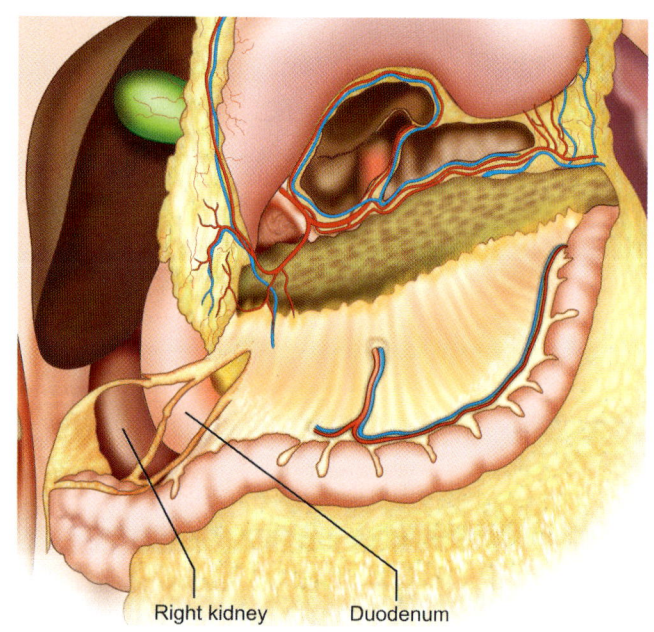

Right kidney   Duodenum

The exposure of superior mesenteric vein tracing the middle colic vein

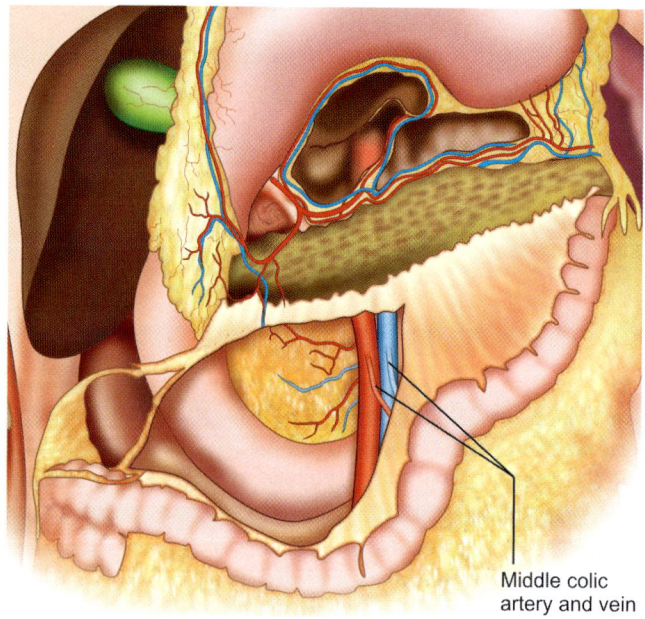

Middle colic
artery and vein

Complete exposure of superior mesenteric vessels and its relation with head of pancreas

Try to become not a man of success, but try rather to become man of value.

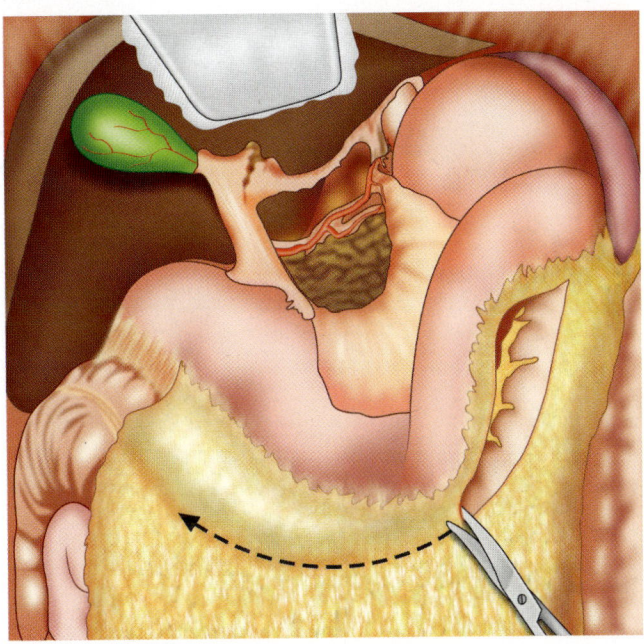

Lesser sac is entered through the greater omentum

Step 3: Portal dissection: Portal dissection begins with gallbladder in a fundus first fashion. The cystic duct is not divided. The anterior peritoneum is divided over the hepatoduodenal ligament and identify the hepatic triad:

1. Common hepatic duct and bile duct
2. Portal vein: Posterior to the bile duct
3. Hepatic artery: Left of bile duct
4. Take stay suture on both the sides of common hepatic duct (CHD) and transect, remove the previously placed biliary stent, if any.
5. Now, the portal vein is exposed. Overlying peritoneum is divided. The common hepatic artery and gastroduodenal artery (GDA) are dissected in a retrograde fashion and tissue freed with lymphnodes resected en bloc with the specimen.
6. GDA is ligated and divided after occluding the GDA to see that arterial inflow to the liver is intact. The loose areolar and connective tissues anterior to portal vein are divided in caudal direction to the junction of portal vein and the neck of the pancreas.
7. The superior mesenteric vein is identified and developed the tunnel between the SMV and the neck of pancreas. Ligate all small veins and arteries at the time of dissection.
8. Continuous dissection in this plane frees SMV and portal vein. The tunnel behind the neck of pancreas marks the pancreatic transaction line.

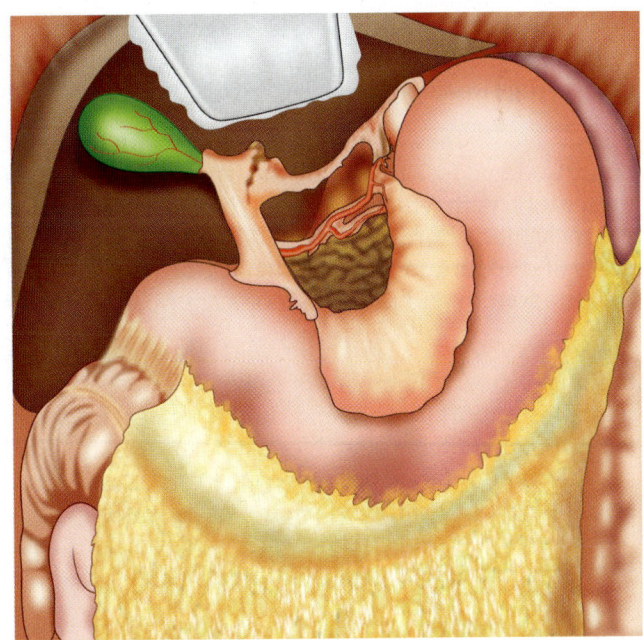

Dissection of hepatoduodenal ligament and identification of the hepatic triad

A valuable man is much more important than a successful man always.

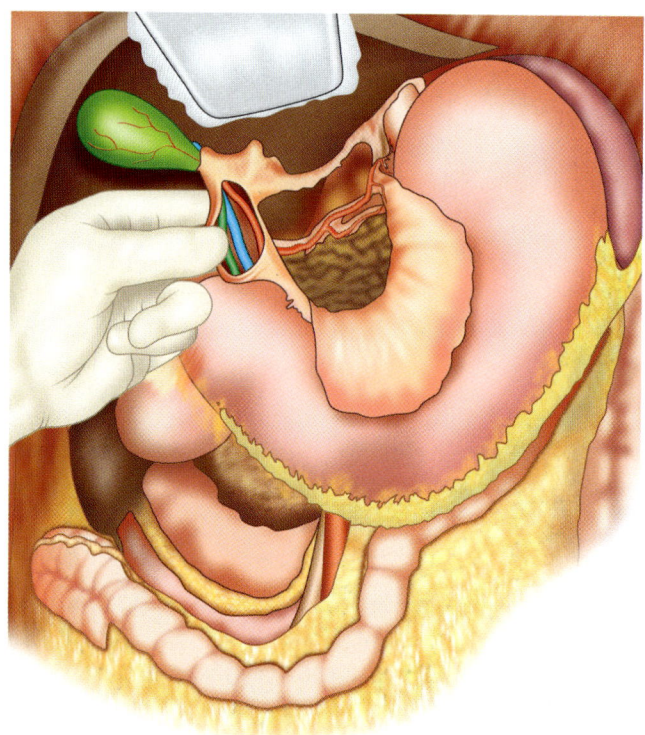

Complete exposure of portal structure

Step 4: Distal gastrectomy: Stomach is mobilized now to do the distal gastrectomy. The line of resection is at the level of third or fourth transverse vein in the lesser curvature and at the confluence of gastroepiploic veins on the greater curvature. The lesser omentum is divided on to the lesser curvature ligating the vessels running parallel to the gastric wall. The greater omentum is divided at the level of the greater curvature transection. Divide the stomach with GIA 75 (linear cutter stapler) with green demarcation.

Step 5: Dissection of ligament of Treitz and transaction of jejunum: Localize the ligament of Treitz in the paraduodenal fossae. Divide the jejunum 10 cm distal to the ligament with GIA 55, taking care of the inferior mesenteric vein which is located to the left of paraduodenal fossae. Dissect, ligate and divide the mesentery at the mesenteric border of jejunal limb with sequential elevation of the proximal jejunum and fourth and third parts of duodenum. The duodenal attachment (mesentery) is similarly divided to the level of aorta and then the duodenum and jejunum loops are pushed gently under the mesenteric vessels to the right.

Step 6: Pancreatic transection and removal of the specimen: Complete the dissection of the uncinate process to make it free. If ligament of uncinate process is present, ligate and divide it along with small vessels on the way. It is important to spend time to dissect uncinate process and carefully make it free from portal vein and superior mesenteric vein. Now stay sutures are placed on either side of the planned transaction line, on the superior and inferior borders of the pancreas. Now, transect with the cautery the head and neck of pancreas at the level of portal vein. Hemostasis is achieved by under running bleeding pancreatic vessels. Tissue in between right border of SMV, PV and pancreatic head ligated and divided serially to deliver the specimen, SMA is exposed and ultimate process is dissected off the proximal part of SMA and the specimen is removed.

Step 7: Reconstruction with pancreas, biliary tree and the stomach: Reconstruction proceeds in a counter-clockwise direction.

Richness is not earning more, spending more or saving more. Richness is when you need "NO MORE".

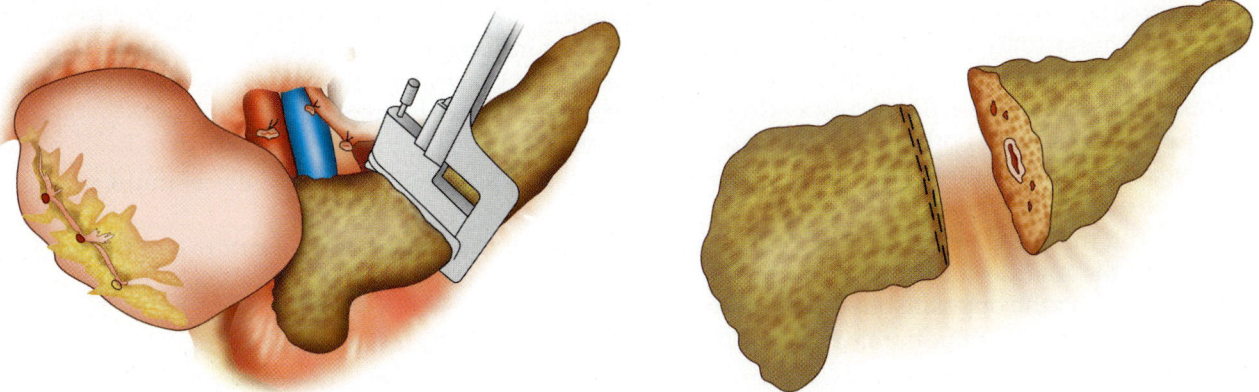

Division of pancreas at the junction of neck and body

i. *Pancreaticojejunostomy:* Pancreatic remnant is mobilized from retroperitoneum and splenic vein for a distance of 3 cm. The transected jejunum is brought through the rent of transverse mesocolon to the left of middle colic vessels, in retrocolic fashion.

A two-layer, end to side, duct to mucosa pancreaticojejunostomy is performed with 4-0 PDS. Complete the posterior row with 4-0 PDS and now make a opening in the jejunum. The anastomosis between the pancreatic duct and small bowel mucosa is done with 4-0 PDS. Each stitch will take a good bite of the pancreatic duct and a full thickness bite of the jejunum. A small silastic stent may be placed and the duct to mucosa anastomosis performed over it; however, it has not been shown to be beneficial.

The posterior row knots will be inside and lateral and anterior knots will be outside. (When the pancreatic duct is not dilated and pancreatic tissue is soft, not fibrotic, the dunking procedure may be performed. Two layers anastomosis that invaginates the cut end of the pancreas into the jejunum. Here, the jejunum is opened for a length equal to the transverse diameter of the pancreas. The pancreatic remnant now sewn to the jejunum with 4-0 PDS, and the anastomosis is to be completed with placement of seromuscular suture with 4-0/5-0 PDS.)

An alternate to pancreaticojejunostomy is pancreaticogastrostomy.

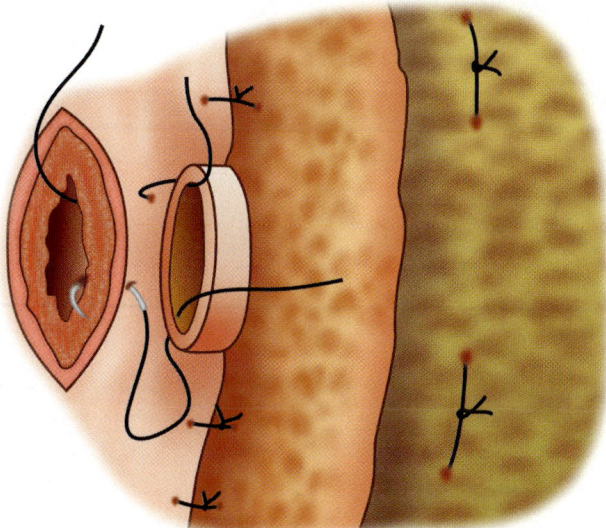

Pancreaticojejunostomy: duct mucosal anastomosis

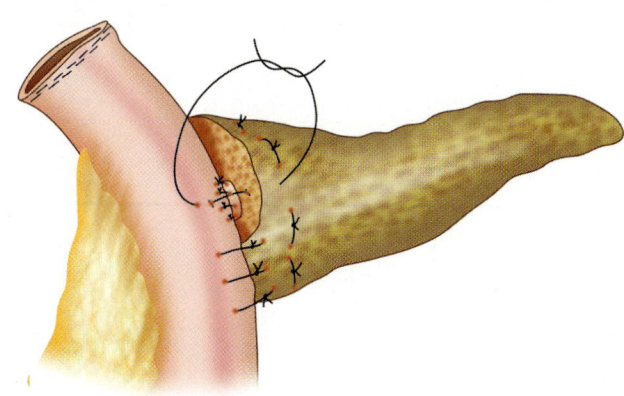

Buttressing of pancreas into the anterior wall of jejunum

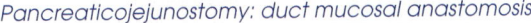

You cannot change how people feel about you, so do not try just live your life what you feel the best.

ii. *Hepaticojejunostomy:* A single layer hepaticojejunostomy is performed with 4-0 PDS. The hepaticojejunostomy is performed using a single layer of interrupted 4-0 PDS sutures. At one corner of the duct, take the suture from outside-in and then inside-out (like conel), the same suture to take outside-in and then inside-out at the corresponding corner of the jejunum. The same "box" stitches to be repeated to the other corner of both the bile duct and the jejunum.

Now, a suture to take at the middle of the posterior wall of both the bile duct and the jejunum and keeps it in the middle as a guide.

Now, hold the "box" suture at one corner and take full thickness posterior wall suture one by one 1mm apart till the middle suture kept as a guide. Repeat the same thing on the opposite site of the middle suture holding the opposite box suture at the corner.

(*Remember:* Mucosa of both the duct and jejunum to be taken in the suture invariably).

Now, start tying the suture, one by one, from one corner to another corner. Thus, the knots of the posterior layer will be on the inside. The first and middle and the middle and last sutures are held to steady the anastomosis. Now, cut the middle suture which has been kept as a guide but keep both corner suture long.

The anterior wall anastomosis: Assistant will hold the corner suture and the surgeon will take through and through suture in both the anterior wall of the bile duct and jejunum 1 mm apart. Throughout the anterior wall of both, ensuring that post wall anyway is not taken during anterior wall anastomosis.

Now, tying all sutures one by one and the knots of the anterior wall be on the outside.

Lastly, cut both the corner suture and the anastomosis is completed.

iii. *Gastrojejunostomy:* An anticolic, isoperistaltic, end-to-side gastrojejunostomy to be done in two layers.

iv. *Feeding jejunostomy (Witzel)*

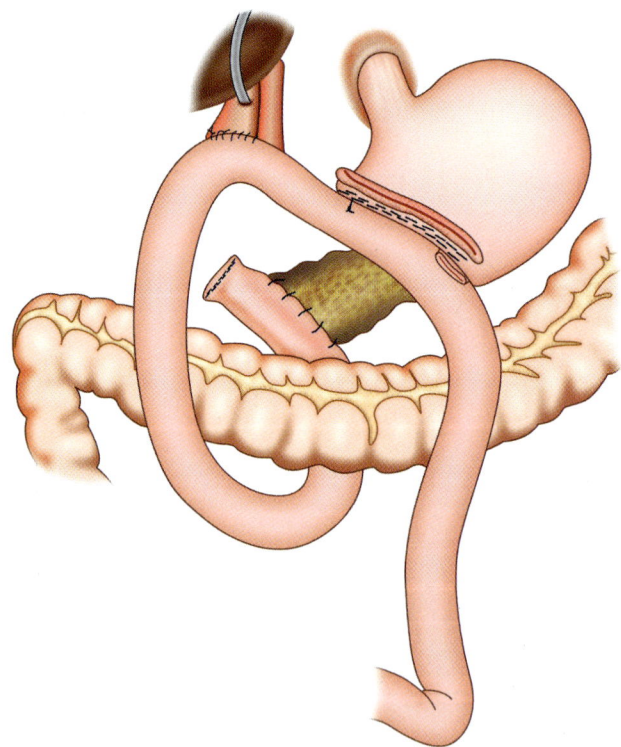

Reconstruction after Whipple's surgery—pancreaticojejunostomy, hepaticojejunostomy and gastrojejunostomy

---

Some people come in your life a blessing, some come in your life as lesions.

1. Select a loop of proximal jejunum approximately 15 cm from the ligament of Treitz (distal to one peristaltic segment of jejunum).
2. Make a stab wound in the abdominal wall and insert the catheter.
3. Take a purse string suture with 3-0 silk/vicryl and make a small incision on the jejunal wall inside the purse string and insert the catheter (12/14 F Foleys) and tighten the purse string suture around the catheter.
4. Create a seromuscular tunnel 5–6 cm in length and fix the catheter using interrupted 4-0 silk suture.
5. Fix the tunnel to the parietal wall too at least three points keeping the direction of the catheter tip downward.
6. Fix the catheter to the skin properly.

Step 8: Achieve complete hemostasis, wash the abdominal cavity with warm normal saline. Place two drains, anterior and posterior, to the pancreaticojejunal anastomosis, in such a way that it will cover all the anastomoses. Close the abdomen in layers.

Postoperative care: Apart from intravenous (IV) fluids and injectable antibiotics, injectable proton pump inhibitor (pantoprazole 40 mg IV BD)

1. Injection octreotide 100 mg IV TDS/5 days in order to prevent pancreatic anastomotic leak. Its role is controversial.
2. Keep nasogastric (NG) tube for 4–5 days.
3. Keep the drain 8–10 days and send the drain fluid for amylase on PO D$_3$.
4. Maintain adequate intake and output
   - Feeding jejunostomy (FJ) starts on bowel movement
   - Maintain nutrition.

Complications

- Postoperative hemorrhage
- Leakage from pancreatic anastomosis
- Biliary anastomosis
- Postoperative sepsis
- Acute pancreatitis
- Hepatic failure
- Postoperative bleeding.

6.1.2 LATERAL PANCREATICOJEJUNOSTOMY

Indications

1. Chronic pancreatitis with intractable pain not responding to medical treatment.
2. Dilated pancreatic duct more than 5 mm in diameter with intract pain in chronic pancreatitis.

Pitfalls

1. Overlying of
   - Portal hypertension
   - Carcinoma pancreas
2. Pancreatic fistula.

Procedure

1. General anesthesia
2. Supine position
3. Incision: As above.

Happiness does not obey the laws of mathematics. When you start "dividing" it among others, it actually multiplies.

Step 1: Explore the abdomen, through the gastrocolic omentum enter into the lesser sac and explore whole length of pancreas. Divide the peritoneal attachments between the pancreas and the posterior wall of the stomach.

Step 2: Palpate the main pancreatic duct, if not palpable, aspirate pancreatic juice and locate the duct. (Usually, the duct is located about one-third of the distance of the superior to inferior margin of pancreas.) Once the pancreatic duct is identified, open it by making the incision along the anterior wall and should open the entire duct from the head to tail with Potts scissors. Hemotasis to be achieved in every step with cautery or with fine absorbable suture. (If any stricture is there in the duct, insert a probe through the strictured area and incise the anterior wall of the duct with a knife over the probe. Remove all calculi or debris from the duct.)

Step 3: Roux-en-"Y" jejunostomy: Prepare the Roux loop as described above (steps 2, 3 of cystojejunostomy) (in place of cyst write pancreas).

Step 4: Now prepare for side-to-side duct jejunal anastomosis. The cut end of the jejunum would be anastomosed with the tail side of the pancreas.

Incise the antimesenteric border of the jejunum over a length equal to the incision of the pancreatic duct. With 3-0/4-0 PDS/vicryl, anastomose the posterior wall of the duct jejunum. Pass the needle through the fibrotic parenchyma of pancreas and through the duct and then the needle to be inserted through both mucosa and seromuscular part of jejunal wall. Tie the suture with the knot inside the lumen of the duct (many surgeons like to take continuous suture throughout the whole length) for the anterior layer full thickness of jejunum and the duct including the parenchyma. The knot will be outside.

Step 5: Jejunojejunostomy: Make a 3–4 cm window, approximately the same diameter of jejunal opening in the anterior cyst wall. Perform one layer anastomosis, the jejunal and cyst window. Insert 3-0/4-0 absorbable suture interruptedly. Now, fix the mesocolon to the jejunum with 3-0 vicryl where the jejunum passes through the mesocolon.

Step 6: Close the mesenteric window with 3-0 vicryl and fix the jejunal wall which is passing through it. Hemostasis to be achieved completely and place a drain below the pancreaticojejunal anastomosis. Close the abdomen in routine fashion.

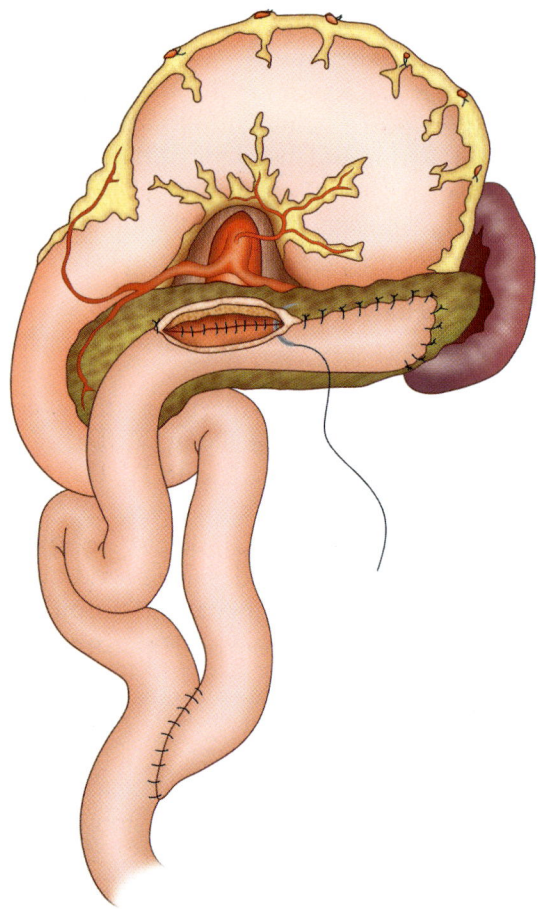

Lateral (side-to-side) pancreaticojejunostomy and end-to-side jejunojejunostomy

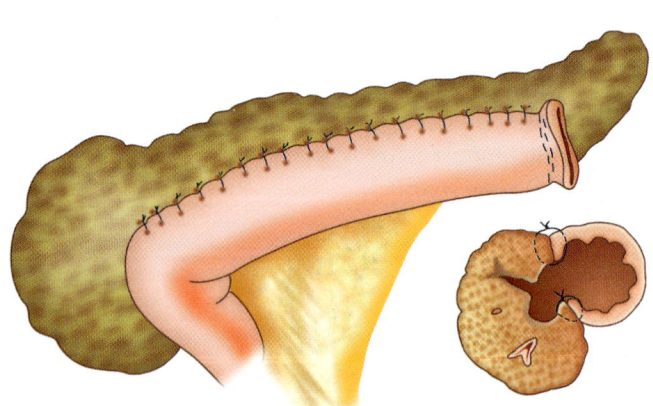

Lateral pancreatic jejunostomy completed

Postoperative Care

- Keep the drain for 5–6 days. On 5th day, send the drain fluid for amylase to exclude leak.
- Keep the NG for 1–3 days
- Antibiotics as usual.

Complications

- Pancreatic fistula
- Acute on chronic pancreatitis
- Infection, etc.

6.1.3 INTERNAL DRAINAGE OF PANCREATIC PSEUDOCYST

CYSTOGASTROSTOMY

Indications

- Pseudocyst just lying behind the stomach.
- When pseudocyst is moderate in size, i.e. where the chance of dependent part is less after drainage.
- Matured pseudocyst more than 5 cm in size.

Pitfalls

- Anastomotic leak
- Hemorrhage in both intraoperative and postoperative periods
- Chance of misdiagnosis of cystadenocarcinoma as pseudocyst
- Associated aneurysm.

Preoperative Preparation

The diagnosis of "pseudocyst" to be confirmed.

- Rule out cyst adenocarcinoma
- Rule out the gallstone and bile duct obstruction
- Preoperative nasogastric (NG) tube placement and antibiotics.

Procedures

- General anesthesia
- Supine position
- *Incision:* Long midline incision.
- Just below xiphisternum to just below the umbilicus
- Alternatively, rooftop incision is preferable.

Step 1: Explore the abdomen and identify the pseudocyst and its attachment with posterior stomach wall. (If the cyst is not adherent to the stomach wall, perform a Roux-en-"Y" cystojejunostomy as leakage from the cystogastrostomy is much more dangerous than cystojejunostomy.)

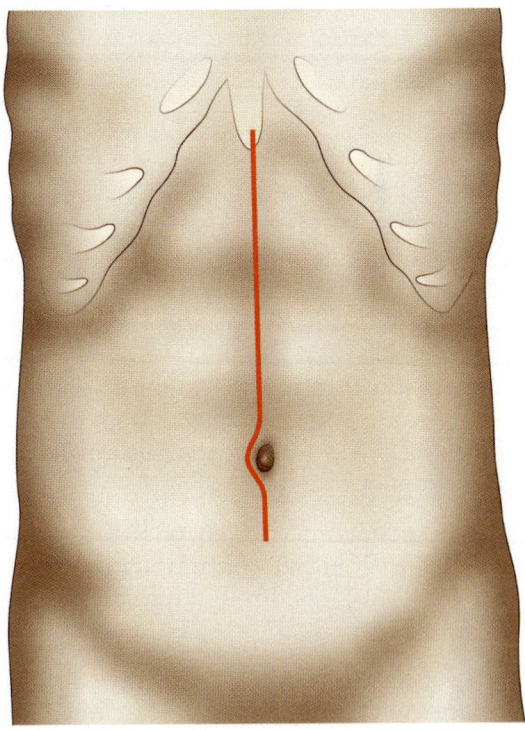

Long midline incision

As you get older you will understand more and more that it is not about what you look like or what you own, it is all about the person you have become.

Step 2: Take two stay sutures and make a 6–8 cm longitudinal anterior gastrostomy in between the stay sutures and opposite to the most prominent portion of the retrogastric cyst. Aspirate the cyst with 18 gauge needle through the posterior wall of the stomach to confirm and localize the cyst and rule out the presence of fresh blood.

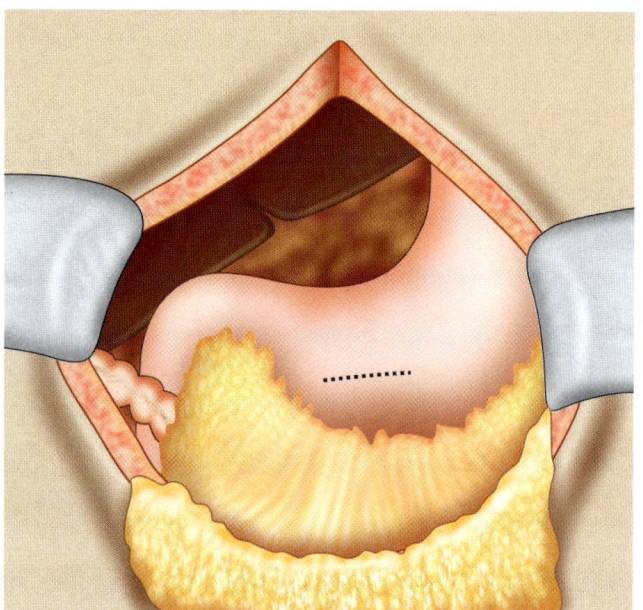

Incision of the stomach wall over the cyst

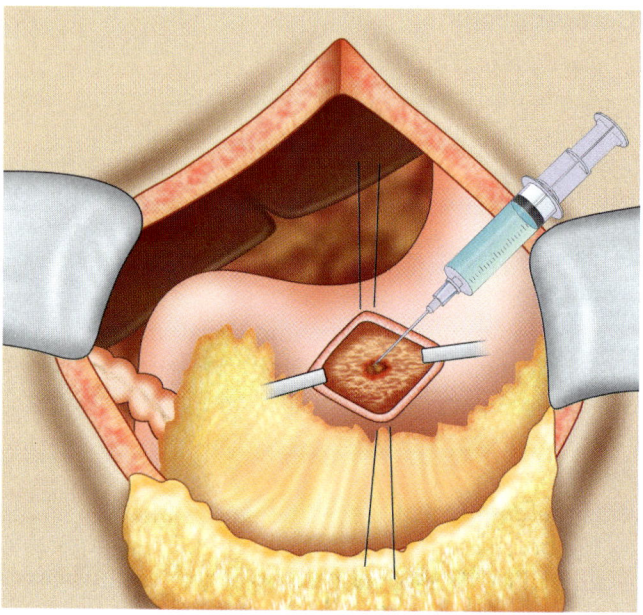

Opening of the anterior wall of the stomach to reach to posterior wall over the cyst

Step 3: Assess the thickness of the cyst wall. (If the cyst wall is thin, hold the suture, insert a Silastic catheter and take it out through a stab wound in the left upper quadrant.) Now, take a deep stay suture in the posterior stomach wall and 3–6 cm incision is made through the posterior wall of the stomach and continue the incision through the anterior wall of the cyst. (Excise some portion of tissue from the anterior wall of the cyst and send for frozen section, if any suspicion of cystadenocarcinoma.)

Step 4: Approximate the cut edges of the stomach and the cyst with either continuous or interrupted 3-0 absorbable sutures through the full thickness of both the walls.

Step 5: Closure of anterior gastric wall. The NG tube is placed within the stomach. The clouse is done either by stapler or by hand sewn technique.

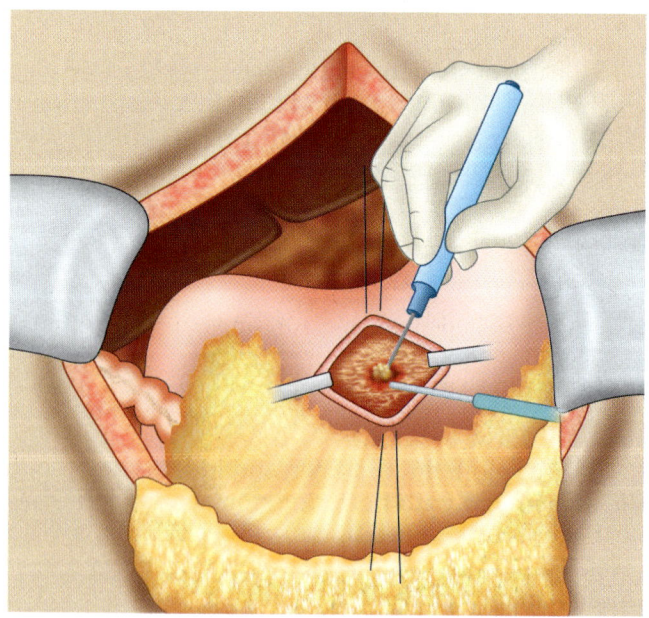

Opening of posterior wall of the stomach and the cyst wall

Generosity is to find one's own satisfaction in the satisfaction of others.

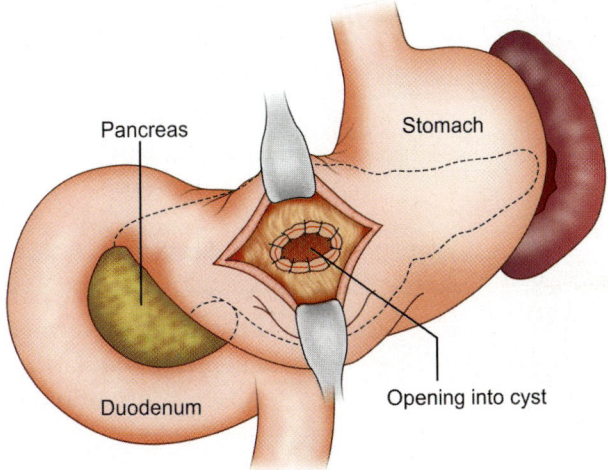

Cystogastrostomy with the full thickness of both the stomach and cyst wall

Step 6: The closure of abdominal wound and skin is as usual fashion.

6.1.4 ROUX-EN-Y CYSTOJEJUNOSTOMY

- *Indication:* Matured, large pseudocyst
- General anesthesia
- Supine position.

Procedure

Incision: As above.

Step 1: Explore the abdomen and confirm the size and site of the cyst. Expose the anterior wall of the cyst by dividing the omentum over it.

Step 2: Prepare a segment 15 cm away from duodenojejunal flexure and divide the jejunum with GIA 55. The 45–60 cm length of distal jejunal segment, i.e. the Roux loop is taken to the cyst without any tension.

Step 3: Make a small window through an avascular part of transverse mesocolon and take the distal jejunal segment into the supracolic space. Now prepare for cystojejunostomy either end to side or side to side.

Step 4: Anastomosis for cystojejunostomy: Make a 3–4 cm window, approximately the same diameter of jejunal opening in the anterior cyst wall. Perform one layer anastomosis the jejunal and cyst window. Insert 3-0/4-0 absorbable suture interruptedly. Now, fix the mesocolon to the jejunum with 3-0 vicryl where the jejunum passes through the mesocolon.

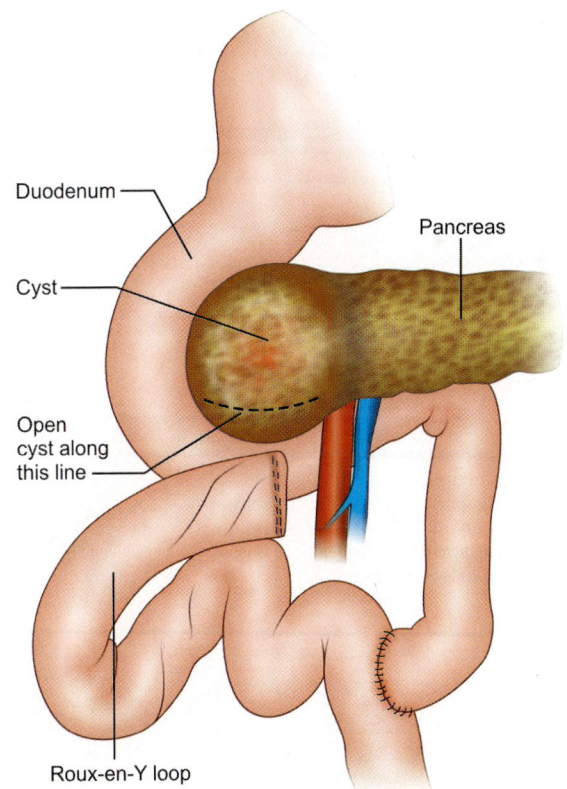

Roux-en-Y loop for cystojejunostomy

Step 5: Jejunojejunostomy: The jejunojejunostomy is now performed at 45–60 cm away from the cysto-jejunostomy.

Step 6: Hemostasis to be achieved. Drain may or may not be placed. Abdominal wound and skin is closed as usual fashion.

Complications

- Acute on chronic pancreatitis
- Postoperative intragastric bleeding
- Persistent fistula
- Abscess formation in the dependent portion, etc.

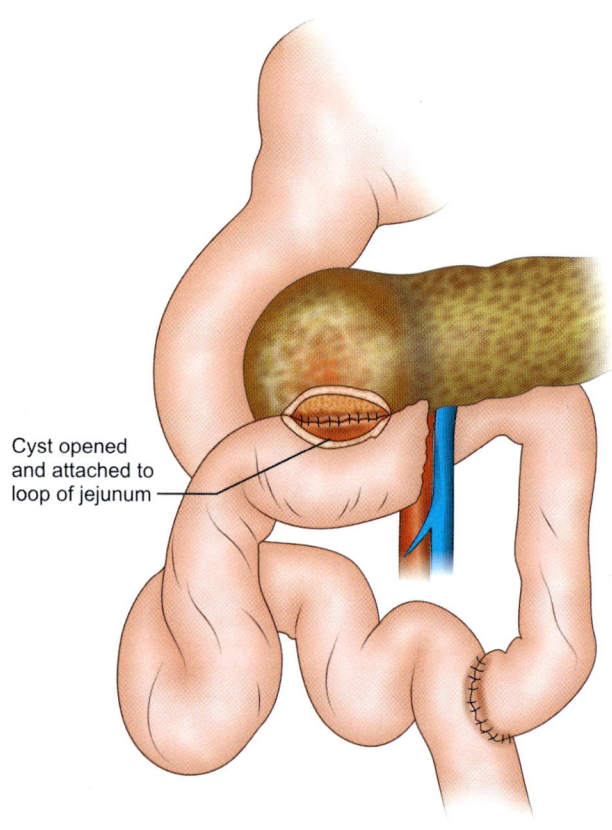

Cyst opened and attached to loop of jejunum

Cystojejunostomy with jejunojejunostomy

6.2 STOMACH

6.2.1 GASTRECTOMY

Surgical Anatomy

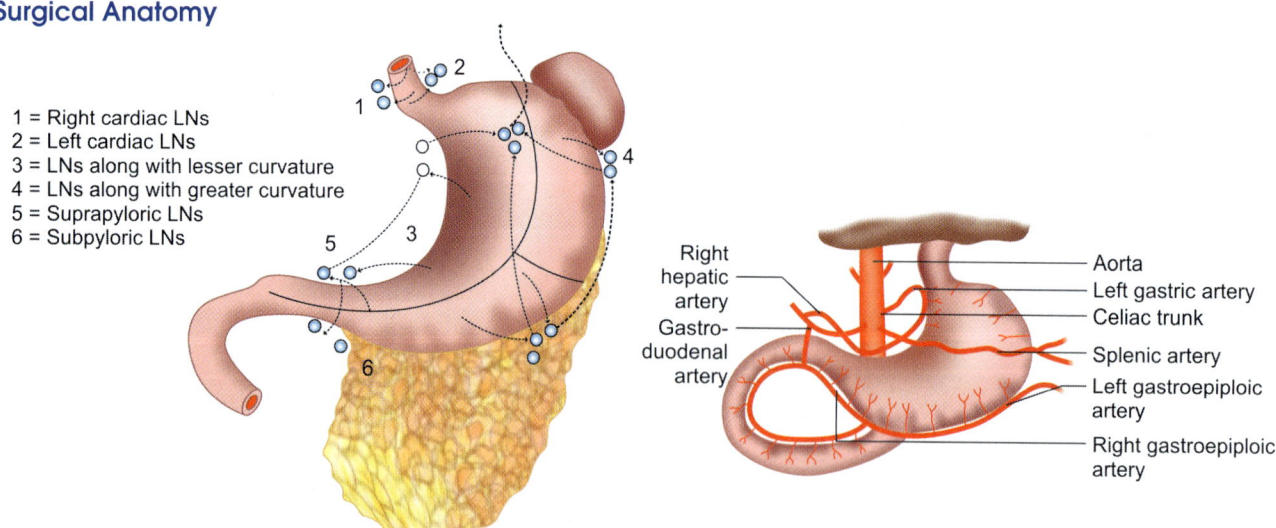

1 = Right cardiac LNs
2 = Left cardiac LNs
3 = LNs along with lesser curvature
4 = LNs along with greater curvature
5 = Suprapyloric LNs
6 = Subpyloric LNs

Right hepatic artery
Gastro-duodenal artery

Aorta
Left gastric artery
Celiac trunk
Splenic artery
Left gastroepiploic artery
Right gastroepiploic artery

Many people come in your life as lessons, but only few people come as blessings.

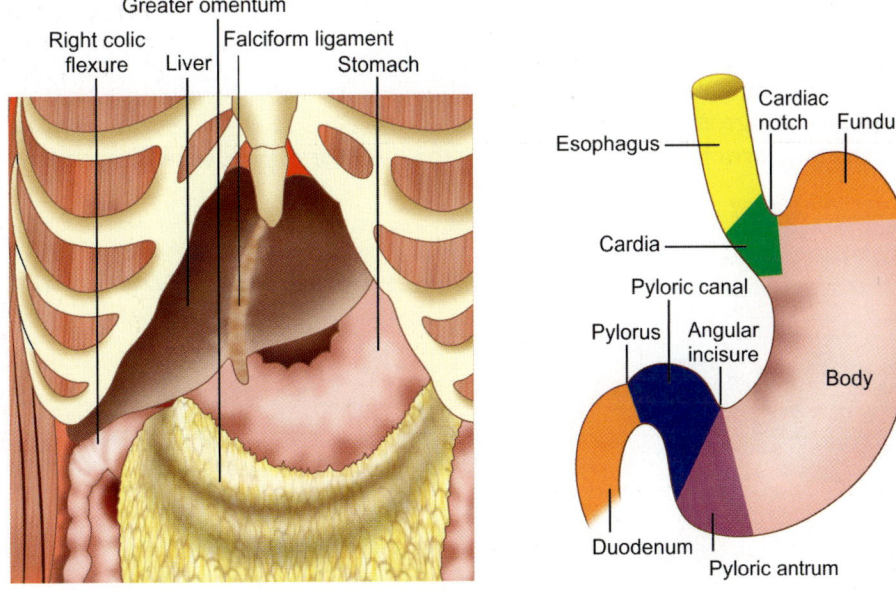

Upper abdominal anatomy

6.2.2 PARTIAL DISTAL GASTRECTOMY

Indications

- Distal gastric carcinoma as a radical procedure
- As a part of Whipple's procedure
- Pyloric or duodenal stenosis
- Uncontrolled bleeding, duodenal or gastric ulcer, where endoscopic procedure fails
- GIST distal stomach, etc.

  Steps for partial distal radical gastrectomy for distal carcinoma stomach have been described below.

Surgical Steps

1. Supine position
2. General anesthesia
3. Operation proper

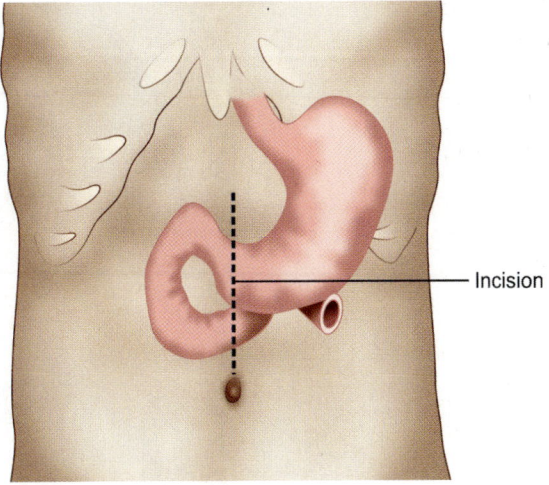

Upper midline incision

To work for your perfection, the first step is to become conscious of yourself.

Staging laparoscopy to rule out peritoneal and surface liver mets.

Step 1: Laparotomy through linea alba. Diagnosis to be confirmed operability to assess by observing extent of growth involvement of adjacent structures and lymphnodes, look for distant spread to liver, peritoneum, omentum pelvic deposits and gross ascites.

Now, you divide the falciform ligament and elevate the liver for exposure of lesser omentum.

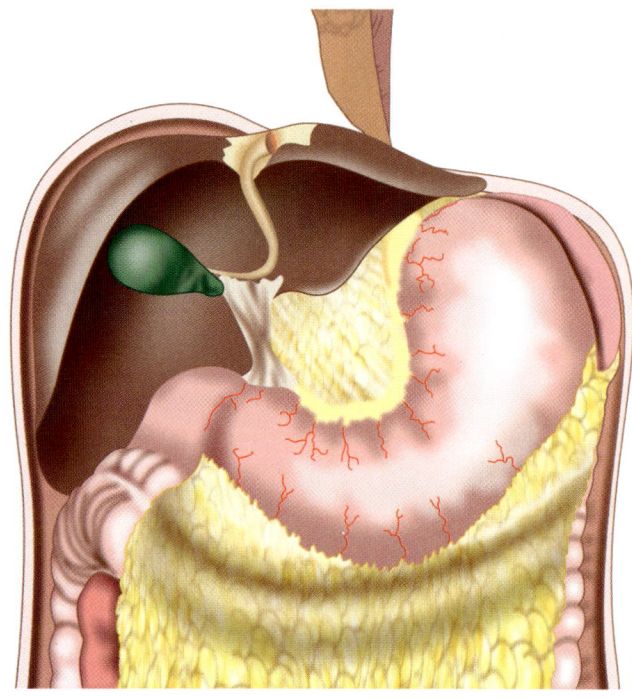

Assessment of stomach, liver, peritoneum, omentum, pelvic deposits and gross ascites

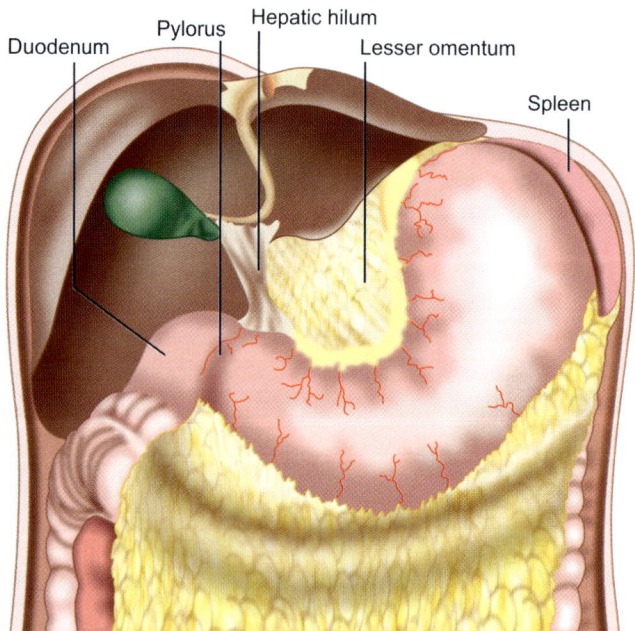

Exposure of lesser omentum after elevating the liver

It is not money that makes a man happy, but rather an inner balance of energy, good health and good feelings.

Step 2: Mobilization of omentum and vessles ligation: Division of greater omentum from transverse colon at the avascular plane 1 cm above detachment will be well beyond first part of duodenum.

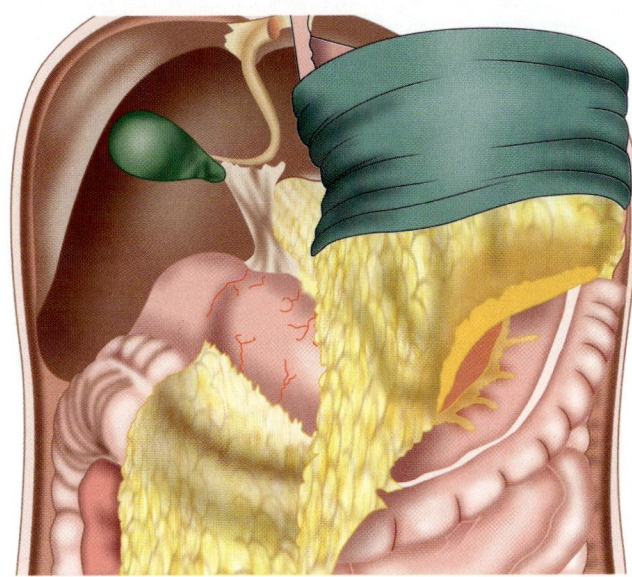

Anterior layer of transverse mesocolon is incised and stripped up to the anterior surface of pancreas

Ligation and division of right gastroepiploic vessels: Division and ligation of lesser omentum, gastrohepatic ligament, close to porta hepatis. Right gastric artery is ligated and divided close to its origin from hepatic artery. Division of gastroduodenal artery may be required during mobilization of duodenum.

Exposure of gastric vessels along the lesser curvature after dissection of lesser omentum and the gastric vessels along the greater curvature are exposed after taking off the greater omentum from transeverse colon.

Step 3: Kocherization of duodenum, mobilization of hepatoduodenal ligament, division of duodenum and closure of duodenal stump carefully in two layers. (First layer with 3-0 polyglactin sutures and second layer with 3-0 mersilk, linear stapler is the alternative way. Better to under run the staple line by 3-0 silk.)

Step 4: Lymphnodes dissection: Divided stomach is lifted up and along the lymphnodes to be dissected from stomach bed, hepatic artery up to its origin along the splenic artery up to its hilum and lymphnodes along the left gastric artery to be resected en bloc.

If you truly loved yourself, you could never hurt another.

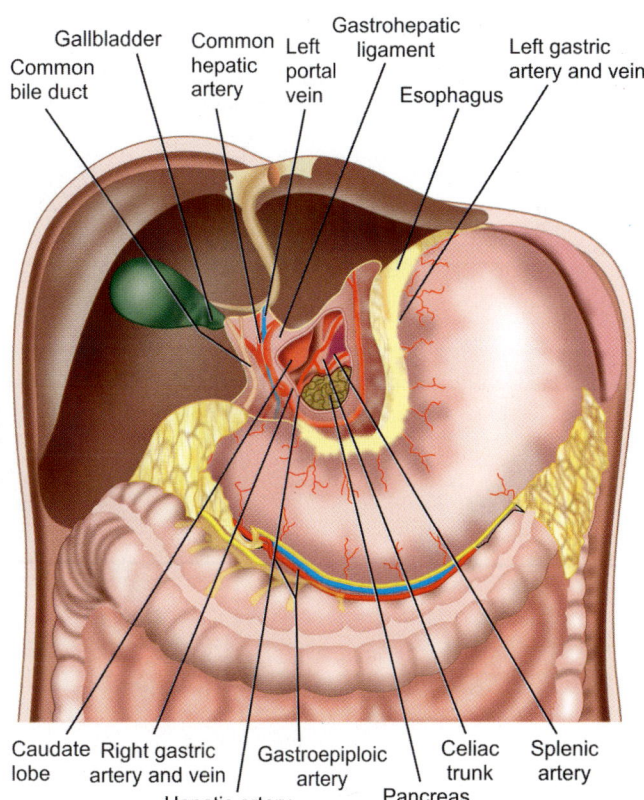

Vascular supply of stomach and related anatomy

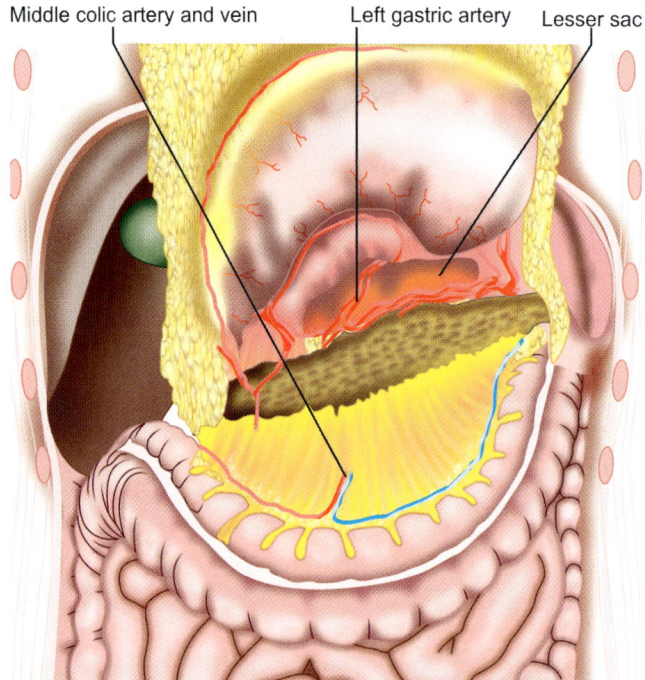

Middle colic artery and vein   Left gastric artery   Lesser sac

Complete mobilization of greater omentum elevates the stomach and exposes the lesser omentum clearly

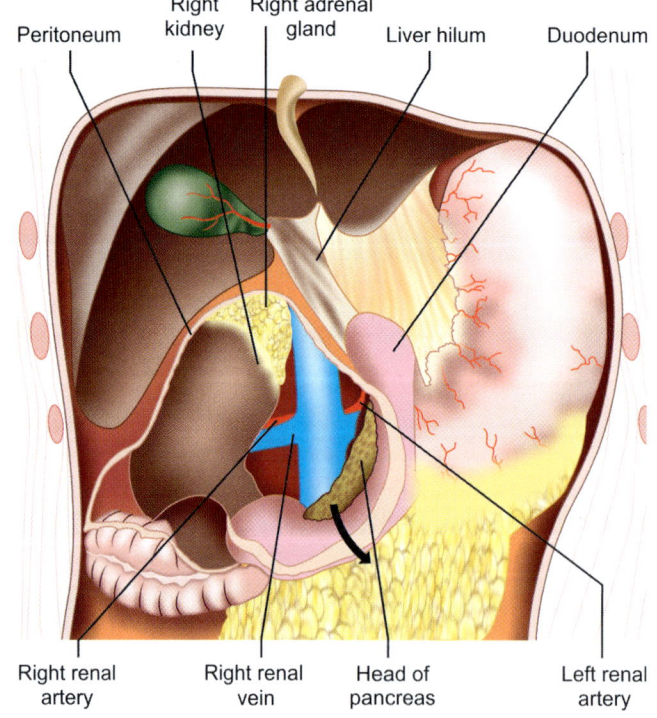

Right kidney   Right adrenal gland

Peritoneum   Liver hilum   Duodenum

Right renal artery   Right renal vein   Head of pancreas   Left renal artery

Kocherization of duodenum done till the left-sided renal vein is seen

The things you do for yourself are gone when you are gone, but the things you do for others remain as your legacy.

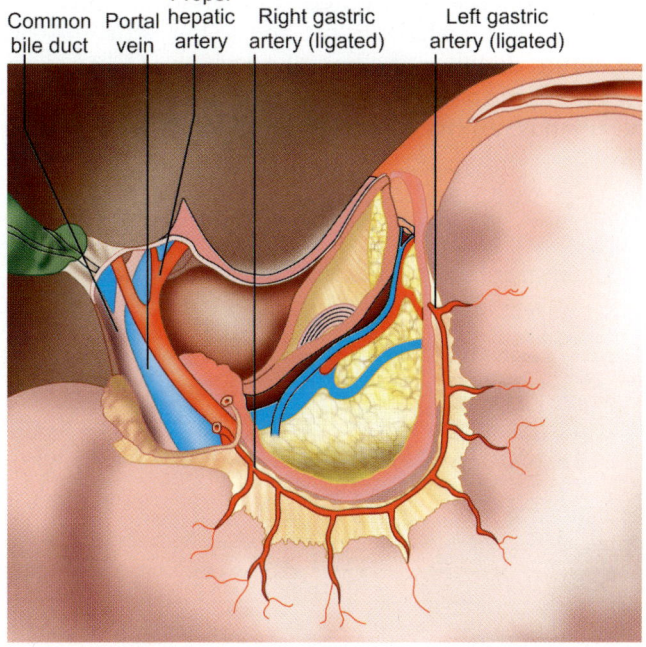

Common bile duct | Portal vein | Proper hepatic artery | Right gastric artery (ligated) | Left gastric artery (ligated)

Detachment of hepatoduodenal ligament and exposure of hepatic artery proper and right gastroepiploic artery

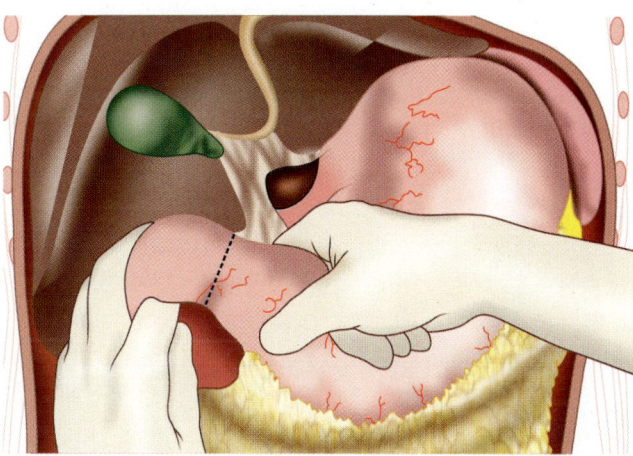

Division of duodenum either by scissors or by stapler just distal to the pyloric vein of Mayo

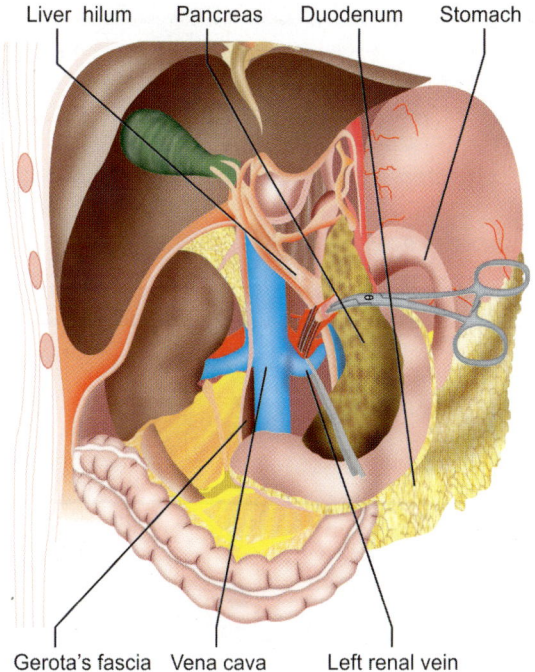

Liver hilum | Pancreas | Duodenum | Stomach

Gerota's fascia | Vena cava | Left renal vein

After clearance of all lymphnodes

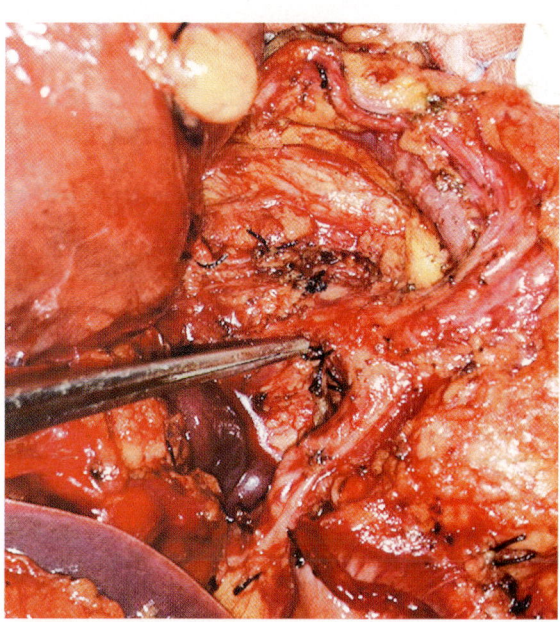

D2 Lymphnodes dissection (Courtesy: Dr Durgatosh Pandey)

Time is the costliest thing which can never be purchased by anyone. If someone spends it on you it shows the depth of care they have for you.

Step 5: After transaction, stomach is lifted up and left gastric vessels ligated and divided. There is devascularization of greater curvature by ligating and dividing left gastroepiploic and lower short gastric arteries. Apply occlusion clump proximally and crushing clump distally. The line of resection is just below the last short gastric artery and which is minimum 5 cm proximal from the tumor margin (alternately the stomach may be divided by GIA linear cutter stapler). Specimen is removed containing stomach with tumor, greater omentum, lesser omentum along with lymphnodes.

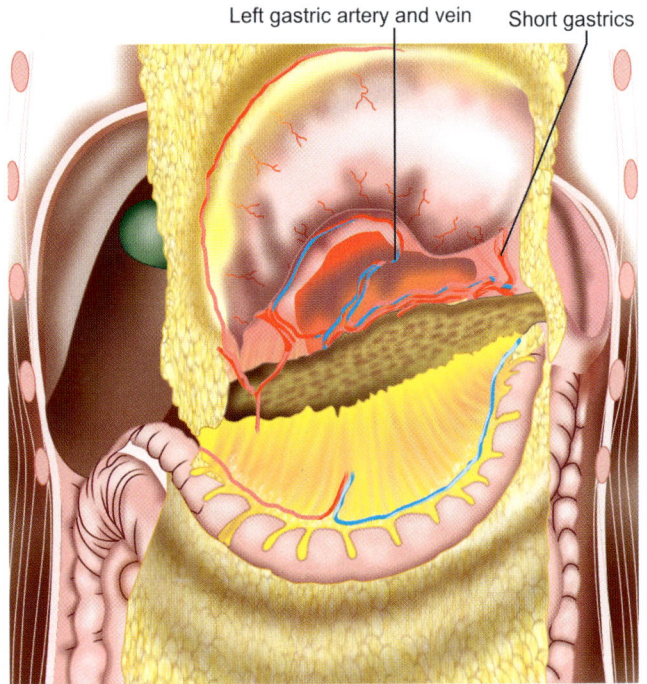

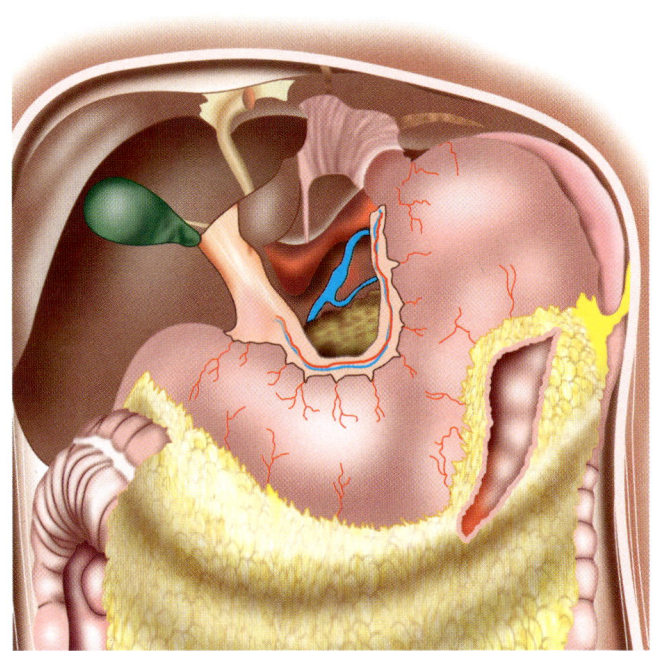

Left gastric and short gastric vessels are ligated and divided   Mobilization of greater curvature and devascularization

Step 6: Gastrojejunal anastomosis: The ideal criteria of gastrojejunostomy are:

1. Retrocolic
2. Isoperistaltic
3. Short loop or no loop
4. Without any tension and
5. Vertical stoma with good vascularity. Identifying the proximal jejunum and bring it to the site of the stomach in an anticolic fashion. The gasrtojejunostomy may be in loop or Roux-en-Y fashion.

Place the antimesenteric border of jejunum in a position with the posterior wall of the stomach. Take a stay suture

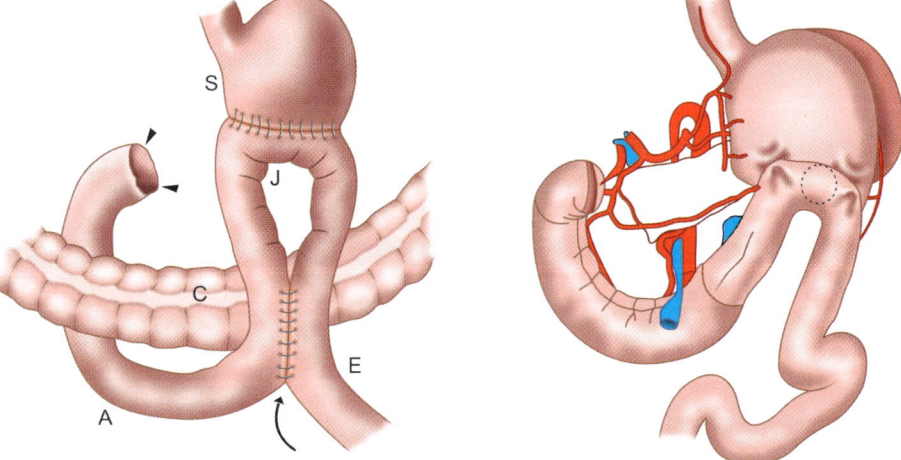

Anticolic gastrojejunostomy

approximating the antimesenteric border of jejunum to the greater curvature of the stomach, minimal 3 cm proximal to the staple line or suture line and one suture at the tip of the stapler. Then with electrocautery make a stab wound in the posterior wall of the stomach and in the jejunum. Insert a linear cutter stapler one in the gastric lumen and one in the jejunum. Be sure that there is no extraneous tissue between the walls of two structures. Lock the stapler and fire. If any bleeding in the staple line, coagulate it or insert 4-0 vicryl suture. Now, close the staple aperture with hand sewn or by a 55 linear stapler/TA 60 stapler.

Close the defect in the mesocolon intermittently with 3-0 vicryl.

- To stabilize the anastomotic site, the stomach wall may be fixed to the margins of the rent in mesocolon.
- Hemostasis to be achieved completely.
- Drain to be placed at renal pouch of Morrison close to the duodenal stump.
- Abdomen to be closed in layers.

6.2.3 TOTAL GASTRECTOMY

Greater omentum to be separated from transverse colon and continued in the upward dissection of greater omentum with ligation of upper short gastric vessels.

Gastric mobilization is required from gastroesophageal junction to the distal portion of first part of duodenum.

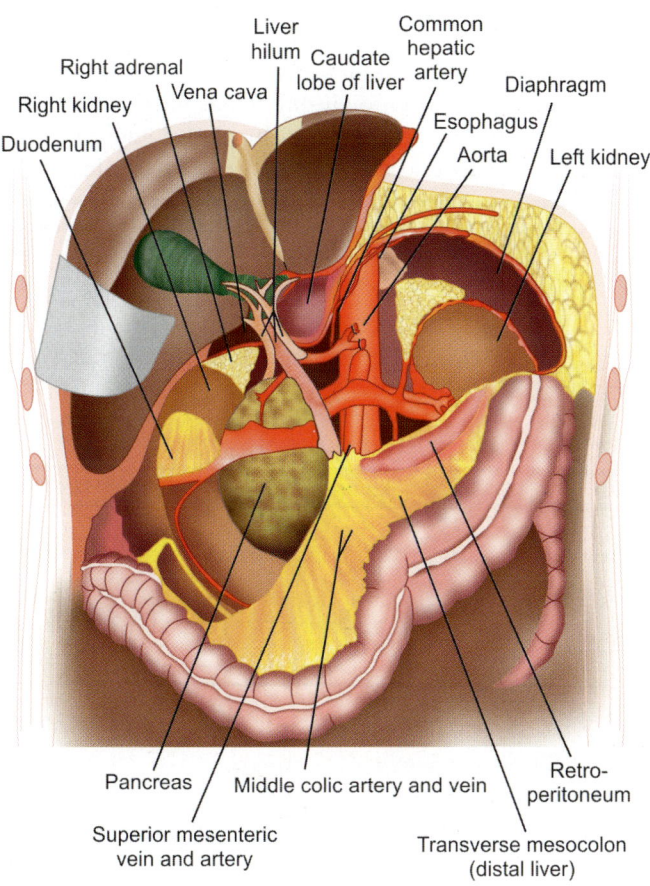

Anatomical appearance after total gastrectomy

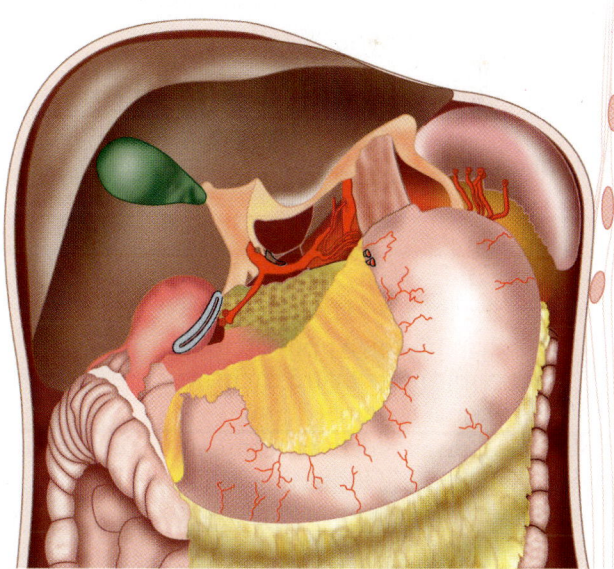

For esophagojejunal anastomosis, after total gastrectomy, the lower part of esophagus is mobilized and line of dissection is determined

---

In an unshakable faith lies all our hope.

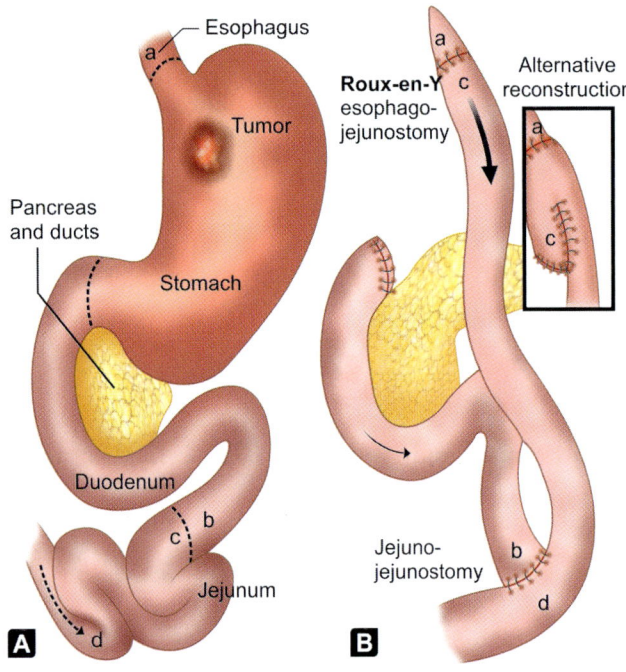

After total gastrectomy "Roux-en-Y" esophagojejunostomy and jejunojejunostomy

On the greater curvature, remaining short gastric vessels to be ligated as close to the spleen hilum. It is sometimes required to remove spleen and even pancreatic tail en-bloc in resected specimen along with lymphnodes (if the tumor extension is there).

Truncal vagotomy, both anterior and posterior vagus nerves to be identified and removed a segment of the nerves after skeletonize the abdominal part of esophagus. Esophagojejunal anastomosis to be done end-to-side or end to end either hand sewn or with 27 mm end-to-end anastomosis (EEA) stapler.

6.3 COLON

6.3.1 RIGHT HEMICOLECTOMY

Surgical Anatomy

Indications

* Malignancy in:
  - Cecum
  - Ascending colon
  - Hepatic flexure
  - Less common: Appendicular carcinoma more than 3 cm mass
  - Carcinoma terminal ileum
* Benign causes, such as terminal ileal hyperplastic tuberculosis not responding to treatment or causing recurrent obstruction.

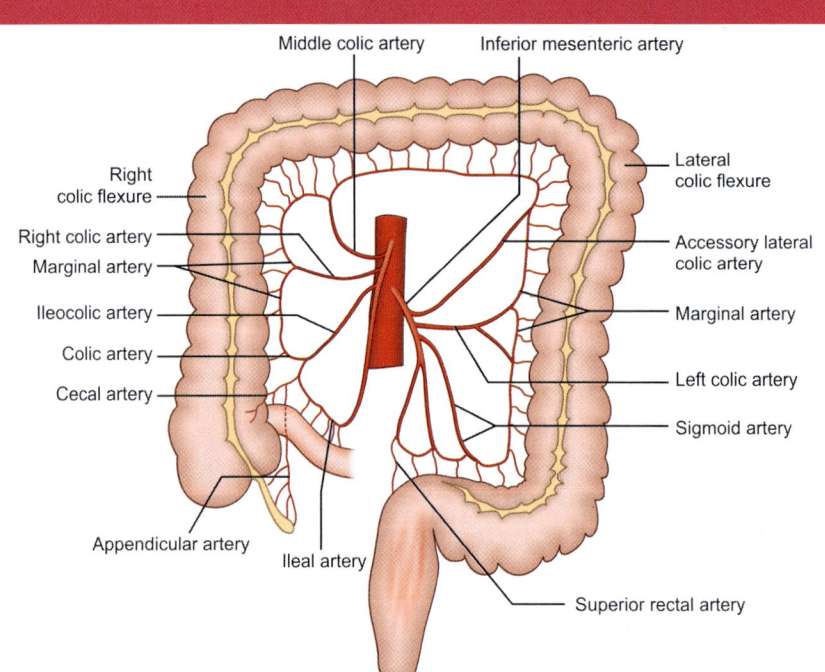

Anatomy of whole colon—vascular supply and lymphatic drainage to the right colon

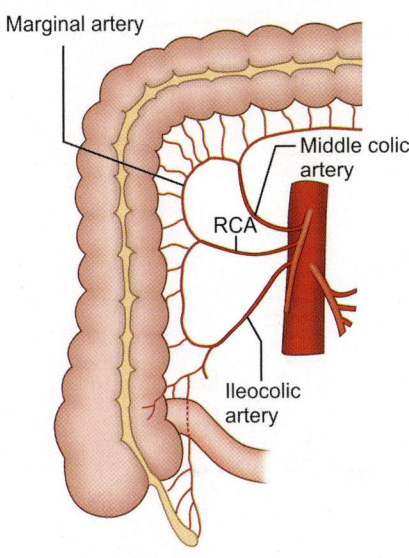
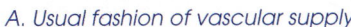

A. Usual fashion of vascular supply

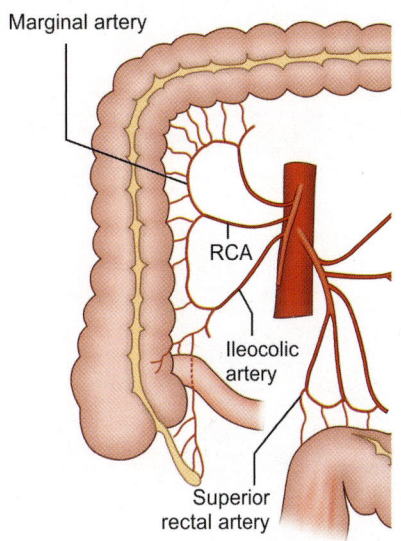

B. Unusual pattern—the marginal artery may be incomplete (X)

Pitfalls

- Inadvertent ligature to superior mesenteric vessels or injury to it.
- Injury to duodenum
- Injury to right ureter
- Failure of anastomosis.

Preoperative Preparation

- Full length colonoscopy and biopsy
- Contrast-enhanced computed tomography (CECT) abdomen
- Bowel preparation
- Prophylactic antibiotics.

Operative Procedure

- Supine position
- General anesthesia.
- *Incision:* Midline from mid-epigastrium to midpoint between symphysis pubis and umbilicus.

Step 1: After opening the abdomen, have a sincere look at the pathology, i.e. the growth, extension of the growth, liver lesion if any lymphnodes involvement, ascites and over all resectability. Pack the coils of small intestine to left side of the abdomen.

Step 2: Detach the greater omentum through the avascular plane from the right one-third of transverse colon, if the growth is located at cecum or ascending colon up to 10 cm. If the growth is at upper part of ascending colon, hepatic flexure, the omentum to be detached just distal to the gastroepiploic arcade of the stomach, caring for the blood vessels and dividing them between ligatures.

One tree makes one lac matchsticks, but one matchstick can burn 1 lac trees. A single negative thought can kill HUNDRED DREAMS, so be positive always.

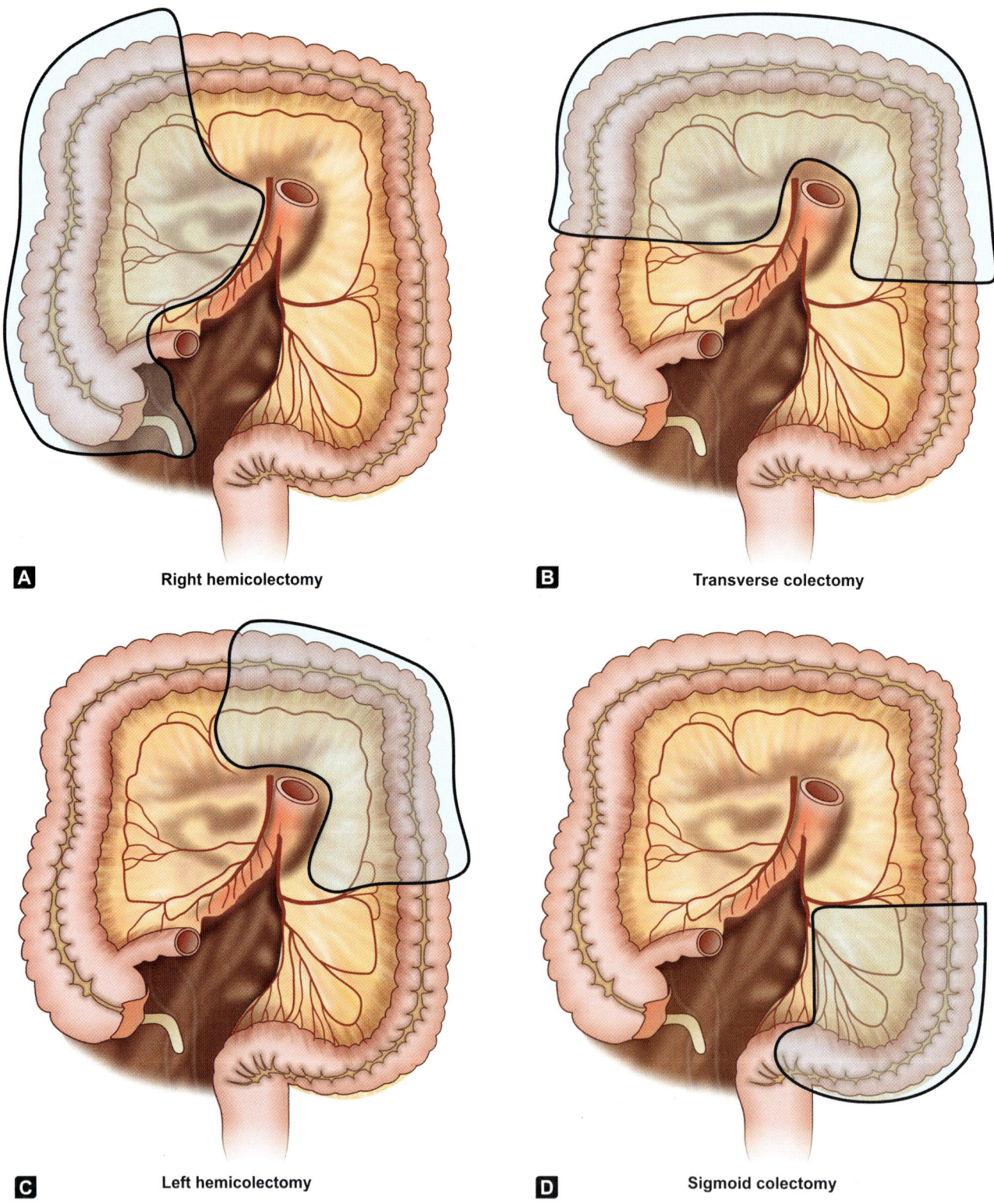

A Right hemicolectomy	**B** Transverse colectomy
C Left hemicolectomy	**D** Sigmoid colectomy

Different types of hemicolectomy

Never tell a lie: absolute condition for safety on the path.

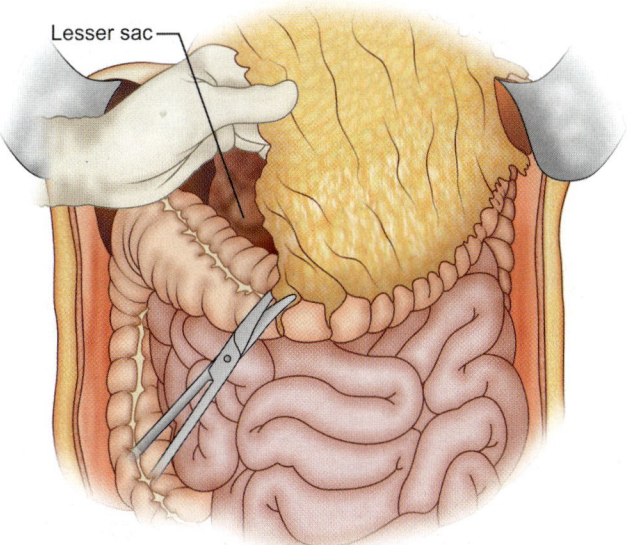

Lesser sac

Dettachment of greater omentum from the transverse colon at avascular plane

Step 3: Mobilize right colon: Incising the peritoneal reflection from the lateral side of the ascending colon, i.e. the white line of "Toldt". This is the plane for entering the plane between mesentery and true retroperitoneal structures. The incision is carried from cecum to hepatic flexure.

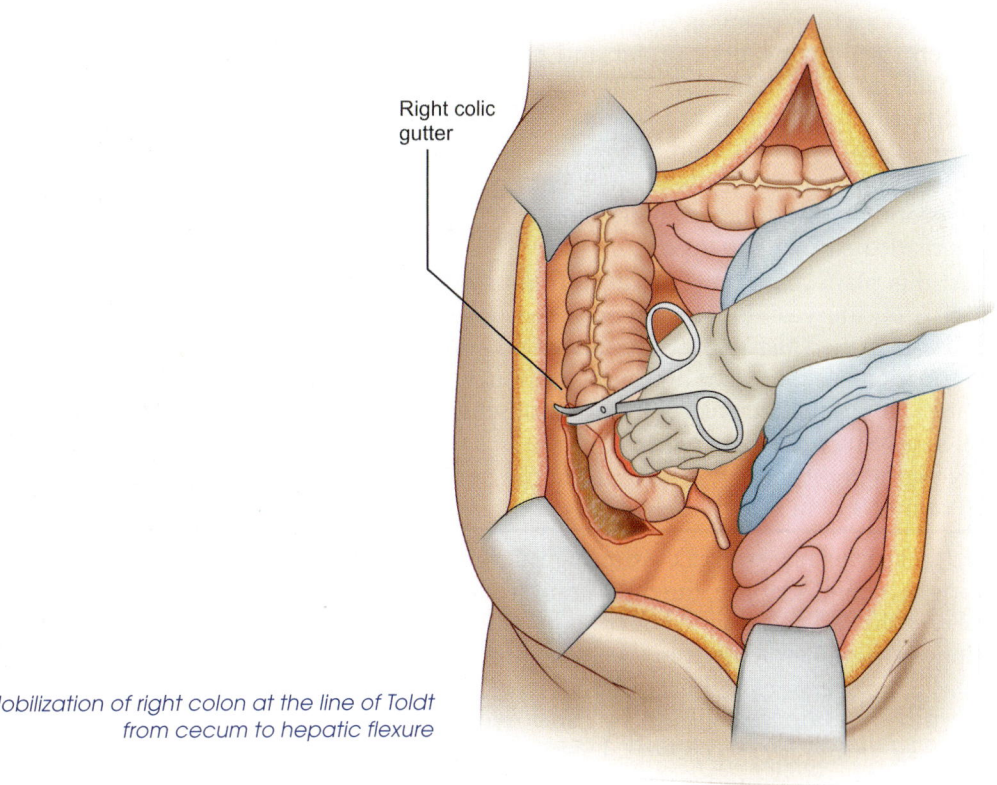

Right colic gutter

Mobilization of right colon at the line of Toldt from cecum to hepatic flexure

Honesty is the best protection.

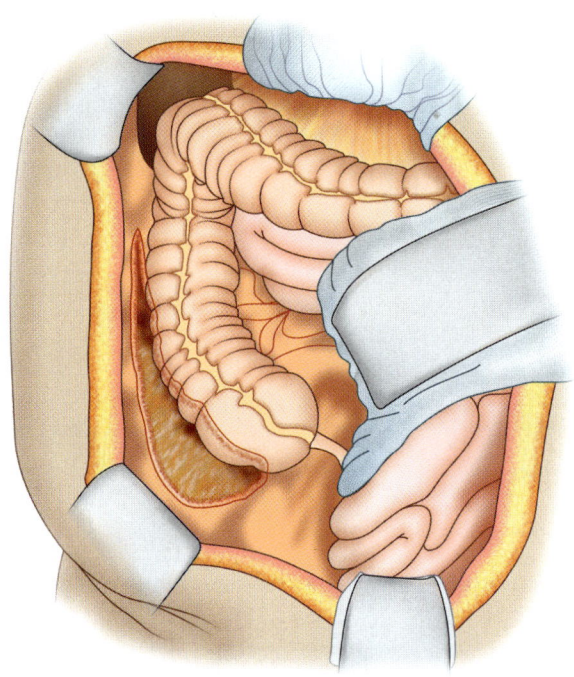

Complete mobilization of hepatic flexure done

This avascular plane is followed medially by sharp dissection, allowing both ureter and gonadal vessel to fall back into the right place. Ureter to be protected by pulling a tape around it. The gonadal vessel may be ligated, if any injury is there.

Deep dissection: As the dissection is continued medially, the second part of duodenum and the anterior surface of pancreatic head will be exposed.

At this plane, care must be taken to prevent injury to small, delicate vessels. The superior mesenteric vessels will be identified just below the pancreas where they enter the root of mesentery. The line of separation of mesentery is lateral to the main trunks of superior mesenteric vessels which is to be preserved carefully.

Now the right colon will be only hanging by the single leaf of mesocolon with blood vessels and lymphatics.

Step 4: Ligation of vessels: Division of middle colic vessels for right hemicolectomy, the right branch of middle colic artery is ligated and divided beyond its bifurcation. (For extended right hemicolectomy, i.e. when the growth is at hepatic flexure, or early part of transverse colon, dissect the middle colic vessels up to the lower border of pancreas, caring for the collateral vein that connects the inferior pancreaticoduodenal vein with middle colic vein.

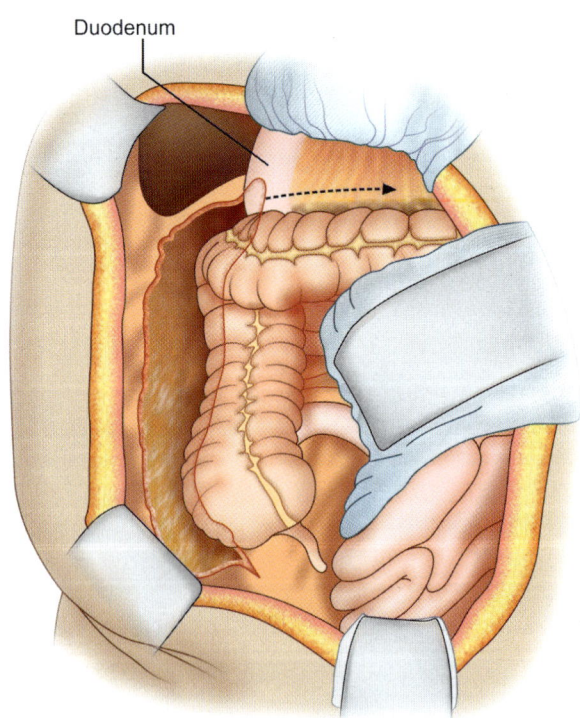

Duodenum

Exposed duodenum and marked the line of resection

Difficult does not mean impossible, it simply means you have to work hard.

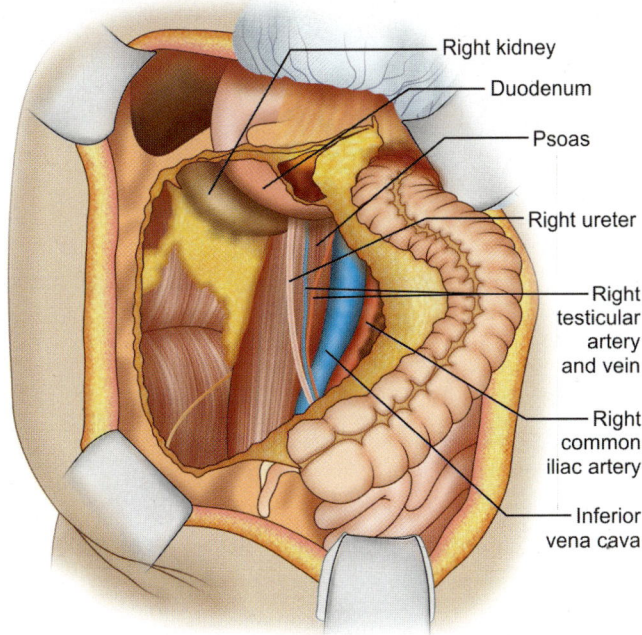

Complete mobilization of right colon

Now, ligate the middle colic artery at the origin and site of resection will be at the junction of right two-thirds and left one-third of the transverse colon, but usually it is extended up to upper one-third of descending colon as splenic flexure is vulnerable for avascularity.)

Next, the right colic and ileocolic vessels are double ligated close to the origins and divided. Sweep any lymphnodes down toward the specimen side too.

Step 5: The mesocolon of the mobilized is divided in a line, starting from the point, where the middle colic vessels are divided, gradually being through the points of right colic and ileocolic vessels are divided, to the terminal ileum 15–20 cm and above to the junction of right one-third and left two-thirds of the transverse colon.

Step 6: Division of the bowel and anastomosis: Divide the ileal mesentery 10–15 cm ileum away from the ileocecal junction, placing an intestinal clamp distal and proximal to the selected sites, either by stapler or by knife. Divide the transverse colon at the selected site, placing the intestinal clamp both proximal and distal to the selected site, either by stapler (GIA or TA 55) or knife (when stapler not available). (In the opened bowel, clean both the sides with suction and gauze. And end to end anastomosis can be done.) Now, the ileocolic anastomosis without tension is performed.

- Side-to-side: Most popular one
- End-to-end
- End-to-side.

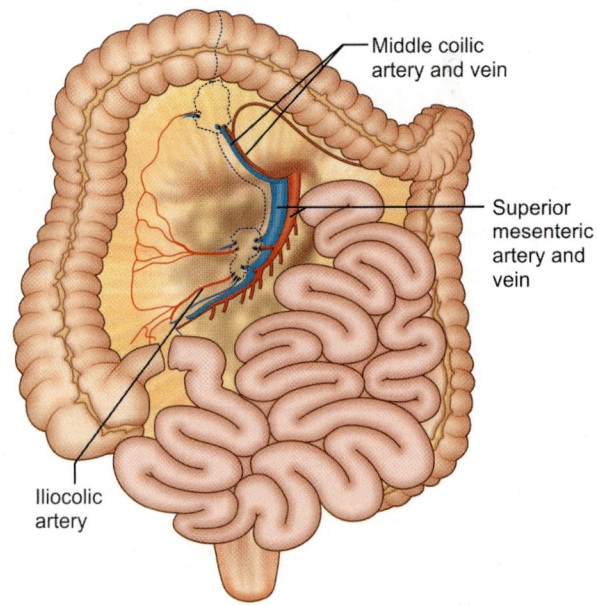

Right branch of middle colic, right colic and iliocolic arteries is ligated and divided

---

Pain is the key that opens the gates of strength; it is the high-road that leads to the city of beatitude.

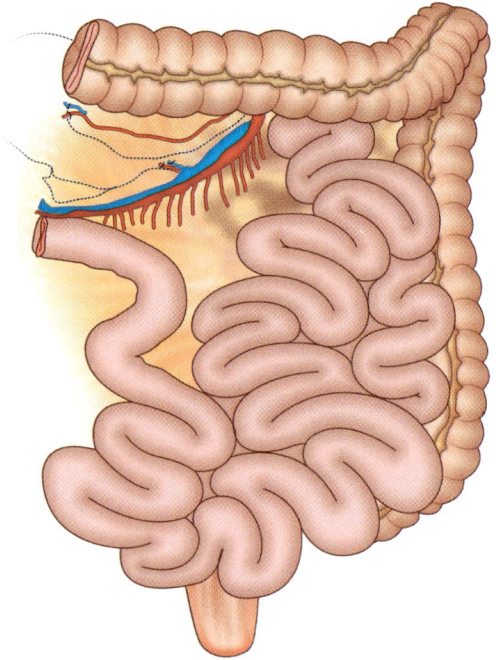

Divided mesentery is closed

Either by stapling device or hand sutures in two layers, i.e. through and through and Lembert seromuscular and cover with omentum. Approximate the divided mesentery.

Step 7: Wound closure: Change the gloves and discard all used instruments. Ensure the hemostasis, once more clean the abdomen with warm normal saline. A drain may or may not be placed. Close the abdomen in routine fashion.

Variations in Steps of Surgery

Some surgeons prefer to do the "no touch technique", i.e. they ligate the vascular pedicle before mobilizing the right colon. The lumen of terminal ileum and transverse colon are occluded with tape both proximal and distal to the tumor. Vessels are ligated at their origin from superior mesenteric artery and vein to isolate the lymphovascular tree. But, this variation has no proven oncological advantage.

Remember: A mobile tumor is always better to be resected than bypassed, even if the tumor is considered inoperable, to avoid unavoidable complications, like bleeding, obstruction.

In operability includes:
- Multiple liver metatases in different segments or both lobes
- Secondaries to para-aortic nodes, etc.

The present day recommendation is to perform single stage metastasectomy of the solitary liver metastasis. Even you can do the segmentectomy for multiple metastases in one segment of the liver, along with colectomy.

Postoperative Care

- Continuous NG suction 1–3 days
- Usually, oral sips to start on 5th–6th postoperative day
- If ileus persists more than 6 days, do ultrasonography (USG)/CECT abdomen to exclude collection, abscess, leak or any obstruction.

True enthusiasm is full of a peaceful endurance.

Complications and Its Management

i. *Leakage from the anastomotic site:* It may manifest as peritonitis, colocutaneous fistula, localized infected collection or abscess.

Management of spreading peritonitis
Relaparotomy and exteriorization of both ends of anastomosis, proximal end as temporary end ileostomy and colostomy as a mucous fistula
- Systemic antibiotics
- Correction of fluid, electrolytes
- Reanastomosis to be done after 6 weeks.

ii. *Localized collection and sepsis:* Subhepatic, subphrenic or pelvic collection may get infected and developed sepsis.

Management
- Percutaneous drainage, like pigtail drainage
- Systemic antibiotics, usually take care.

iii. *Wound infection:* There is a fair chance of development of surgical wound infection, if proper wound care is not taken.

Management
- Remove the overlying skin sutures to allow wide drainage
- Regular wound cleaning with normal saline
- Secondary suturing when the wound is healthy after 10–12 days.

6.3.2 LEFT HEMICOLECTOMY

Indications

- Malignancy in distal transverse colon,
- Splenic flexure,
- Descending colon, and
- Sigmoid colon.

Pitfalls

Injury to:
- Spleen
- Ureter
- Third part of duodenum
- Anastomotic leak.

Few Important Points to Remember

Radical left hemicolectomy implies the resection of the bowel, includes left one-third of transverse colon, splenic flexure, descending colon, sigmoid colon and upper one-third of rectum, i.e. in the vicinity of inferior mesenteric arterial supply. And colorectal anastomosis is done.

But, all the time, total radical left hemicolectomy not required. Minimum 5 cm margin on both the sides of tumor is acceptable and resection area is depended upon the site of the tumor.

Good life means smile open, dream big, put efforts more, laugh a lot and more over you realize how blessed you are for what's all already you have.

- To avoid injury to the spleen and pancreas, splenocolic, phrenicocolic, pancreaticocolic ligaments to be divided carefully.
- To avoid injury to ureter, always identify and put a tape around it.
- Avoid injury to third part of duodenum, which almost always, covers the origin of IMA and its downward continuity. So careful dissection of inferior mesenteric artery (IMA) is required to prevent injury to the third part of duodenum.
- No touch technique, i.e. ligation of vascular pedicle before mobilization the colon is more difficult in left colonic lesions.

Procedures of Radical Total Left Hemicolectomy

- Supine position
- General anesthesia
- Cleaning, draping
- *Incision:* Midline incision from a point of 4 cm below the xiphoid to 4 cm above the pubis. May be extended as per requirement.

Step 1: Open and explore the abdomen and assess the growth and operability. Exteriorize the small intestine and pack it with a wet OT towel and keep it to the patient's right. Place a Thompson/Omnitract retractor to expose the area clearly. Umbilical tape ligatures may be applied to occlude the colon proximal and distal to the tumor.

Step 2

- Stand at the left of the patient.
- Greater omentum to be detached from the desired length of tranverse colon.
- Make a long incision, peritoneum in the left paracolic gutter, between the descending colon and the white line of "Toldt".
- Elevate the peritoneal layer with left index finger and incise the peritoneum till the right-angled curve of the splenic flexure is reached.
- Similarly, the incision to be extended caudally and detach the sigmoid colon from its lateral attachment up to rectosigmoid junction.

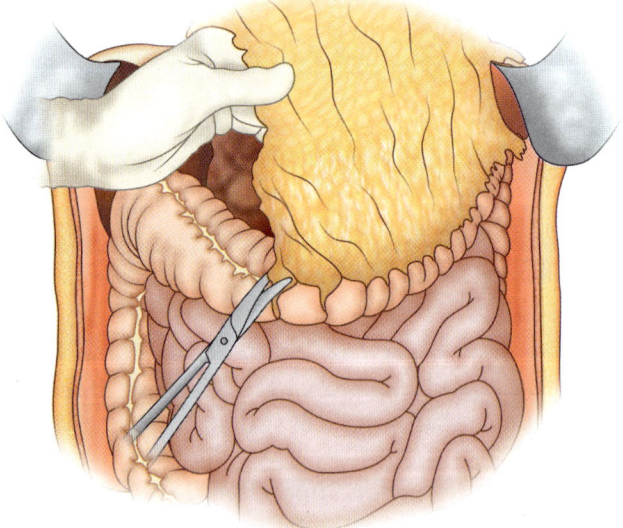

Dettachment of omentum from the tranverse colon at the avascular plane

Happiness of a person shows the internal beauty of soul. Thoughts show the status of mind and behaviour shows the language of heart.

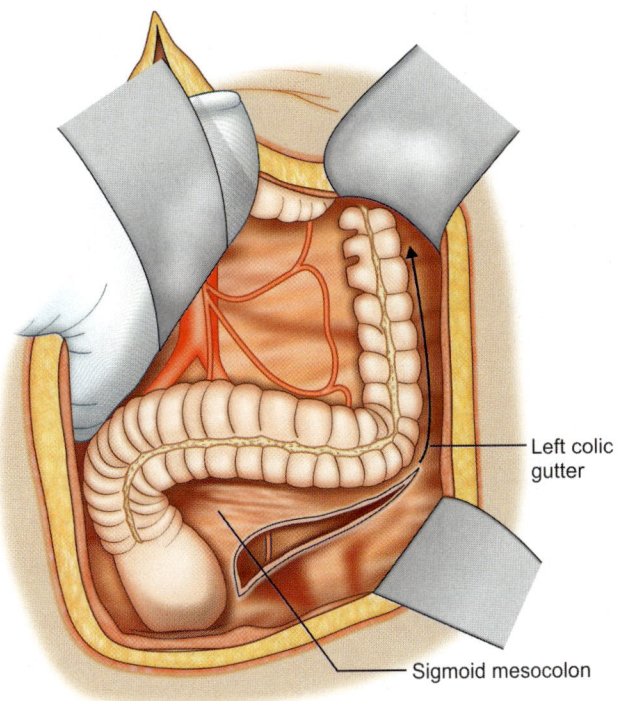

Left colic
gutter

Sigmoid mesocolon

Mobilization of left colon, incising along the line of Toldt

Step 3: At the splenic flexure, the phrenicocolic ligament is divided between the ligatures. The greater omentum, which is attached to the left part of the transverse colon, 10–12 cm, is divided between the fat of appendice epiploicae and the more lobulated fat of the omentum. (If the growth is at distal transverse colon or at the splenic flexure, divide the omentum just outside the gastroepiploic arcade.)

Step 4: Next divide the renocolic ligament, after retracting the descending colon medially, taking off from the psoas major muscle.

Now, left ureter and gonadal vein are exposed. Put a tape around the ureter and trace it down to its entrance into the pelvis. Next, look for further medially located pancreaticocolic ligament, an avascular structure. It is an upper extension of transverse mesocolon. After the division of this ligament, the distal transverse colon and splenic. Flexure will be free. Hemostasis is very important in each step.

Step 5: By gauze dissection, the whole of the left colon is elevated from its bed and swept medially on its mesocolon, carrying the blood vessels and lymphatics. At this stage

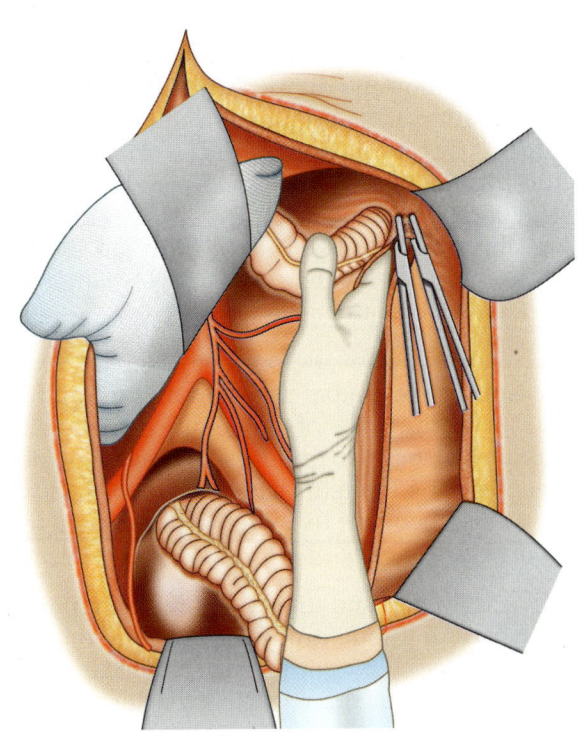

Mobilization of splenic flexure

The secret of happiness lies within you, not outside.

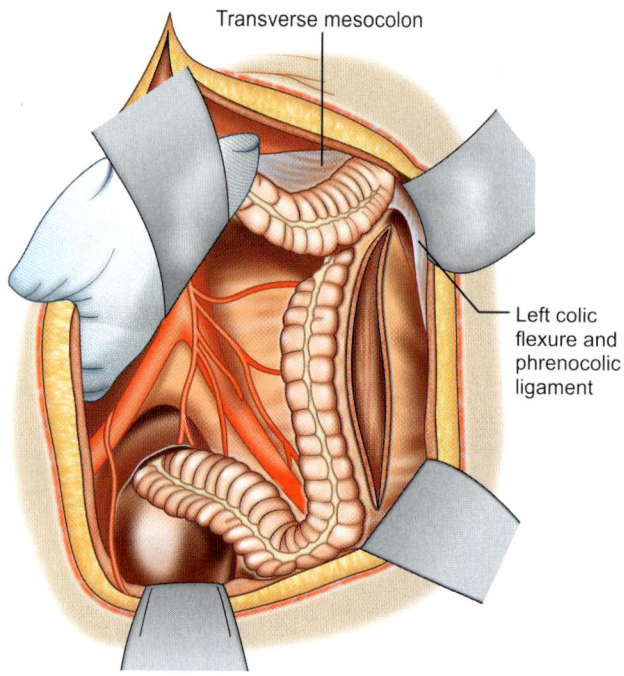

Transverse mesocolon

Left colic flexure and phrenocolic ligament

Mobilize left colon is deviated medially, taking off from psoas

too, care to be taken duodenojejunal flexure, the left kidney and ureter, and left gonadal vessels.

Step 6: Ligation and division of IMA: Identify the IMA by palpating at its origin from the aorta. Sweep the lymphatics and lymphnodes in this vicinity downward, toward the specimen. Skeletonize the IMA and ligate double with 2-0 silk, 1.5 cm away from the aorta and divide it. Now, divide the inferior mesenteric vein. The vein passes behind the duodenojejunal junction and pancreas.

Step 7: Division of mesocolon: Make a "V" shaped incision on the medial aspect of mesocolon from the level of the third part of duodenum down to the sacral promontory or up to the level of resection of the colon. So depending upon the site of the growth, divide the mesocolon between two intestinal clamps. It includes the marginal artery.

Step 8: Ligation and division of mesorectum: Divide the vascular tissue around the upper one-third of rectum covered by peritoneum and clear the areolar tissue and fat at the site, selected for anastomosis, usually 2–3 cm above the sacral promontory.

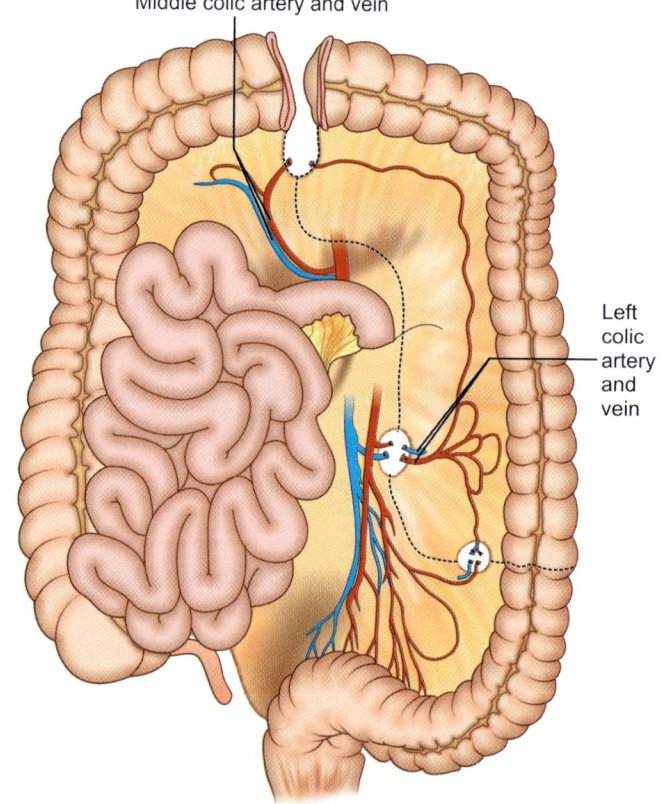

Middle colic artery and vein

Left colic artery and vein

Division of left branch of middle colic artery and left colic vessels along the line of mesenteric resection

Be more concerned with your character than your reputation. Your character is what you really are, while your reputation is merely what others think you are.

Step 9: Division of colon and rectum: At the selected site of colon, cut it by the linear cutter stapler or apply two intestinal clamps both the sides and cut it to avoid contamination. Handle the rectum in same manner and divide the upper rectum and remove the specimen. Suck the spillage and irrigate it properly. Achieve complete hemostasis.

Step 10: Now, the anastomosis is done between transverse colon and upper end of rectum either by 29 mm or 32 mm end-to-end-anastomosis (EEA) [stapler device for hemorrhoids (SDH)] or by hand sutures in two layers. The steps of hand sewn two-layer anastomosis:

1. Ensure adequate blood supply of both the ends of the bowel and there is no unusual tension.
2. Rotate the proximal colon in such a manner that mesenteric border enters at the right lateral margin of the anastomosis.
3. Anastomosis to be done in two layers. Seromuscular suture by 3-0/4-0 silk and second layer is through the full thickness of the bowel by 4-0 vicryl or PDS. (See the anastomosis thrice, do one and teach one, then only you will be able to perform in a patient in a proper manner.)

If anastomosis is not possible due to various factors, do the Hartmann's procedure, i.e. closure of rectal stump and do the temporary end colostomy and anastomosis to be done after 6 weeks.

Step 11

- Closure of the wound
- Change gloves and instruments
- Close the defect in the mesocolon with 3-0 silk or vicryl
- Close the abdomen in the fashion of mass closure with or without placing a drain

Postoperative Care

- Continuous NG suction 1–3 days
- Usually, oral sips to start on 5th–6th postoperative day
- If ileus perrists more than 6 days, do USG/CECT abdomen to exclude collection, abscess, leak or any obstruction.

Complications and Its Management

1. *Leakage from the anastomotic site:* It may manifest as peritonitis, colocutaneous fistula, localized infected collection or abscess.
   Management of spreading peritonitis: Relaparotomy and exteriorization of both ends of anastomosis as a double-barrel colostomy.
   - Systemic antibiotics
   - Correction of fluid, electrolytes
   - Reanastomosis to be done after 6 weeks.
2. *Localized collection and sepsis:* Subhepatic, subphrenic or pelvic collection may get infected and developed sepsis.

   Management
   - Percutaneous drainage, like pigtail drainage
   - Systemic antibiotics, usually take care.
3. *Wound infection:* There is a fair chance of development of surgical wound infection, if proper wound care is not taken.

Relations require real effort even when all of us busy with our own lives, a simple message after a long time will remind that few relation are still alive.

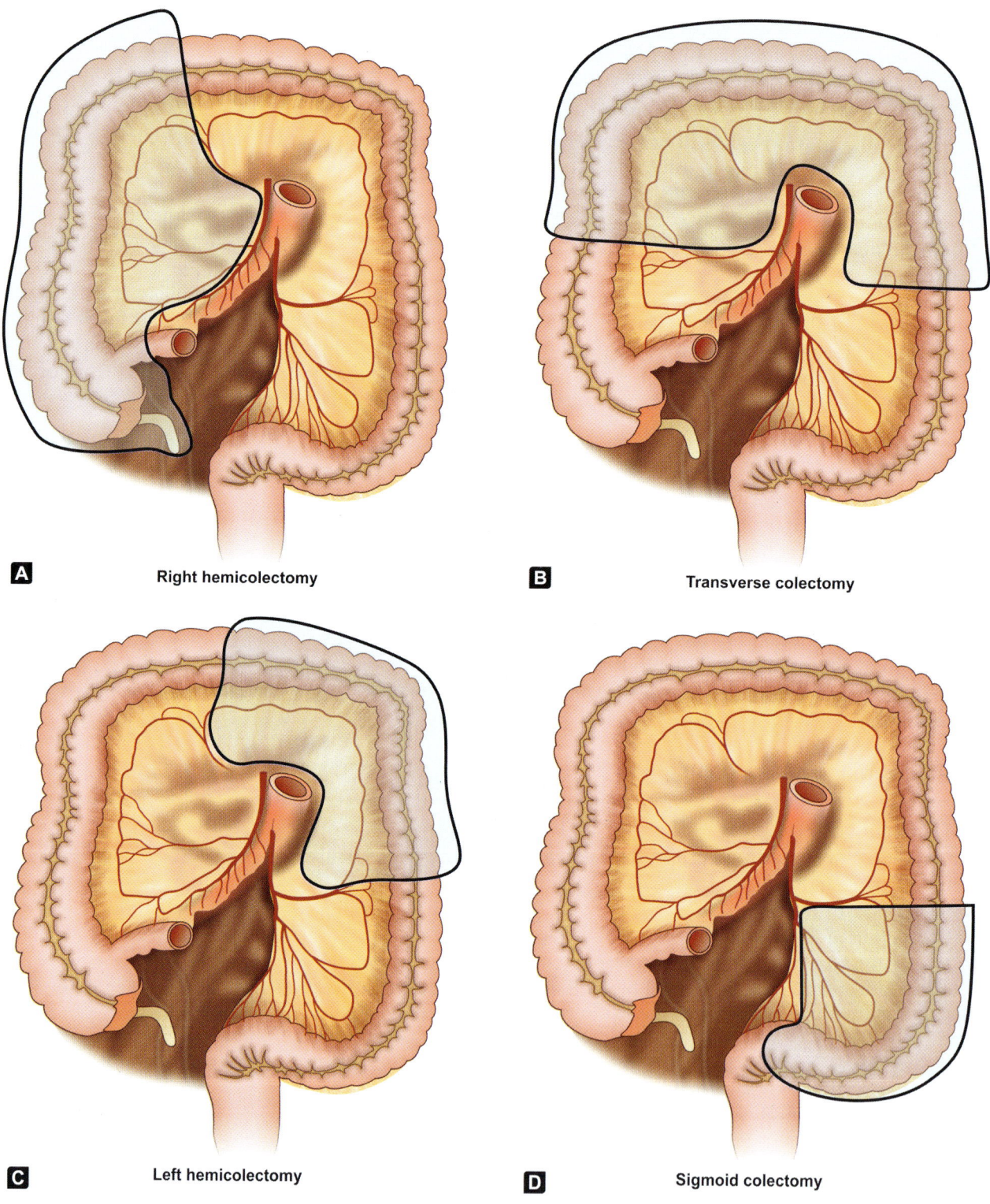

A   **Right hemicolectomy**

B   **Transverse colectomy**

C   **Left hemicolectomy**

D   **Sigmoid colectomy**

Different types of colectomy depending on the site of the growth

Even if we drive fast, we would still find someone ahead. This is true in lives too. We can not get ahead of everyone. So, enjoy the turns and twists in your life.

Management
- Remove the overlying skin sutures to allow wide drainage
- Regular wound cleaning with normal saline
- Secondary suturing when the wound is healthy after 10–12 days.

Points to Remember

i. As the colonic malignant tumor usually grows 1.2 cm longitudinally, so 5 cm margin both the sides of the growth is enough.
   Giving example: The mass is at splenic flexure.
   In this case, you ligate the left branch of middle colic artery and only the left colic artery (no need to ligate the origin of IMA like in total left colectomy).
   And remove the left two-thirds of transverse colon and early 5–7 cm of descending colon and do colocolic anastomosis, i.e. anastomosis between transverse colon and descending colon without tension.
ii. If the diameter of the lumen of one segment is remarkably narrower than the other, make a 2 cm long slit so-called "Cheatle slit" on the antimesenteric border of the narrower segment and anastomose (see once, then you remember only).

6.3.3 ILEOSTOMY

END ILEOSTOMY

Indications

Permanent: At the completion of total colectomy

Temporary:
1. After resection of gangrenous segment of intestine along with mucous fistula.
2. Perforation of any part of large gut-like cecal perforation where primary anastomosis is contraindicated.

Pitfalls

- Stricture and necrosis due to devascularization.
- Ileocutaneous fistula as a result of too deep bite beyond seromuscular layer during refashioning.
- Early fluid and electrolytes loss.
- Lower long-term risk of late adhesion and obstruction.

Procedures

Mark the site: Ileostomy is usually made in the right iliac fossa. Landmark 4 cm below the umbilicus, 5 cm away from midline and 2.5 cm above and medial from anterior superior iliac spine.
- Patient is already under general anesthesia for the definite procedure.
- Make a circular incision with a diameter of 2 cm.
- Reach up to anterior rectus sheath with a disc of skin but without excising the core of subcutaneous fat unless the patient is significantly obese.
- Make a cruciate incision over the anterior rectus sheath.
- Rectus muscle is splited.
- The same incision is extended through the posterior sheath. Parietal peritoneum opened and dilated using two fingers. The opening should not be too tight or too loose.

Do not judge a person by what other say. The person may be true to you, but not to others because the same Sun which melts ice, hardens the clay.

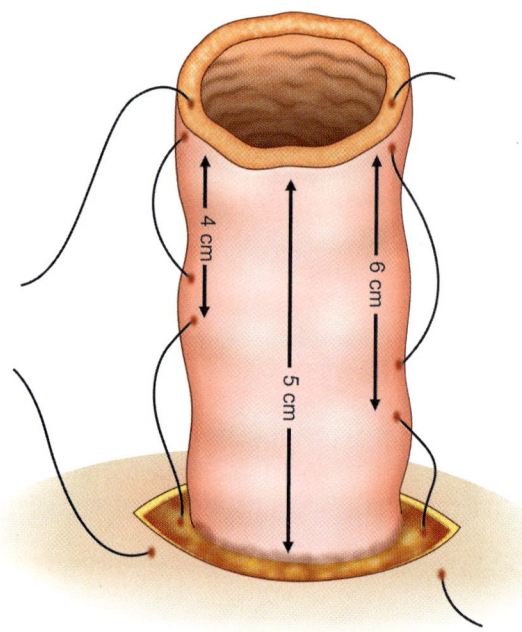

4 cm

6 cm

5 cm

Ideal end ileostomy

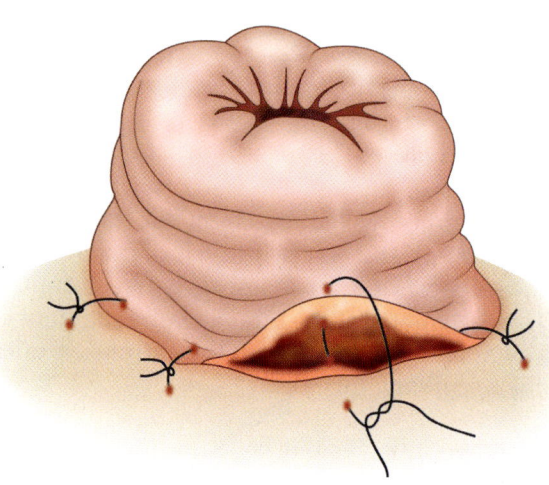

Proper fixation of ileostomy all around

Step 1: Six centimeters ileum to be brought from the level of peritoneum along with some mesentery to maintain vascularity of stoma.

Remember: Distal 2–3 cm of ileum will retain viability even if you remove the mesentery at that portion.

Step 2: 2–2.5 cm spout is enough and the spout is created by an eversion maneuver.

Step 3: The superior everting suture (2-0 Mersilk) starts at one angle at the open edge (seromuscular) and next bite at 6 cm from the edge (seromuscular). The inferior everting suture from another angle of the open edge, if ileum and seromuscular second bite at 4 cm from the edge.

Two lateral sutures with second seromuscular bite 5 cm away from the open edge. Now, all four sutures will be tied with four sides of the anterior rectus sheath. The ideal stoma should face downward.

Step 4: After eversion, further skin mucosal apposition suture is placed between each of the everting sutures.

Step 5: Closure of mesenteric gap with 3-0 vicryl, suture the edge of ileal mesentery to the cut edge of the paracolic peritoneum continuously. This maneuver completely obliterates the mesenteric defect.

Step 6: Hemostasis and viability of the stoma to be ensured. Put the colostomy bag appropriately.

Complications

Early

- Occasional necrosis of the distal ileum
- Peristomal leak
- Infection.

A smile is a language that even a body understands, it costs nothing. It happens in a flash but the memory lasts forever. Keep smiling.

Late

- Prolapse
- Retraction
- Stricture
- Obstruction
- Parastomal skin excoriation
- Peristomal hernia.

LOOP ILEOSTOMY

Indications

- To defunction an empty colon to protect vulnerable distal anastomosis
- As a part of initial treatment of severe inflammatory bowel disease
- When temporary diversion of fecal stream is required, like colonic perforation repair, colonic injury, etc.

Pitfalls

Total fecal diversion may not be accomplished, if the ileum is not transacted at the right site and if the proximal stoma is not made dominant.

Procedures

- Supine position
- General or spinal anesthesia
- Mark the site for ileostomy.
- *Incision:* If it is done as a primary procedure, a middle incision from the umbilicus to 10 cm caudally.

Step 1
- Abdomen opened
- Distal loop of ileum is identified.

Step 2: Excise a coin-sized circle of skin in right iliac fossa. Expose the anterior rectus sheath. Make a cruciate incision over the anterior rectus sheath. Rectus muscle is split. The same incision is extended through the posterior sheath. Parietal peritoneum opened and dilated using two fingers. The opening should not be too tight or too loose.

Step 3: The terminal part of ileum is brought out by a Babcock forceps. Before closure of main wound, the loop is oriented such a manner that the distal limb is inferior and three sutures are placed between the seromuscular coat of the distal limb and the skin edge to confirm orientation. Main abdominal wound closed in layers.

Step 4: A incision is made 3–4 mm above the skin margin of apposition sutures. The superior and first lateral eversion sutures are placed but untied. As soon as the sutures are tied, the proximal stoma everts as a spout. And the distal bowel opening will be visible very close to the skin. Ensure hemostasis. Now, fix the stoma all around with the skin with 3-0 mersilk/nylon.

Step 5: Ensure hemostasis. Irrigate the area with antiseptic solution, like betadine. Properly dry the skin and apply tincture benjoin lightly on the peristomal skin before applying the stoma bag.

Complications

Early

- Occasional necrosis of the distal ileum

The best way of meeting difficulties is a quiet and calm confidence in the grace.

- Peristomal leak
- Infection.

Late

- Prolapse
- Retraction
- Stricture
- Obstruction
- Peristomal skin excoriation
- Peristomal hernia.

Closure of Ileostomy

- Supine position
- General/spinal anesthesia
- Cleaning, draping
- Insert moist gauge at the stoma
- *Incision:* An elliptical incision around the stoma 3–4 mm away from mucocutaneous junction.

Step 1: Skin incision is depended into subcutaneous fat and bowel wall is identified. The plane is followed between the abdominal wall and the bowel wall. Be sure not to incise the wall of the ileum. Continue down to the point where ileum meets anterior rectus sheath.

Step 2: Facial sheath dissections: All around the wall of the ileum dissect the subcutaneous fat off the anterior wall of the sheath. Now, a clean rim of the sheath is visible. Dissect the ileum away from the fascial ring until the peritoneal cavity is entered.

Step 3: Peritoneal dissection: Now with the help of index finger, wall of the ileum to be separated from the adjoining peritoneal attachments. Now wall of the ileum is freed from anterior abdominal wall as well as peritoneal attachments. (If any difficulty in separation, extend the incision laterally for a distance adequate to complete the dissection smoothly.)

Step 4
- Freshening the edge of the ileostomy by excising a rim of 4–5 mm scarred tissue
- Ensure no significant ileum wall injury
- Superficial serosal damages are not significant.

Step 5: Closure of ileum defect by:
- Suture technique in two layers with 3-0 vicryl and mersilk, respectively
- Longitudinal defect to close transversely to maintain adequate patency of the lumen
- Stapler: If the wall of the ileum is not so thick that compressing it to 2 mm produces necrosis, stapling is ideal
- Resection and anastomosis: When the tissue is of inadequate quality for simple transverse closure, resection and anastomosis is preferable.
- Ensure hemostasis.

Step 6: Closure of the abdominal wall. Close rectus sheath with intermittent 1-0 prolene or nylon. Close the skin and subcutaneous tissue also intermittently with 2-0 nylon/prolene, placing a corrugated rubber drain. Irrigate the operative area and apply a proper size stoma bag.

Do not wait for extraordinary opportunities. Seize common occasions and make them great.

6.3.4 COLOSTOMY

LOOP COLOSTOMY

Loop colostomy is possible only in sigmoid or transverse colon because of their mobility due to mobile mesentery. Sometimes, particularly in obese patient, transverse mesocolon is too short to mobilize. So, mobilization of hepatic and splenic flexures is required to get a mobile loop. Sigmoid loop colostomy should be preferred at the junction of descending colon and sigmoid colon as peritoneal fixation of descending colon will protect the proximal stoma from getting prolapsed.

LOOP TRANSVERSE COLOSTOMY

Indications

Diversion of fecal stream when it is required specially after
- Coloanal anastomosis
- To relieve the obstruction of left colon, a standard emergency treatment. To protect the left colon anastomosis called defunctioning loop colostomy.

Pitfalls

Performing colostomy for an error in dignoses, like fecal impaction or pseudo-obstruction.
- In advanced colonic obstruction, cecal rupture or impending cecal rupture to be ensured before deciding a transverse colostomy for this purpose.
- Tranverse colostomy is not a pleasant procedure for the patient as the site is very embarrassing and there is more chance of wound infections and incisional hernia after closure.

Remember: If there should be a leak, the more distal stoma is preferrable as it can provide a better defunction of the anastomosis and reduces contamination from the leak.

Preoperative Preparation

- Confirm the indication for the colostomy. The diagnosis has to be confirmed by CECT, colonoscopy or at least by barium enema.
- Preoperative flat radiograph of the abdomen to identify the position of the transverse colon, relatively to a fixed point, like umbilicus. So, place a coin over the umbilicus and ask to take X-ray.
- Fluid resuscitation and Ryle's tube insertion.
- Preoperative prophylactic antibiotics.

Procedure

- Supine position
- General anesthesia/short GA
- *Incision:* 4–6 cm transverse incision over the lateral part of rectus abdominis muscle at the 2 cm right of the midline.

Note: Incision may be over the middle and lateral thirds of the upper right rectus muscle and ideally the length of skin incision should be equal to the length of the longitudinal incision to be made in the colon (4–6 cm usually).

Step 1: Divide the anterior rectus sheath, split the rectus abdominis muscle and posterior rectus sheath.

Step 2: Deliver the transverse colon, holding with two Babcock forceps, 2 cm apart through a small hole of the omentum and pass Ryle's tube or a plastic rod. (Transverse colon is easily identified by the transversely

---

Do not look for someone who solves your problems; look for someone who can teach you to face them.

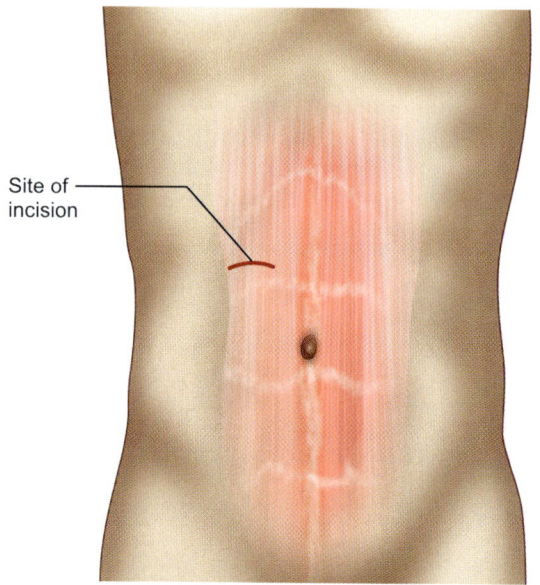

Site of incision for transverse colostomy

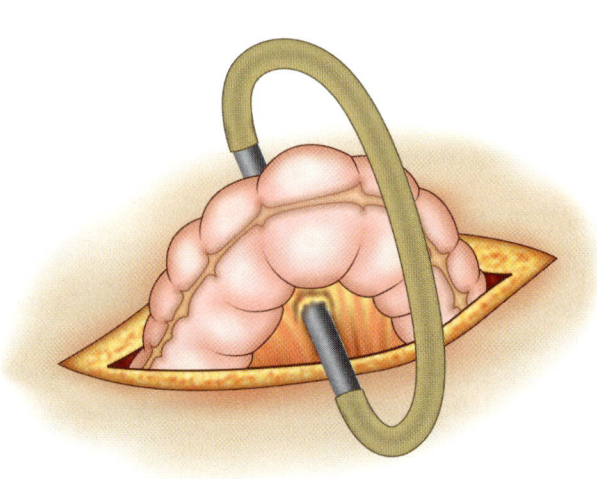

Holding the colon with Ryle's tube or plastic rod

placed taenia by making an incision over the omentum or through the usually thin omentum or by displacing it. And then, insert a 16 guage needle attached to low pressure suction in between two babcocks. Gas will escape and colon can be exteriorized easily.) So that, no tension of the colon is there.

Step 3: Open the colon, making a 4–6 cm longitudinal incision in the tenia, suck the gas and contents of the colon. Fix the colonic seromuscular wall with the rectus sheath at least four sides. Now, the bowel edges are folded back to the skin edges and the skin mucosal apposition is achieved with interrupted 3-0 vicryl suture sparing the stoma bar sites. Left opening is functional colostomy and right one is the mucus fistula.

Step 4: The main abdominal wound is now closed, ensuring complete hemostasis. Irrigate the operative field with normal saline and antiseptics. Apply colostomy bag and advice for nasogastric suction until the colostomy functions.

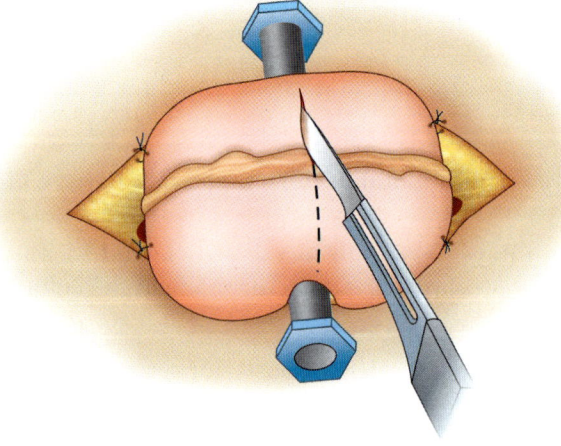

Opening the colon

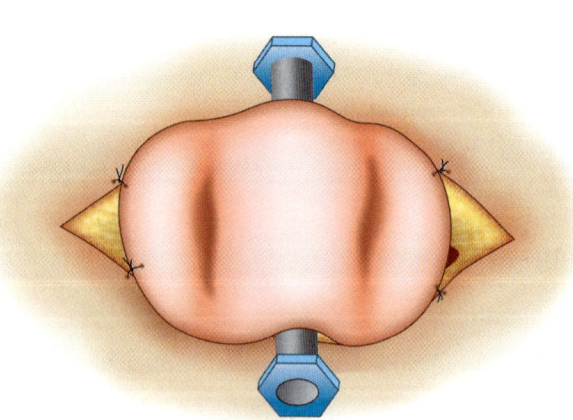

Loop colostomy

Regularity: Indispensable for all serious accomplishment.

END COLOSTOMY

Indications

Permanent

1. When there is no effective distal bowel loop for anastomosis, like after abdominoperineal resection (APR).

Temporary

1. When a restorative procedure is contraindicated, like colorectal anastomoses when the chance of leak is high.
2. As a part of Hartmann's procedure where the proximal end is brought out as an end colostomy and the distal bowel is closed and left in situ.

Procedures

The basic things to be followed are as above, i.e. the position, anesthesia, etc.

- In the vicinity of left iliac fossa, put a mark in ideal place, i.e. at the lateral border of rectus and 2.5 cm away from the anterior superior iliac spine.

Step 1: Excise a round piece of skin with approximately 2.5–3 cm in radius (practically we hold the skin with Allis forcep and around it, skin is excised). Divide or excise the fat and expose anterior rectus sheath.

Step 2: Make a cruciate incision, on anterior rectus sheath, split the muscle and open the peritoneum. Stoma is dilated with two fingers. Now, with the help of a babcock forcep, grasp the proximal end of colon and 4–5 cm of the colon is brought out. Fix the seromuscular colonic wall with the rectus sheath in four sites, using marsilk 3-0 or vicryl too.

Step 3: See the viability of the colon at the edge, if required. Excise the full thickness all around and healthy edges to be fixed with the skin edges, using 3-0/4-0 vicryl without any tension of the colon and without any gap between the skin and the bowel wall.

Step 4: Ensure hemostasis: Irrigate the operative area and apply a proper size colostomy bag.

Complications and Its Management

Prolapse of the defunctionalized limb is fairly common when it is kept for a long time, i.e. months to years.

How to Manage the Prolapse?

1. Resect the prolapse colon and restore the gut continuity.
2. Resect the prolapse part and convert to a new end colostomy. To prevent the prolapse, carefully tacking of the limb at peritoneal level helps to prevent this complication.
3. Peristomal sepsis uncommon with the present era of antiseptics. If develops, local incision and drainage is the first step and in case of uncontrolled local sepsis, colostomy to be moved to an other site.
4. Other complications are:
   - Retraction and stricture
   - Parastomal hernia, etc.

CLOSURE OF COLOSTOMY

A temporary colostomy is usually closed at around 6–8 weeks as by this time the stoma becomes matured and the planes around the stoma become well defined. But in suitably prepared patient, he may undergo the closure as early as 2–3 weeks after surgery.

Let all circumstances, all happening in life be occasions, constantly renewed, for learning more and ever more.

Pitfalls

Suture link leak local or intra-abdominal sepsis.

Preoperative Preparation

- Barium enema: X-ray to exclude any stricture or obstruction in distal colon.
- Nasogastric (NG) tube insertion
- Mechanical and antibiotic bowel preparation (know details about it)
- Saline enema to cleanse inactivated colonic segment
- Correct electrolytes imbalance
- Prophylactic systemic antibiotics.

Procedure of Loop Colostomy Closure

- Supine position
- General/spinal anesthesia
- Cleaning, draping
- Insert moist gauge at the stoma.
- *Incision:* An elliptical incision around the stoma 3–4 mm away from mucocutaneous junction.

Step 1: Skin incision is deepened into subcutaneous fat and bowel wall is identified. The plane is followed between the abdominal wall and the bowel wall. Being sure that not to incise the colonic wall. Continue down to point where colon meets anterior rectus sheath.

Step 2: Facial sheath dissection: All around the colonic wall, dissect the subcutaneous fat off the anterior wall of the sheath. Now, a clean rim of the sheath is visible. Dissect the colon away from the facial ring until the peritoneal cavity is entered.

Step 3: Peritoneal dissection: Now, with the help of index finger, colonic wall to be separated from the adjoining peritoneal attachments. Now, colonic wall is freed from anterior abdominal wall as well as peritoneal attachments. (If any difficulty in separation, extend the incision laterally for a distance adequate to complete the dissection smoothly.)

Step 4
- Freshening the edge of the colostomy by excising a rim of 4–5 mm scarred tissue
- Ensure no significant colonic wall injury
- Superficial serosal damages are not significant.

Step 5: Closure of colonic defect by:
- Suture technique in two layers with 3-0 vicryl and mersilk, respectively. Longitudinal defect to close transversely to maintain adequate patency of the lumen.
- Stapler: If the colon wall is not so thick that compressing it to 2 mm produces necrosis, stapling is ideal.
- Resection and anastomosis: When the tissue is of inadequate quality for simple transverse closure, resection and anastomosis are preferable.

Step 6: Closure of the abdominal wall close rectus sheath with intermittent 1-0 prolene or nylon. Close the skin and subcutaneous tissue also intermittently with 2-0 nylon/prolene, putting a corrugated rubber drain.

Complications

- Wound infection
- Abdominal abscess
- Colocutaneous fistula.

Cleanliness is the first indispensable step toward the supramental manifestation.

6.4 RECTUM

6.4.1 ABDOMINAL PERINEAL RESECTION (APR)

Indications

1. Carcinoma distal rectum which is not amenable to sphincter preservation.
2. Anal cancer where there is residual disease after chemoradiation.

Procedure

1. General anesthesia
2. *Position:* Lithotomy/modified Loyd Davis position lithotomy, Trendelenburg position, sand bag/several folded sheets behind sacrum, slightly flexed and abducted thigh.
3. *Incision:* Just above umbilicus to 2 cm below pubic crest.

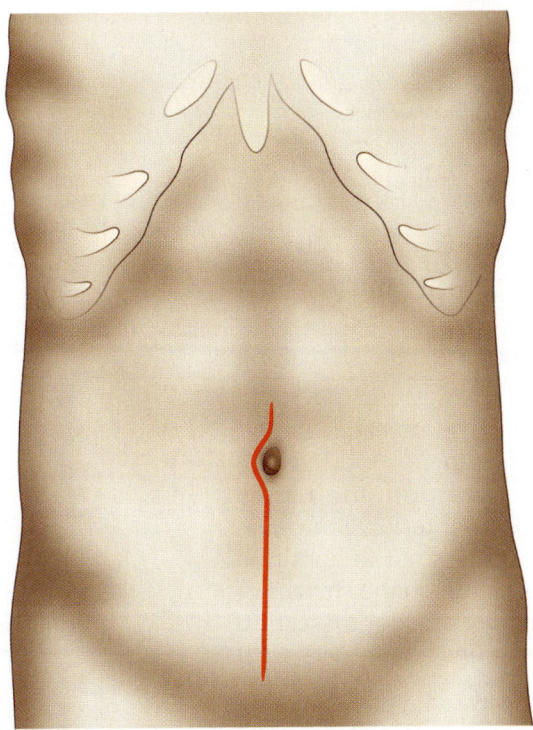

Incision for abdominal perineal resection (APR)

Step 1: Assess the operability, extent of tumor involvement of sacrum, see liver, peritoneum, omentum for metastases and look for free fluid, bladder may be fixed on skin to improve exposure.

Step 2: Mobilization of sigmoid colon: On the right side of sigmoid, the incision should begin at a point overlying the bifurcation of the aorta and continue in a caudal direction along with the line where the mesosigmoid meets the right lateral leaf of peritoneum in pre-sacral space. Right ureter to be indentified and incision to be carried down toward rectovesical pouch.

On the left, retract the sigmoid to patients left. Expose the left lateral peritoneal gutter and divide several congenital attachments between mesocolon and posterolateral parietal peritoneum.

In quietness, you will feel that the divine force, help and protection are always with you.

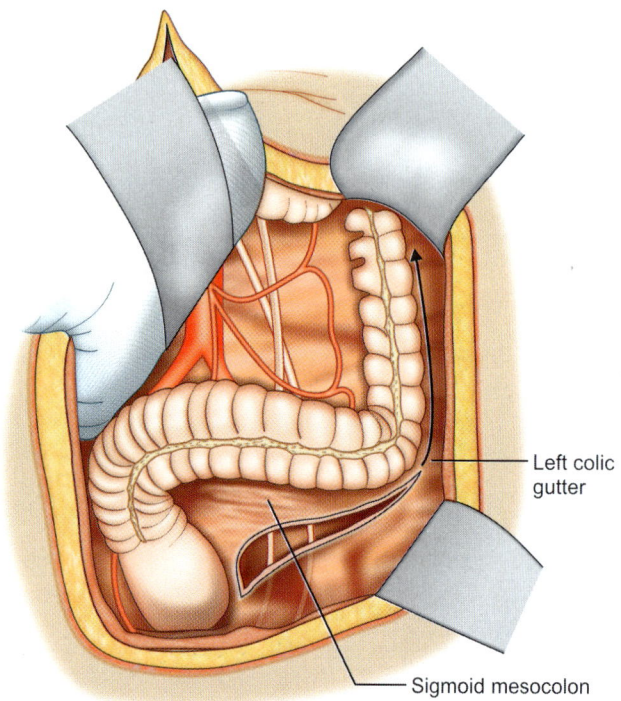

Left colic gutter

Sigmoid mesocolon   *Mobilization of the sigmoid colon and rectum*

Identify left ureter and safeguard it, and gonadal vessels to be taken care off.

Dissection to be confined the peritoneal incision along the left side of the rectum down to the rectovesical pouch.

Rectum mobilization: The plane of dissection is just immediately outside the mesorectum to mobilize the upper and mid rectum. The dissection should be posteriorly first then lateral and lastly anterior. The plane immediately outside the mesorectum is not to continue where it cones in below the mesorectum on the surface of levator ani and at the level of tumors. Posterior dissection should stop at the first point where pelvic floor fuses with Waldeyer's fascia.

Presacral dissection: Posterior dissection is to be ensured first by a upward traction on the band of tissue extending from mid-sacral on to the posterior rectum. Mesorectum will be evident and on either side of it. There is only loose areola tissue. Now, surgeon to insert the hand in presacral space. Blunt + sharp dissection with diathermy to be carried out so that specimen is elevated from the sacrum as far as the lateral ligaments on each side. The wishbone of sympathetic hypogastric nerve will be visible at the pelvic brim posteriorly. Endopelvic fascia should be intact to prevent hemorrhage as presacral veins are beneath the fascia.

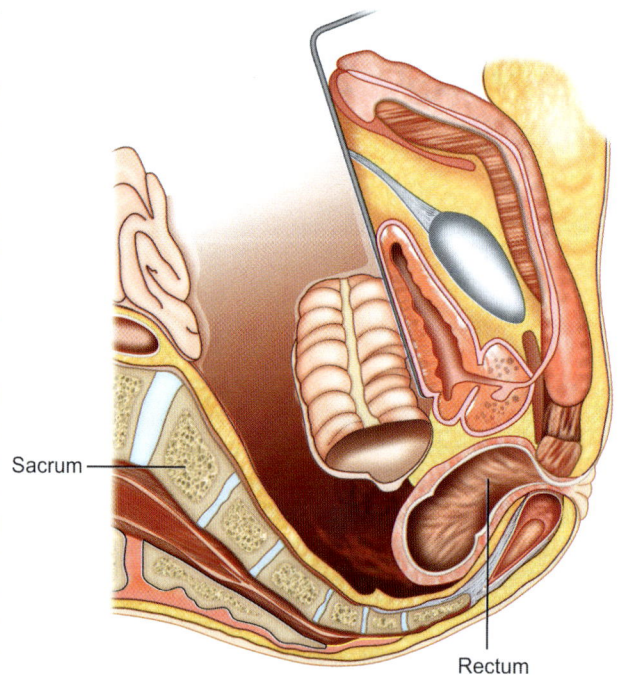

Sacrum

Rectum

Mobilization of rectum from sacrum

Let the sun of aspiration dissolve the clouds of egoism.

Lateral pelvic dissection: The lateral plane on the surface of dissection of mesorectum will allow the hypogastric nerves and then inferior hypogastric plexus to fall back on to the pelvic side wall. Now, the lateral ligaments on both the sides will be divided with ureter intact. The middle rectal artery will require diathermy coagulation or ligation.

Anterior dissection: In male patients, the plane for anterior dissection lies between anterior mesorectal tissue and prostate, seminal vesicles.

Lateral dissection is carried forward on the surface of mesorectum leads round the seminal vesicles. The dissection is kept on the posterior surface of the vesicle.

Dissection to continue down in front of Denonvilliers fascia which comes as a shiny white layer on anterior surface of the distal part of anterior mesorectum. This fascia to be cut at higher level, i.e. before fusing base of prostate prevents injury to neurovascular bundles and prostatic plexus.

In female patient: The plane lies between anterior mesorectum and posterior vaginal wall. Denonvilliers' fascia is not well developed. A cuff of posterior wall of vagina is to be removed along with the specimen, if there is an invasion or tumor is close to it.

Perineal resection: Close the anal orifice with purse string suture of silk, make circumferential perianal incision 3 cm away from closed anus. Both sides the dissection enters the ischiorectal fat.

The blunt and sharp dissection to be carried out posteriorly toward the coccyx ligates inferior middle rectal vessels and other vessels on both the sides. Anococcygeal ligament to be divided both the sides.

A transverse incision in front of tip of coccyx or excising the coccyx to clear the lateral pelvic floor. The levator ani muscle divided.

The midline incision is to go through Waldeyer's fascia for inserting the fingers to supralevator compartment and remove the specimen by dividing the pelvic diaphragm with diathermy.

Lastly, the levator ani muscles are divided completely both the sides and the specimen is delivered through the perineum.

Finally: Division of colon and formation of permanent colostomy to be done now. The pelvic peritoneum should be closed to avoid herniation and obstruction of small bowels. If peritoneum is not enough to close after radical dissection, vicryl mesh to be used to serve the purpose.

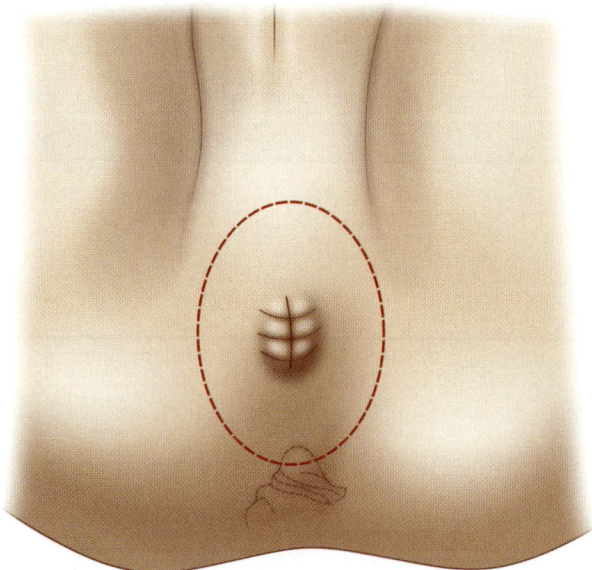

Circumferential perianal incision

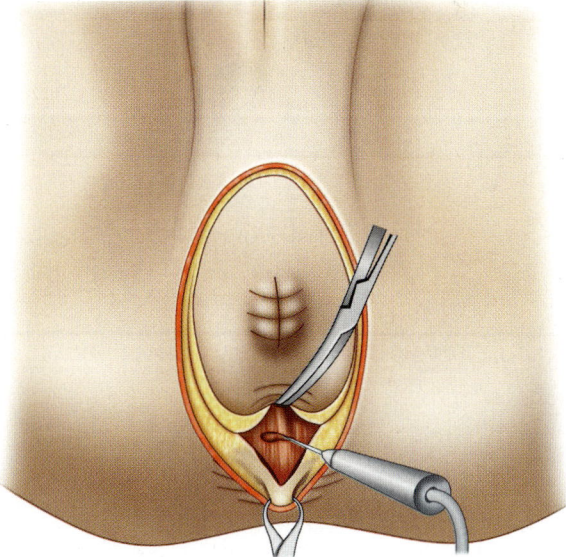

Dissection enters the ischiorectal fat both sides

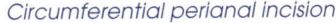

The path is long, but self-surrender makes it short; the way is difficult, but perfect trust makes it easy.

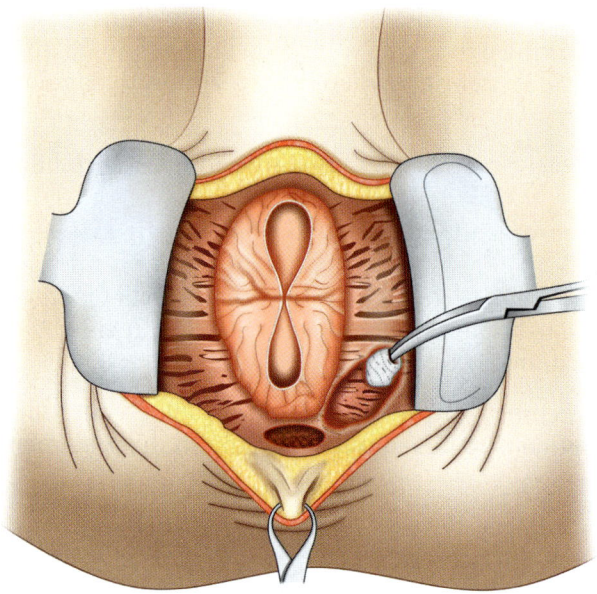

Division of anococcygeal ligament both the sides

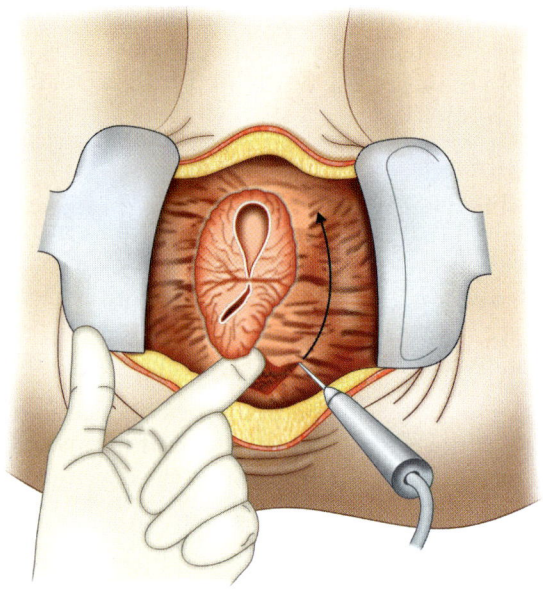

Division of levator ani

If possible, right and left pelvic diaphragms to be approximated. Hemostasis to be achieved meticulously. Close the perineal wound with vicryl 3-0 suture after placing two suction drains and close the skin.

For locally advanced tumors: Radical excision is required including internal iliac nodes, autonomic nerves, seminal vesicle, involved prostate or bladder and in female en bloc hysterectomy.

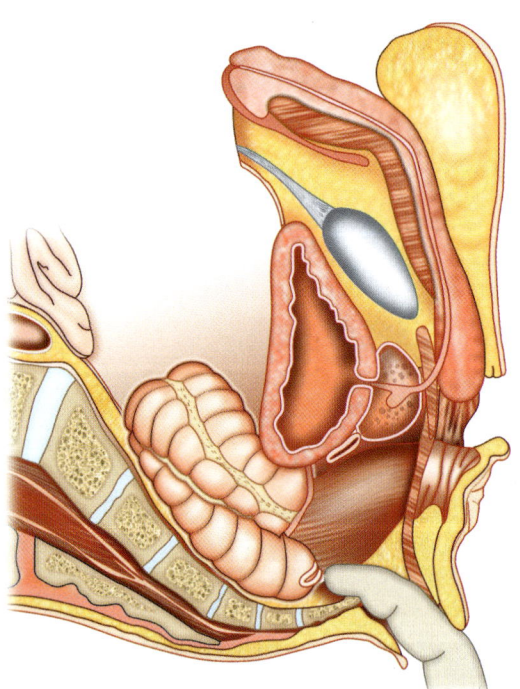

Lateral view to access presacral space

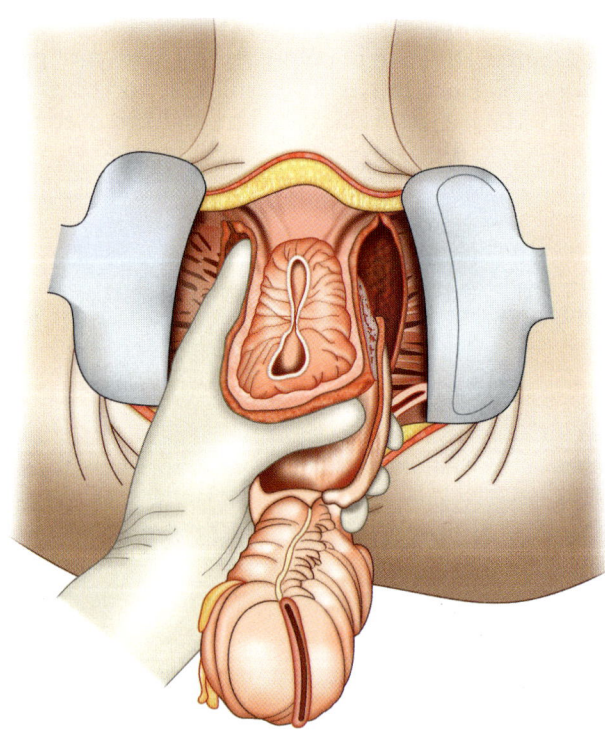

Division of levator ani and delivery of specimen

Stop complaining about the management of the universe. Look around for a place to sow a few seeds of happiness.

6.4.2 ANTERIOR RESECTION (AR) AND LOW ANTERIOR RESECTION (LAR)

The difference between AR and LAR is like this—in AR, colon is anastomosed to the peritonealized portion of rectum and in LAR, the anastomosis is done to the extraperitoneal portion of the rectum.

Indications

- Carcinoma middle and upper third of rectum 6–14 cm from anal verge.
- Selected low rectal cancer where sphincter can be saved, keeping 1 cm healthy margin from the lower edge of the tumor.

Pitfalls

- Anastomotic leak/failure
- Injury to ureter
- Presacral bleeding.

Preoperative Preparation

As in colon cancer.

Procedure

- General anesthesia
- Modified lithotomy position/Loyd Davis position
- Surgeon will stand on patient's left
- *Incision:* Midline incision, starting from few cm above the umbilicus to the symphysis pubis.

Step 1: Stage the disease clinically: Assess the operability of the tumor, fixity to sacrum, peritoneal involvement, ascites, liver metastases.

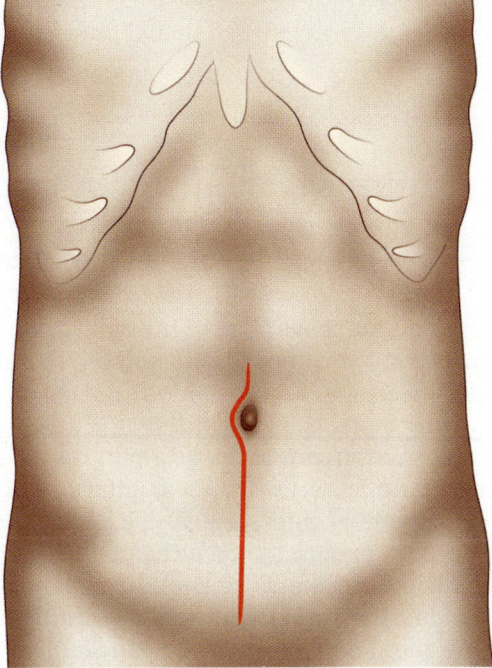

Incision for anterior resection/low anterior resection

No one in this world is pure and perfect. If we avoid people for their mistakes, we will always be alone in this world. Judge less and love more.

Remember: Single liver metastases or multiple liver metastases in the same segment are not contraindications for resection. Along with AR/LAR, do metastasectomy or segmentectomy. Urinary bladder is fixed to the skin to avoid obstruction during pelvic dissection.

Step 2: Mobilization of sigmoid colon: Make a long incision over peritoneum in the left paracolic gutter between the descending colon and the white line of "Toldt".

Elevate the peritoneal layer with left index finger and incise the peritoneum till the right angle curve of the splenic flexure is reached.

Similarly, the incision is extended caudally and detaches the sigmoid colon from its lateral attachment up to rectosigmoid junction. (The little modification is that avoid mobilization of the splenic flexure. The modification depends upon the suitable sigmoid colon for reconstruction.)

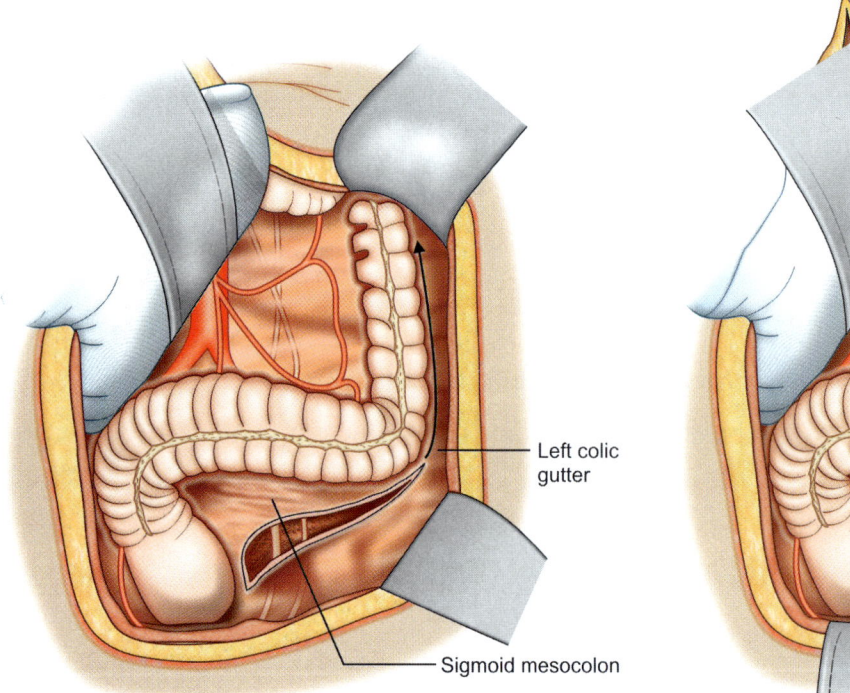

Mobilization of left colon, incising along the line of Toldt

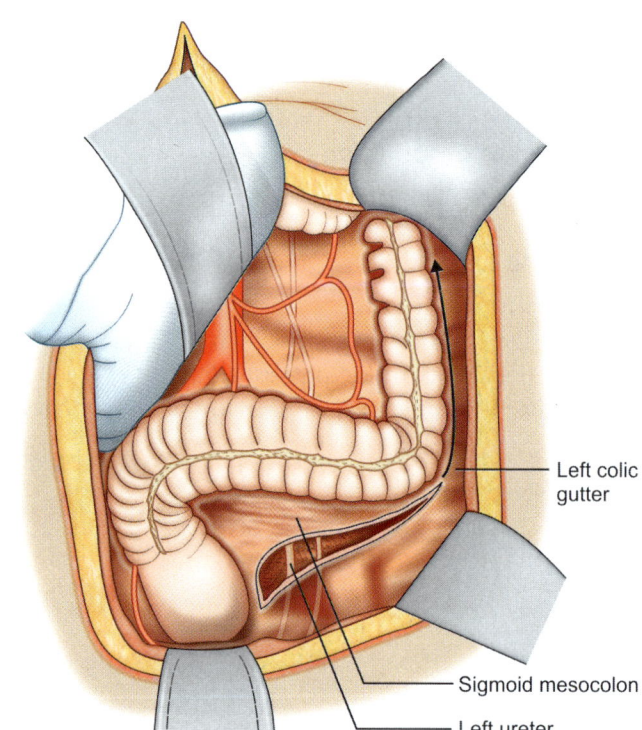

Mobilization of sigmoid colon and upper rectum

Step 3: Lymphovascular dissection: Separate the gonadal vein from the lateral leaf of mesocolon and let it fall posteriorly. Retract the descending and sigmoid colons. Now, palpate the inferior mesenteric artery (IMA) inserting the index finger between the deep margins of mesosigmoid and the bifurcation of the aorta. Vascularity of sigmoid colon may be improved by preserving the left colic artery, arises 2–3 cm away from the origin of IMA. Skeletonize the IMA by incising the peritoneum at the origin of the artery. All fat and lymphatic tissue is to be drawn toward the specimen. In routine cases, the IMA is ligated and divided just distal to its ascending left colic branches. Look at the base of mesentery and see a single division of inferior mesenteric vein as a cord-like structure, preventing the descending colon to reach the pelvic floor. Ligate the inferior mesenteric vein at the lower border of pancreas faciliating the extra mobility of the left colon. Now, the transverse mesocolon is retracted upward and the inferior mesenteric vein is identified. Dissect the flimsy peritoneum on the left side of duodenojejunal flexure and now dissect either side of inferior mesenteric vein which is to be ligated properly and divided. It allows the left colon to come down into the pelvis.

The true mastery is to be master of oneself.

Step 4: Mobilization of rectum: The plane of dissection is just immediately outside the mesorectum to mobilize the upper and mid rectum. The dissection should be posteriorly first then lateral and lastly anterior. The plane immediately outside the mesorectum is not to continue where it cones in below the mesorectum on the surface of levator ani and at the level of tumors, posterior dissection should stop where pelvic floor fusses with, Waldeyer's fascia is first encountered.

In case of male, vesicorectal space to be dissected out to detach the rectum from the bladder and in case of female, rectum to be separated from rectouterine space.

Presacral dissection: Posterior dissection is to be encountered first on steady upward traction. The band of tissue extending from mid-sacral on to the posterior rectum and mesorectum will be evident and on either side of it there is only loose areola tissue. Now, surgeon to insert the hand in presacral space, sharp dissection with diathermy to be carried out so that specimen is elevated from the sacrum as far as the lateral ligaments on each side. The wishbone of sympathetic hypogastric nerve will be visible at the pelvic brim posteriorly. Endopelvic fascia should be intact to prevent hemorrhage as presacral veins are beneath the fascia.

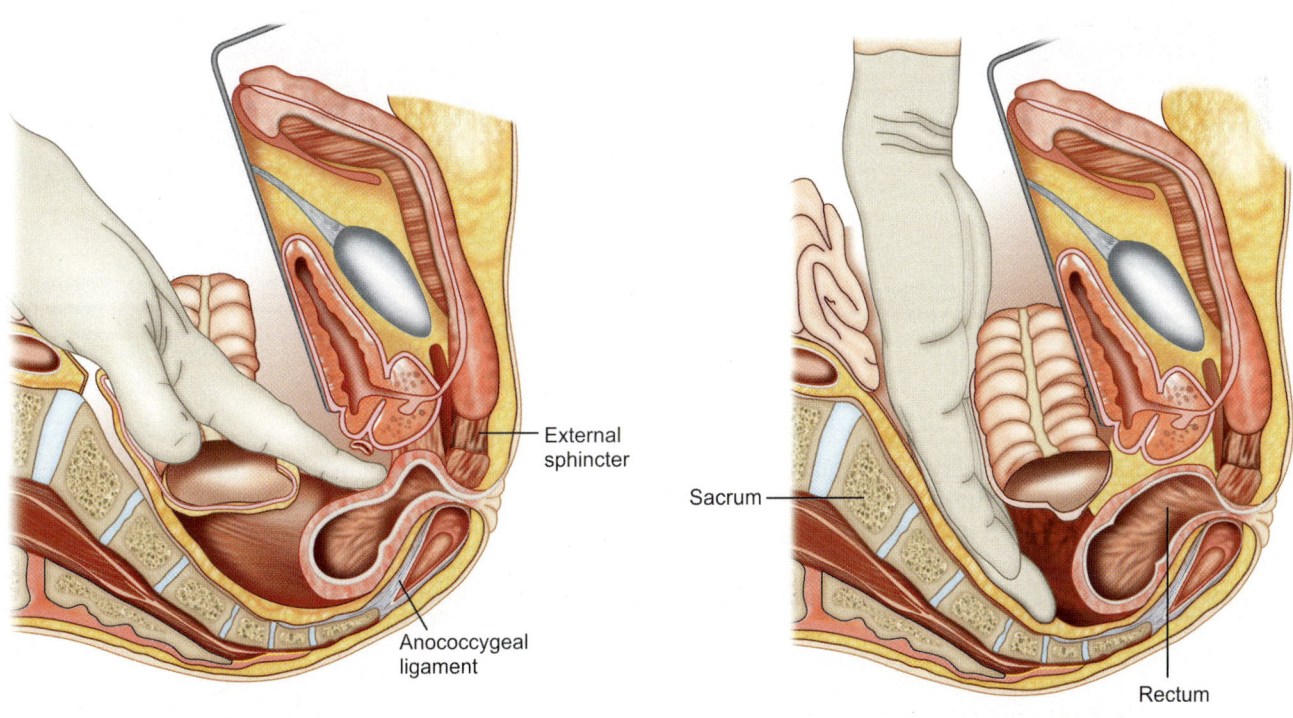

Vesicorectal dissection in case of male

Mobilization of rectum from the sacrum

Step 5: Lateral pelvic dissection: The lateral plane on the surface of dissection of mesorectum will allow the hypogastric nerves and then inferior hypogastric plexus to fall back on to the pelvic side wall. Now, the lateral ligaments on both the sides will be divided with ureter intact. The superior rectal vessels are ligated and divided just distal to the sigmoid arteries. The middle rectal artery will require diathermy coagulation or ligation.

Life ends when you stop dreaming, hope ends when you stop believing and love ends when you stop caring. So dream, hope and love. Make life beautiful.

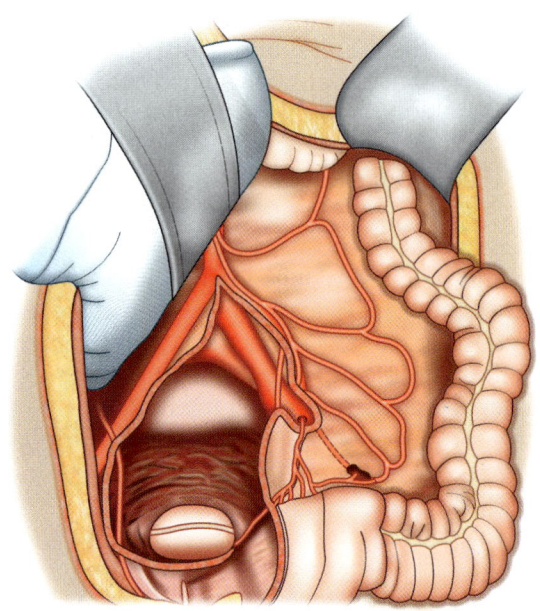

Superior rectal artery ligated and divided distal to sigmoid arteries

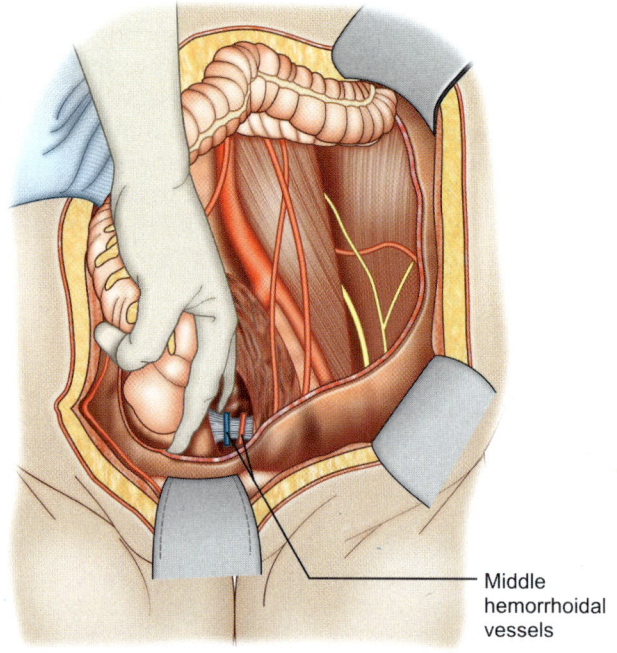

Middle hemorrhoidal vessels

Middle rectal vessels are ligated and divided

Pelvic hemostasis is a very important part of this procedure. Along the lateral wall of pelvis, identified vessels may be clipped. But in presacral area, vessels are thin-walled, thereby application of clips or sponging are not effective. Pointed tip cautery also may convert the bleeding point to a major venous laceration. Ball-tipped electrode is safer to coagulate the bleeder. Profuse presacral bleeding localized at a single formen, use thumbtack to control the bleeding. When multiple points of bleeding are there, should be covered with topical hemostatic agent, pack large gauze over it and apply pressure. (Usually, it stops the bleeding. If it does not keep the pack for 24–48 hours and then remove it under GA.)

Step 6: Preparation of rectal stump: After complete mobilization of rectum en-bloc with mesorectum along the tumor, divide at least 2 cm distal to the lower edge of the tumor with TA 30/45 or with a similar linear stapler. (In the present era of chemo-radiotherapy, minimum 1 cm healthy margin from the distal edge of the tumor is acceptable to save the sphincter function.)

In middle rectal tumor, although total mesorectal excision (TME) performed, the mesorectum is drawn up as the stapler is closed and a short cuff of distal rectum is left for colorectal anastomosis in lower third cancer, the stapler has to be closed beyond the distal margin of the mesorectum to clear the tumor with adequate healthy margin.

Remember: In case of upper third tumor, evidence indicates that TME is not required.

Catch hold of a peace deep within and push it into the cells of the body. With the peace will come back the health.

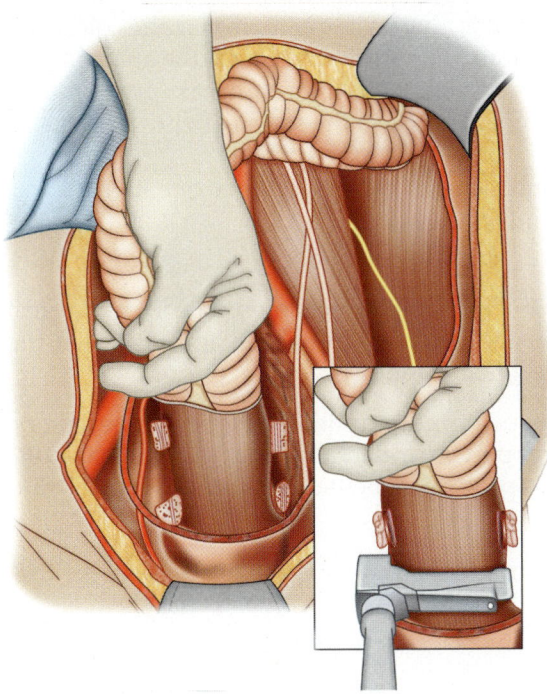

Resection of rectum 2 cm approximal (minimum 1 cm) to the sphincter

Step 7: *Proximal resection of bowel:* The general agreement is that descending colon, rather than sigmoid, used for colorectal anastomosis, as the leak rate is reduced with this. In such case, splenic flexure to be mobilized completely to bring the descending colon to the anastomotic site. So, resect total length sigmoid colon along with the specimen with linear cutter GIA/NTLC 55/60. (But if you could spare the upper branches of sigmoid artery, then you resect the partial length of sigmoid colon and anastomose provided the cut margin of sigmoid colon having the good vascularity.)

Note: After completion of complete left colon mobilization along with the splenic flexure, if still the length is insufficient. What we can do is;

1. Transilluminate the mesentery and see the suitable site for ligation of vessels.
2. Mobilize whole of the right colon from the lower part of the cecum to hepatic flexure and transverse colon so that the middle colic artery can be rotated downward.
3. If the length is not still adequate, divide the origin of middle colic artery. The mobilized cecum, like a clock pendulum, is moved downward and now tension free anastomosis is possible.

For low colorectal anastomosis with circular device: To use the circular stapling device for low colorectal anastomosis, the patient with Loyd Davis position put a sand back below the sacrum. For a lower third tumor 6–9 cm from anal verge, it is required to dissect the rectum down to the levator ani which requires complete division of Waldeyer's fascia posteriorly, dissection of anterior rectum away from the prostate (in male) to the level of urethra and the division of lateral ligaments down to the levators. And the limit of the dissection is puborectalis muscle.

Irrigation of rectal stump: If the bowel preparation is not satisfactory. Clean the rectum, inserting a Foley's or Ryle's tube in the rectum, with normal saline. This irrigation not only removes retained fecal matter but also lyses any shed tumor cells.

Step 8: *Select the anastomotic technique and anastomose:* Use a side-to-end or suture end-to-end technique for a low colorectal anastomosis (like hepaticojejunostomy). Or use SDH (EEA) circular stapler 29 or 33 mm. A purse string suture (1-0 prolene) is inserted at the edge of enterotomy and tightened it after inserting the anvil and cut the suture. Now, the head of stapling device introduced through the anus and now two portions of the device are locked together and the bowel ends are anastomosed. Open the stapler, check the anastomosis and both the "doughnuts" [some surgeons make a "J" shaped colonic pouch (7 × 7 cm) with GIA 75. About 6 cm enterotomy is made on the antimesenteric border from the close bowel end. Now with EEA circular stapler, colorectal anastomosis

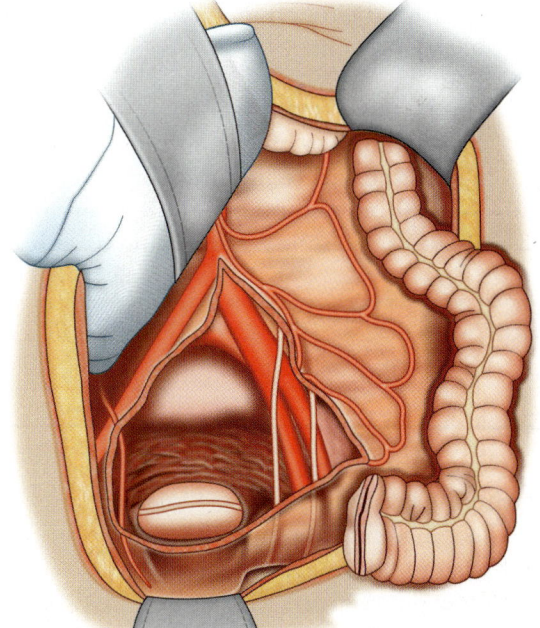

Picture after resection of the specimen

The will to win, the desire to succeed, the urge to reach.

is made]. If there any doubt about the technical part of anastomosis, it is always better to protect the colorectal (or coloanal) anastomosis by a temporary defunctioning loop ileostomy or colostomy. Check the anastomosis by introducing 200 mL of air per anus. Bubbles appear and in the fluid filled pelvis indicate a leak (preoperative chemotherapy/radiotherapy also make the anastomosis vulnerable). And close the stoma after 6–8 weeks. A delayed clouser is ideal.

The use of LAR in middle rectal and selected low rectal tumors has been increased for two main reasons.
1. Double-stapled technique has permitted a simpler and lower anastomosis.
2. The acceptance of 2 cm (even 1 cm minimal) distal margin has enabled lower tumor to be resected by LAR.

Double-stapled technique: Use (1) when the rectum is unusually thick or large to accommodate by the largest circular stapler cartridge; (2) as it is much simpler to apply at a significantly lower level and (3) use in the patient who had undergone Hartmann operation requires colorectal anastomosis.

Step 9: Wound closure and drainage: Change the gloves and do not use all contraminated instruments. Irrigate the abdomen thoroughly and wound with betadine. Place a drain at pelvis (presacral drainage) or left paracolic gutter. Close the abdomen in layers, mass closer with loop nylon/prolene, subcutaneous with vicryl 2-0 and skin with 3-0 nylon or stapler.

Postoperative Care

- Nasogastric suction for 3–5 days
- Nothing per oral (NPO) for at least 4 days
- Continue IV antibiotics for 3–5 dyas
- Keep the catheter for 6–7 days
- Drainage catheter to be kept 4–5 days or till the significant drainage volume.

Complications

i. *Presacral bleeding:* The most important complication.
ii. Bladder dysfunction may follow LAR. Usually normal function resumes after 6–7 days of continuous bladder drainage.
iii. *Pelvic sepsis:* Secondary to anastomotic leakage is the most serious complication following low colorectal anastomosis. Usually 6–9 postoperative days, patient presents with fever and having ileus and passing loose stool. On investigation, presence of leukocytosis. Digital per rectal examination (DRE) reveals a gap in the suture line and confirm it by computed tomography (CT) scan and managed by intravenous (IV) antibiotics and CT-guided percutaneous catheter drainage.
iv. *Sexual dysfunction:* In men and usually due to extensive dissection in presacral space, lateral ligament, etc.

6.5 OTHERS COMMON ABDOMINAL OPERATION

6.5.1 EXPLORATORY LAPAROTOMY WITH REPAIR OF PEPTIC PERFORATION

Steps

- General anesthesia
- Supine position
- Cleaning and draping
- Incision: Midline incision.
  Halfway between umbilicus and xiphisternum to halfway between umbilicus and symphysis pubis.

Step 1: Exploratory laparotomy: Confirm the perforation and locate the site. Look other common sites for perforations, like gastric, ileal or rectal perforations, etc. Usually, first part of duodenum is the most common

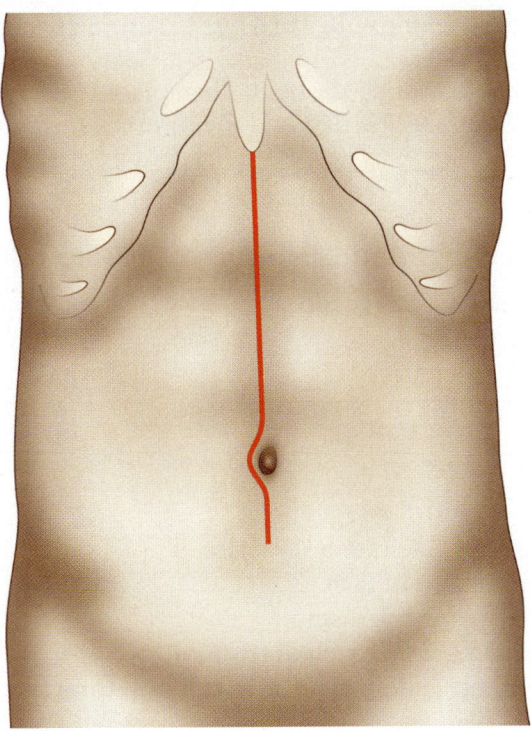

Midline abdominal incision

site for a perforation. In case of perforated gastric ulcer, a biopsy to be taken from the ulcer margin to exclude malignancy. If no perforation is seen in anterior wall of duodenum and stomach, the whole small intestine, colon, appendix and rectum are to be examined meticulously, before you come to a decision that there is no perforation. Small perforation may be sealed also.

Step 2: Aspirate the peritoneal fluid and thorough peritoneal lavage to be done with normal saline.

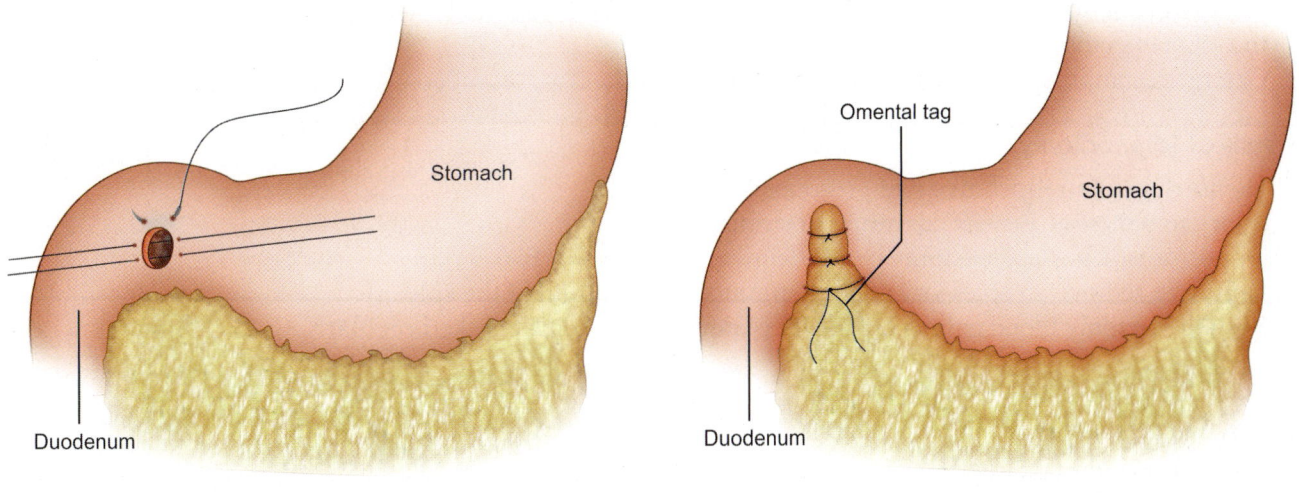

Placement of suture in duodenal perforation   *Graham patch repair*

Physical education is meant to bring into the body, consciousness and control, discipline and mastery, all things necessary for a higher and better life.

Step 3: The closure of the perforation is done with 3 or 4 bite of suture depending upon the size of perforation, with interrupted 3-0 vicryl suture.

First place the central sutures but do not tie the knot. Then place the side sutures one by one. Now, tie the knots one by one. Both corner sutures are tied first and the central suture to be tied last.

Step 4: Now, place a tag of omentum over the site of perforation and again sutures are tied over the omentum called Grahm patch repair.

Step 5: After closing the perforation, the meticulous peritoneal toileting to be done (all the sites, i.e. paracolic gutter, subdiaphragmatic spaces, pelvis, etc.) with normal saline. Place a drain at right subdiaphragmatic space. Abdomen is closed in usual fashion. Skin is closed by interrupted nylon or polyamide sutures.

6.5.2 SPLENECTOMY

Indications

- Trauma
- Spontaneous splenic rupture
- Malignancy in adjacent organs, like carcinoma stomach
- Left-sided portal hypertension (sinistral PHT)
- Overactive enlarged spleen, like hypersplenism
- Portal hypertension with enlarged spleen to avoid rupture
- Enlarged spleen causing discomfort and pressure effects like in tropical splenomegaly, malaria, kala-azar, chronic myeloid leukemia, etc.
- Splenic cyst, abscess
- Primary splenic tumor
- Staging for Hodgkin's disease (not done nowadays)

Preoperative Preparation

1. Arrange adequate quantity of blood.
2. Immunize the patient's minimum 2 weeks prior to surgery against Pneumococcus, Meningococcus, *Haemophilus influenzae* to avoid overwhelming postsplenectomy sepsis (OPSI).
3. In case of emergency splenectomy, immunization to be delayed until 2 weeks after the operation to obtain the most effective immune response.
4. Gastric decompression, prophylactic antibiotics are other important considerations.

Pitfalls of Splenectomy

- Hemorrhage: Intraoperative and postoperative
- Injury to pancreas, greater curvature of stomach
- Opportunistic postsplenectomy overwhelming infection (OPSI)
- Failure to remove an accessory spleen (common site is hilum of the spleen)
- Postsplenectomy blood counts especially platelet counts to be checked regularly.

Steps

1. Supine position
2. General anesthesia
3. Incisions
   - Left subcostal or midline

In order to be truly happy in life, one must love work.

- Left subcostal to reach up to
- Left anterior axillary line for mild to moderate splenomegaly. Sometime Kher extension of subcostal incision is required which is up to the middle to the xiphocostal junction
- For massive splenomegaly or where costal arch is narrow, midline incision is preferable.

Step 1: Abdomen is opened. Pathology confirmed. Surgeon's left hand to be placed at the lateral surface of the spleen to lift the spleen forward and medially and posterior layer of linorenal ligament is divided. It allows spleen to move adequate.

Step 2: Now clamp, incise and ligate the left part of gastrocolic ligament, left gastric artery and vein to be ligated and divided, if require. This will provide access to the lesser sac. Incise the avascular portion of the gastrohepatic ligament along the middle of the lesser curvature and elevate the stomach to expose the upper border of pancreas.

Step 3: Look at the superior border of pancreas and locate splenic artery to be doubly ligated as distally as possible. Clamp, divide and ligate short gastric arteries and veins one by one.

Step 4: Mobilize the spleen by dividing several ligaments with scissors. Spleen to be separated from renal and from linorenal ligaments by sharp and blunt dissection. Splenocolic, splenophrenic ligaments are now divided and ligated.

Step 5: Elevate the spleen, tail and part of the body of the pancreas, being very careful with the tail of pancreas which is to be preserved. Spleen is now mobilized maximum.

Step 6: At the hilum, ligate and divide all branches of splenic artery. Splenic vein and its tributaries to be ligated and divided in continuity with 2-0 silk and spleen is removed.

Step 7: Search for accessory spleen and invert the greater curvature completely. Hemostasis to be achieved. Inspect the stomach, if suspicion of any damage and the sites of bleedings, etc. From subdiaphragmatic surface continuing to greater curvature of the stomach, pancreatic tail, gastrosplenic, splenorenal, splenocolic and othe ligaments and splenic bed. If any oozing, pack for 5 minutes and ensure complete hemostasis.

Postoperative Complications

- Postoperative pancytopenia, specially thrombocytopenia
- Hemorrhage reactionary and secondary
- Opportunistic postsplenectomy infection (OPSI)
- Subphrenic abscess
- Gastric fistula
- Acute pancreatitis
- Venous thrombosis.

6.5.3 ADRENALECTOMY

Surgical Anatomy

A pair of very important endocrine glands hypofunction lead to situation, like Addison's disease and hyperfunction causes retention of fluid and salt and a situation like Cushing's disease and involving the medulla causing pheochromocytoma.

They are made up of two parts; outer cortex is of mesodermal origin which is responsible for number of steroid hormones and inner medulla of neural crest origin, made up of chromaffin cells and produce adrenalin, noradrenalin and catecholamines.

Let us always do the right thing and we shall always be quiet and happy.

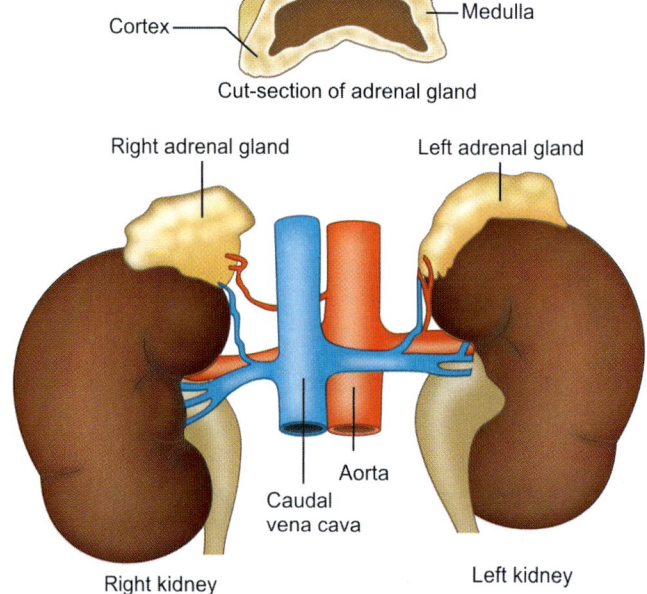

Anatomy of adrenal glands

Each gland located at the upper pole of the kidney in the epigastrium, in front of the crus of the diaphragm, surrounded immediately by loose areolar tissue containing fat and outside, it is covered by renal fascia.

Right Adrenal Gland

It is triangular or pyramidal in shape and left gland is semilunar. Each gland measures 50 mm in height, 30 mm in breadth and 10 mm in thickness.

For all practical purposes, each adrenal gland has only two surfaces: (1) anterior and (2) posterior. The relations of right adrenal gland are as follows:

a. *Anterior surface:* Superiorly, the "bare area" of liver, inferiorly, peritoneum and sometimes the first part of duodenum.
   - Medially: Inferior vena cava (IVC)
   - Laterally: Part of the "bare area" of liver
b. *Posterior surface*
   - Superiorly: Diaphragm
   - Inferiorly: Anteromedial aspect of right kidney.

Left Adrenal Gland

a. *Anterior surface*
   - Superiorly: Peritoneum and stomach
   - Inferiorly: Body of pancreas
b. *Posterior surface*
   - Medially: Left crus of diaphragm
   - Laterally: Medial aspect of left kidney

There are unique moments in life that pass like a dream. One must catch them on the wing, for they never return.

Vascular Supply

a. *Remember:* All India Radio (AIR)
   i. Aortic branch: Suprarenal artery for medial part
   ii. Inferior phrenic branch: A group of 6–8 arteries for superior part
   iii. Renal artery branch: For inferior part of adrenal gland.
b. *Veins:* On the right, the single adrenal vein drains into IVC and on the left, the vein drains into left renal.
   Specialty: The adrenal vein does not accompany the arterial supply.

The left vein passes downward over the anterior surface of the gland and is joined by the left inferior phrenic vein before entering the left renal vein. The right adrenal vein passes obliquely to open into IVC posteriorly. Occasionally, accessory adrenal vein enters the inferior phrenic vein.

Remember: The adrenal vein on the right side is very short and mostly it drains into IVC. So, it is to be tackled very carefully.

Right Adrenalectomy: Open

Steps

1. Supine position
2. General anesthesia
3. *Incision:* Midline from xiphoid process to lower midline or bilateral subcostal (Chevron incision like in Whipple's) and open the abdomen (in case of pheochromocytoma, more longer midline incision is required).

Step 1: Mobilization of right adrenal gland: The anterior approach to the right adrenal gland begins with mobilization of hepatic flexure. Postadhesions between liver and peritoneum are divided. Vessels particularly hepatic veins in medial attachment to be taken care off.

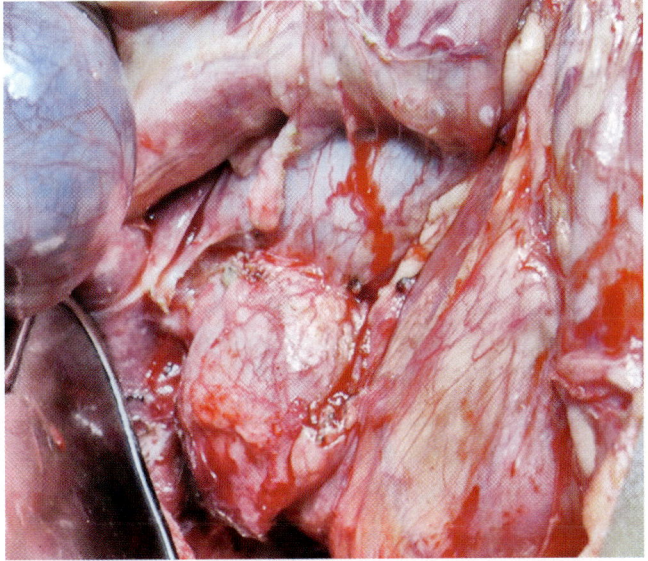

The right adrenal mass (Courtesy: Dr Durgatosh Pandey)

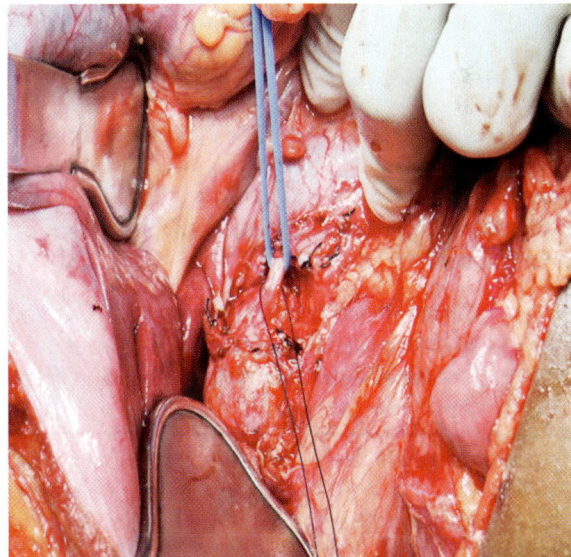

Looping the right adrenal vein (Courtesy: Dr Durgatosh Pandey)

Friendship is association of two persons who may not be equal in qualification, experience and talent but equal in their commitment to understand each other.

Step 2: Kocherization of duodenum: After mobilization of colon, duodenum is exposed. Now, kocherization of duodenum is done by dividing the lateral avascular peritoneal reflection. IVC, right adrenal gland along with upper pole of right kidney are now exposed. Common bile duct (CBD), gastroduodenal artery may be visible in this area and to be saved. Duodenum, second part to be retracted medially.

Step 3: Adrenal gland dissection and vessels ligation: Right adrenal gland to be dissected downward with finger carefully. After dissection of liver and IVC, identify right adrenal vein which leaves the gland on its anterior surface and enters the vena cava on its posterior surface. The vein should be handled very gently and ligated very carefully. (To avoid hemorrhage from IVC or adrenal vein, the IVC to be freed far enough to ensure a space for an angle clamp.)

Step 4: Removal of the gland: After proper ligation of all vessels, retract the superior pole of right kidney inferiorly. Then the posterior surface to be separated from underlying fatty tissue. When the apex of the gland is reached liver to be retracted upward. Lateral border to be separated then the medial margin and remove the gland.

Step 5: After removal of the gland, look for any injury to the diaphragm and inspect for any air leak, if any, close the leak with absorbable suture.

Ensure hemostasis completely. Place a drain and close the wound in layers.

Left Adrenalectomy: Open

Steps

1. Supine position
2. General anesthesia
3. Incision: Midline from xiphoid process to lower midline or left subcostal incision extended toward the right and open the abdomen (in case of pheochromocytoma, more longer midline incision is required).

Step 1: Exposure and mobilization of left adrenal gland: The procedure starts with the posterior parietal peritoneum lateral to the left colon, divide the splenorenal ligament avoiding injury to spleen, splenic vessels and pancreatic tail which are covered by splenorenal ligament. (Opening of lesser sac through gastrocolic omentum is another approach to the left adrenal.)

Step 2: Now, the peritoneum under the lower border of pancreas is incised halfway along the tail. Retract the pancreas up gently, the left adrenal along the upper pole of left kidney will be exposed. Covering the fascia of Gerota.

Incise the renal fascia, caring for aorta, renal artery and vein, the left adrenal gland will be exposed and adrenal vein is accessible.

Step 3: Ligation of adrenal vessels: Adrenal vein which emerges from the medial aspect of the gland and runs obliquely downward to enter the left renal vein should be ligated. (In case of pheochromocytoma, it is logical to ligate adrenal vein first to prevent release of catecholamines into the circulation.) All arteries to be ligated one by one—inferior phrenic, adrenal and branch from renal artery as in right-sided adrenalectomy.

Step 4: Now, the dissection to continue at the inferolateral aspect of the left adrenal gland and then superiorly. Retract the gland superiorly and separate it from inferior attachment caring for left renal vessels. Now, remove the left adrenal gland.

Step 5: Ensure complete hemostasis: Look for any surrounding organ injury, especially the spleen. Close the abdomen in layers.

Success is almost totally dependent upon drive and persistence. The extra energy required to make another effort or try another approach is the secret of winning.

Thoracoabdominal Approach

Indication

Large tumor in a single gland: Incision to be started at the angle of 8th to 10th ribs and extend it across the midline to the mid-point of contralateral rectus muscle; just above the umbilicus. Remove the 10th rib, open the pleura and incise the diaphragm from above. Next follow the procedure of anterior approach. Nowadays, laparoscopic adrenalectomy is becoming popular day by day.

6.5.4 APPENDICECTOMY/APPENDECTOMY

Indications

1. Acute appendicitis
2. Recurrent appendicitis
3. Mucocele of appendix
4. Carcinoid appendix less than 3 cm.

Others

1. Early carcinoma not involving base
2. Endometriosis, diverticulosis, etc.

Pitfalls

1. Sepsis
2. Portal pyemia.

Procedure

1. General anesthesia/spinal/epidural
2. Supine position
3. Cleaning, draping
4. *Incision:*
   - McBurney's gridiron incision
   - An oblique, approx 6–7.5 cm incision at McBurney's point at right angle to the spinoumbilical line 2–2.5 cm above and 4–5 cm below.

Step 1: Skin and subcutaneous tissue are incised in the same line. External oblique aponeurosis is incised along the direction of its fibers.

Step 2: Spliting of conjoint tendon split the junction of internal oblique and transversus abdominis with straight artery forcep along the direction of their fibers.

Step 3: Opening of peritoneum: Preperitoneal fat will be visible with underlying peritoneum. Now hold the peritoneum with two hemostatic forceps, lift up and incise it along the line of skin incision.

Step 4: Identification of appendix and cecum: Identify the pathology and decide for the extent of surgery. Hold the cecum with Babcock's forceps. (Cecum is cone-shaped pale looking, having taenia but no mesentery.) And deliver it out of the wound. Appendix will follow it. (If any turbid fluid or pus-like liquid is found, please send it for culture sensitivity.)

Step 5: Division of mesoappendix: Hold the appendix parallel to abdominal wall with two Babcock's forceps. Now the mesoappendix is ligated, part by part, and divided toward the side of the appendix along with the appendicular artery.

If a 5 seconds smile can make a photograph beautiful, imagine how beautiful your life will be if you always keep smiling.

Step 6: Division of base of appendix: Base of appendix is crushed with artery forceps, ligate the base or transfix the base of appendix and divide it 5 mm away. Baz the visible mucosa and leave it inside the abdomen. (Some surgeons like to bury the base by purse string suture.) (One should not crush the base, if it is perforated edematous and gangrenous.)

Step 7: Look for Meckel's diverticulum: Minimum 2 ft of terminal ileum to be taken out to check for associated Meckel's diverticulum. (If it is there, partial resection of ileum along with the diverticulum and anastomosis to be done.)

Step 8: Ensure hemostasis and wound is to be cleaned and closed in layers.

(Retrograde appendicectomy to be done when tip of appendix is not accessible easily. So, start dividing it from the base and proceed towards the tip and remove the appendix.)

LAP APPENDICECTOMY

Procedure

1. General anesthesia
2. Supine position: Head down, right up
3. Ports placement

Ports to be made:
1. 10 mm infraumbilical port for telescope and camera
2. 5 mm port in right iliac fossa
3. 10 mm port in left iliac fossa/5 mm port at suprapubic region.

Author prefers three ports:
1. 10 mm epigastric port for telescope and camera
2. 12 mm supraumbilical port for dissection and stapling
3. Infraumbilical port for retraction.

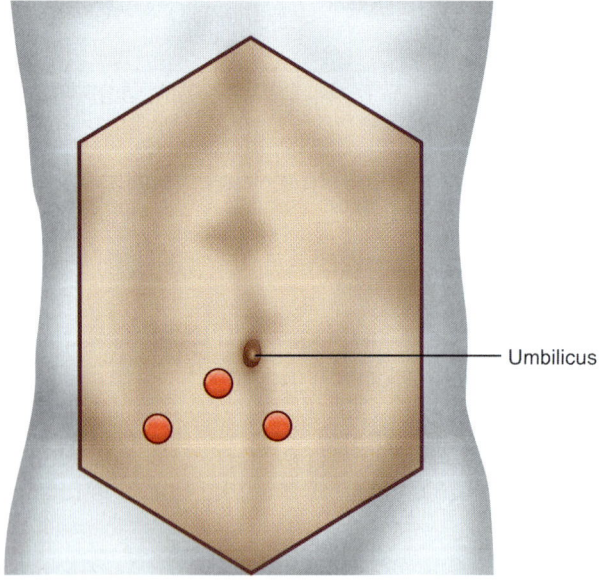

Ports placement

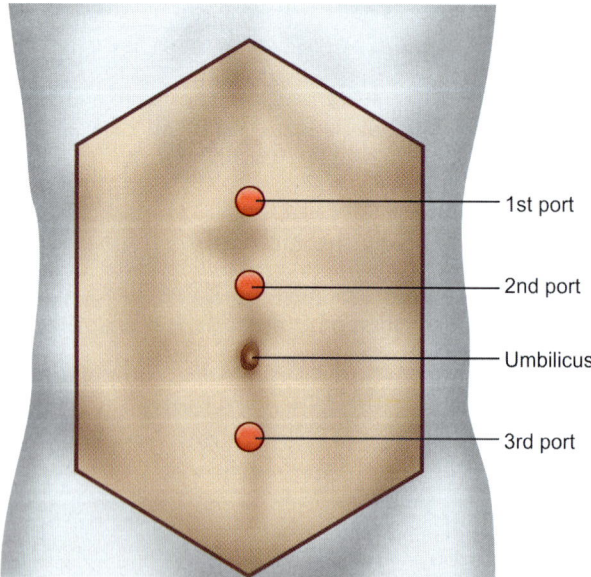

Infraumblical ports for retraction

Daring ideas are like chessmen moved forward, they may be beaten, but they may start a winning game.

Step 1: Identify the pathology of appendix and adhesiolysis.

Step 2: Hold the appendix in antimesenteric border with babcock. Ligate the appendicular artery or divide it with harmonic. Separate the appendix from mesoappendix with harmonic or cautery.

Step 3: Apply endo-gastrointestine (GI) stapler at the base of the appendix or use endoloop at the base and divide it. Remove the specimen through 12 mm mid-port.

Step 4: Hemostasis ensure
- Rectus sheath to be closed in 12 mm and 10 mm ports.
- Skin is closed 3-0 nylon/stapler.

6.6 CHOLECYSTECTOMY

6.6.1 OPEN CHOLECYSTECTOMY

Surgical Anatomy

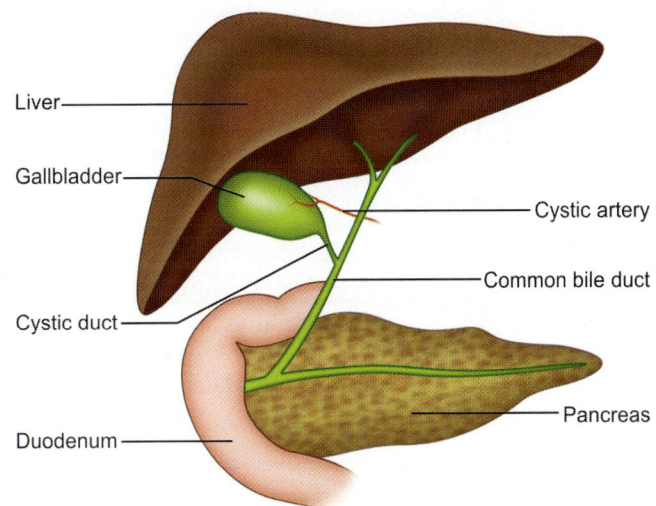

Anatomy of gallbladder for its dissection

Indications
- Chronic symptomatic cholecystitis.
- Acute cholecystitis not responding to conservative management or gangrenous cholecystitis
- Symptomatic acalculus cholecystitis
- Precancerous lesions, like porcelain gallbladder, stone more than 3 cm in size, polyp more than 1 cm, etc.
- Mucocele gallbladder, empyema gallbladder, etc.
- Part of different procedures, like Whipple's pancreaticoduodenectomy, radical cholecystectomy, etc.

Procedures
1. Supine position: Place sand bag beneath the right lower chest wall
2. General anesthesia
3. Incision: Kocher's right subcostal incision from midline 2–3 cm below and parallel to costal margin.

No one in this world is pure and perfect. If we avoid people for their mistakes, we will always be alone in this world. Judge less and love more.

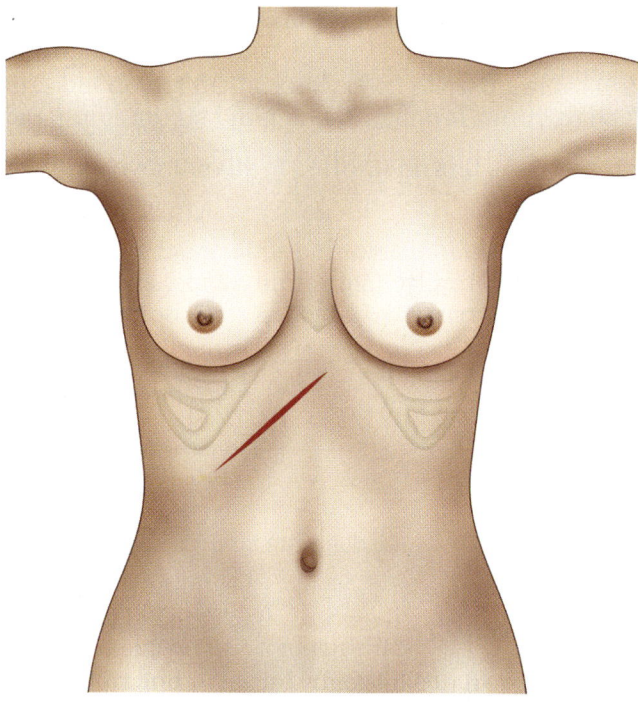

Kocher's right subcostal incision

Step 1: External oblique, internal oblique, transversus abdominis muscles are divided and peritoneum is opened. Assessment of the pathology and spread in case of malignancy palpate CBD at free margin of lesser omentum to exclude calculi.

Placement of packs: Good exposure is an essential part. One mop to place at hepatorenal pouch to retract hepatic flexur and right kidney downward. Second one is to place to retract duodenum and transverse colon and the third mop to place medially to retract the stomach.

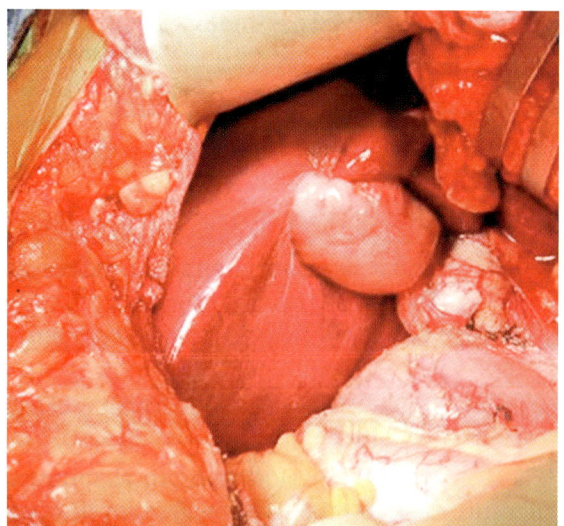

After opening the abdomen, the pathology of gallbladder noticed

---

Control over what one says is more important than complete silence.

Step 2: Retrograde method of dissection (most commonly done): Give a traction to Hartmann's pouch and dissect Calot's triangle. Cystic duct and artery to be dissected, ligated/clipped and divided. Cystic artery often runs anterior to the cystic duct and lymphnode of Lund is the guide for the artery. Artery and duct to be ligated with 1-0 silk after the peritoneum covering the cystic artery and duct is snipped off or clipped with liga clips.

Dissection of gallbladder from the liver bed: Gallbladder is to be retracted in different directions, peritoneal reflection is divided and gallbladder is gradually lifted up from liver bed and separated.

[Fundus first method: It is indicated when (1) dense adhesion at Calot's triangle, (2) anatomy of Calot's triangle and CBD not cleared.
- Fundus is separated from liver
- Dissect medially towards the neck
- Identify cystic duct and artery dissect, ligate and divide.

Remember: Excessive traction of gallbladder to avoid preventing injury to CBD and right hepatic artery. In unavoidable case, gallbladder may be ligated at the neck.

Step 3: Hemostasis and drainage: Hemostasis to be achieved completely up to complete satisfaction limited hot moist mop compression and warm saline wash may control all minor points of bleeding. Drain to be placed in subhepatic space and abdomen is closed in layers.

6.6.2 LAPAROSCOPIC CHOLECYSTECTOMY

This is the gold standard for today's cholecystectomy.

Indications

1. Chronic symptomatic cholecystitis
2. Acute cholecystitis not responding to conservative management or gangrenous cholecystitis
3. Symptomatic acalculus cholecystitis
4. Precancerous lesions like porcelain gallbladder, stone more than 3 cm in size, polyp more than 1 cm, etc.
5. Mucocele gallbladder, empyema gallbladder, etc.
6. Part of different procedures, like Whipple's pancreaticoduodenectomy, radical cholecystectomy, etc.

Procedures

1. Supine position
2. General anesthesia
3. Cleaning and draping.

Step 1: Creation of pneumoperitoneum by close or open method. 10 mm transverse incision is made below umbilicus. Hold the anterior abdominal wall up and either Veress needle is inserted into the abdominal cavity carefully or 10 mm trocar and cannula inserted and trocar is removed. Through the cannula telescope is inserted and pneumoperitoneum is created. Abdomen and pelvis to be inspected along with gallbladder.

(Note Veress needle is safer for the beginner. After inserting the needle into the abdomen, it is to be confirmed by injecting 5 mL NS. If it goes smoothly, it means it is in correct place. Alternately drop test can be done few drops of saline placed at the back end, it will be immediately sucked in then CO_2 insufflator is connected to this needle or telescope side connector. The abdominal pressure to be kept 12–14 mm Hg. Telescope is either 0° or 30° attached to the video camera.)

Step 2: Placement of 2nd, 3rd and 4th ports: These three ports to be made under vision. Second port is 10 mm port and made at epigastrium just below xiphisternum and slightly right to the midline so that falciform

---

The most important surrender is the surrender of your character, your way of being, so that it may change.

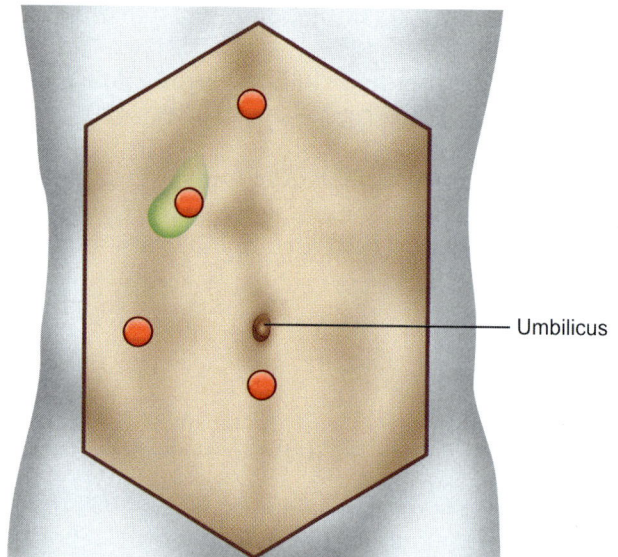

Conventional four ports sites for laparoscopic cholecystectomy

ligament is spared during insertion. Now ask to right up and head up of the patient, 3rd port is 5 mm port and made at midclavicular line just below the costal margin and 4th port is 5 mm made at right anterior axillary line at the level of umbilicus.

Remember: Upper two ports for the surgeon and lower two ports for the assistants).

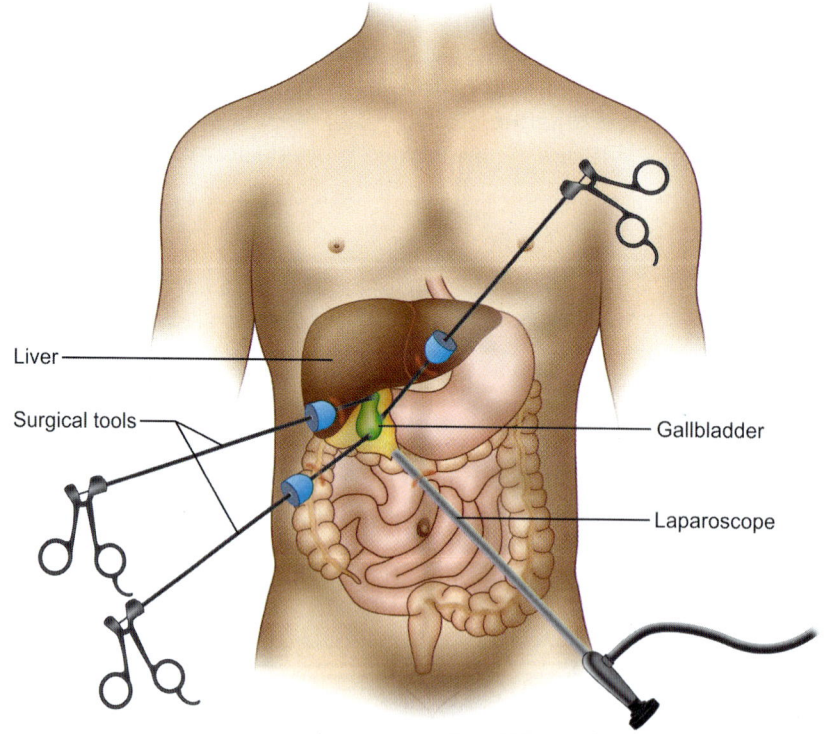

Four ports and their uses

Two lower ports: Below umbilical port for telescope and anterior axillary port for holding the toothed grasper. With this grasper, the gallbladder fundus will be retracted toward the right shoulder to expose the Calot's triangle. Left hand of the surgeon will hold another grasper to hold the Hartmann's pouch through midclavicular port for necessary retraction during dissection. Through epigastric port, surgeon will dissect with Maryland dissector attached to diathermy.

Step 3: Dissection of Calot's triangle: Any adhesion is divided first, posterior dissection of Calot's triangle is very important in early step. Folds of peritoneum are stripped off. Anterior dissection of Calot's triangle is done. Cystic duct and artery to be dissected, clearly make a wide gap in between these two. Cystic duct and artery clipped and divided respectively. Two clips at bile duct side and one at gallbladder side in each structure.

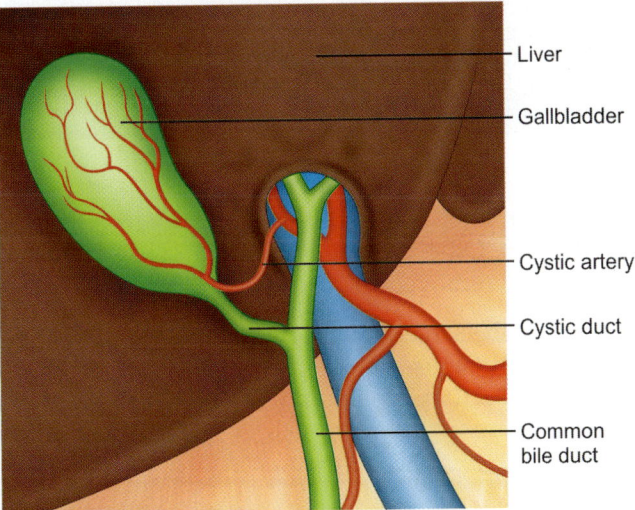

    — Liver

    — Gallbladder

    — Cystic artery

    — Cystic duct

    — Common bile duct

Anatomy of gallbladder and Calot's triangle for dissection

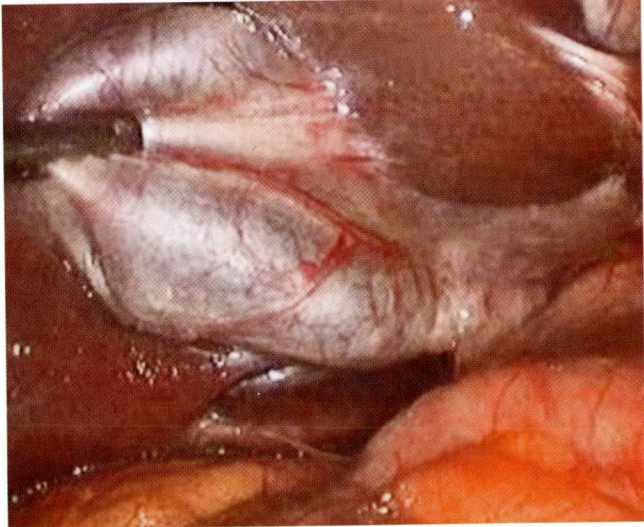

Retraction of gallbladder during dissection

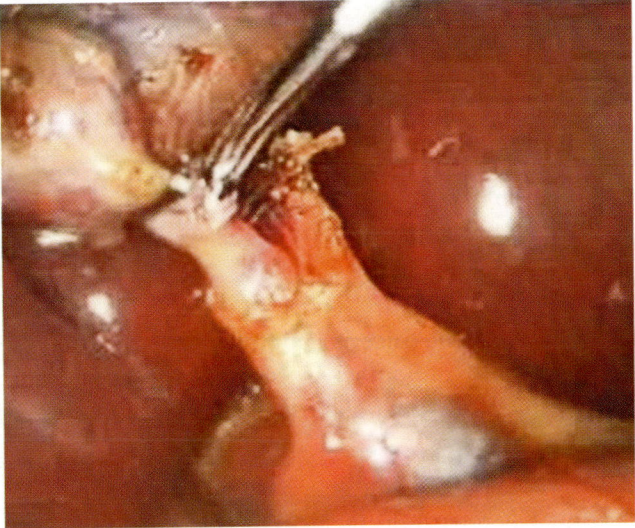

Separation of gallbladder from liver bed

Reflection cannot be seen in boiling water, truth cannot be seen in a state of anger. So, analyze before you finalize.

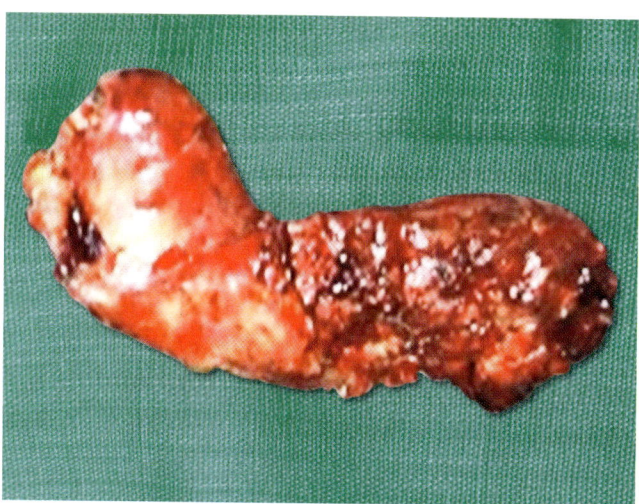

Specimen of gallbladder

Step 4: Separation of gallbladder form liver bed with the help of diathermy. The gallbladder is dissected in between gallbladder wall and the liver. Otherwise either gallbladder will be leaked or bleeding will be there from liver capsule. Gallbladder is now removed through epigastric port.

Step 5: Now irrigate the liver bed and check bleeding points and hemostasis to be achieved completely. Drain may or may not be put as per the quality of dissection. Closure of ports after withdrawl of all cannulas allows pneumoperitoneum to be resolved. The 10 mm ports will be better closed after repairing the rectus sheath with 1-0 polyglycocolic acid (vicryl) suture.

Complications

- *Immediate:* Injury to bile duct and vessels
  - Hemorrhage
  - Rupture of gallbladder and spillage of bile
  - Postoperative bile leak
  - Biliary fistula
  - Waltman Walter syndrome [owing to subdiaphragmatic collection of bile causing pressure over IVC and leading to (1) upper abdominal discomfort, (2) chest pain, (3) low blood pressure (BP) and (4) tachycardia
- Late: Bile duct stricture—post-traumatic or inflammatory

6.6.3 ROUX-EN-Y BILIARY-ENTERIC BYPASS: HEPATICOJEJUNOSTOMY

Indications

- Following bile duct resection for any reason like in Whipple's procedure.
- For reconstruction of severed or stenosed bile duct followimg iatrogenic injury.
- Common bile duct obstruction due to nonresectable tumor, chronic pancreatitis or surgical injury.

Pitfalls of the Procedure

- Injury to surrounding structures, like duodenum
- Injury to hepatic duct, hepatic artery, portal vein
- Necrosis of jejunal loop due to inaccurate division of the mesentery, anastomotic leaks, biliary fistula, etc.

Life's the most deepest feelings are often expressed in silence and the one who can read volumes from your silence is your true friend.

Procedure

- General anesthesia
- Cleaning and draping
- Incision: Long right subcostal or long midline incision and open the abdomen as usual.

Step 1: Adhesiolysis: Make the peritoneal adhesion free from anterior abdominal wall and the underlying structures (if any).

Step 2: Kocherization of duodenum: Mobilize the duodenum by incising the lateral peritoneum. Palpate the duodenum, head of pancreas and distal common bile duct. The supraduodenal part of the duct is lying in the free border of lesser omentum. Mobilization of duodenum and head of pancreas is to be carried out as far as the left side of inferior vena cava (IVC). Kocherization is completed when the left renal vein is seen.

Step 3: Dissect 2–3 cm of CBD distal to cystic duct stump. The peritoneum over the supraduodenal part of CBD is incised. Place 4-0 vicryl as stay suture medial and lateral aspect of the cleaned common bile duct. Aspirate the CBD to make sure that you are not dealing the portal vein (do not incise the CBD now).

Step 4: Now, fashion of Roux loop: The jejunum is divided 10–15 cm away from duodenojejunal flexure. The divided distal end forms the apex of the conduit and this Roux loop is brought to the anastomotic side. To bring it at the anastomotic site, some mesenteric division, and ligating of jejunal vessels are required to get a standard length of 40–45 cm to prevent the reflux of luminal contents from reaching at the apical anastomosis. The end is brought up through a window in the transverse mesocolon to the right of the middle colic vessels.

Step 5: Hepaticojejunostomy: The hepaticojejunostomy is performed using a single layer of interrupted 4-0 PDS sutures.

i. At one corner of the duct, take the suture from outside-in and then inside-out (like Conel) the same suture to take outside-in and then inside-out at the corresponding corner of the jejunum. The same "box" stitches to be repeated to the other corner of both the bile duct and the jejunum.

ii. Now, a suture to take at the middle of the posterior wall of both the bile duct and the jejunum and keep it in the middle as a guide.

iii. Now, hold the "box" suture at one corner and take full thickness posterior wall suture one by one 1 mm apart till the middle suture (kept as a guide). Repeat the same thing to opposite site of the middle suture holding the opposite box suture at the corner.

   Remember: Mucosa of both the duct and jejunum to be taken in the suture invariably.

iv. Now, start tying the suture, one by one, from one corner to another corner. Thus, the knots of the posterior layer will be inside. The first and middle and the middle and last sutures are held to steady the anastomosis. Now, cut the middle suture which has been kept as a guide but keep both corner sutures long.

v. The anterior wall anastomosis: Assistant will hold the corner suture and the surgeon will take through and through suture in both the anterior wall of the bile duct and jejunum 1 mm

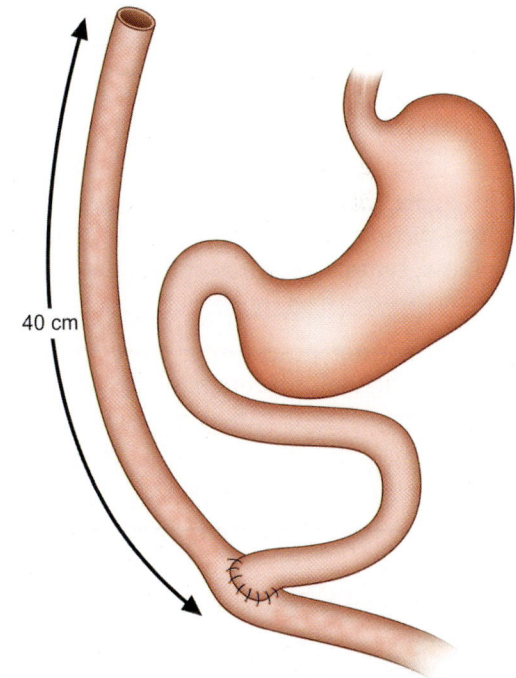

Forty centimeters jejunal loop is brought for apical anastomosis to prevent reflux

Happiness is a delicate balance between "what I want and what I have". It is an inner joy that can be "Sought and Caught", but can never be "Taught and Bought".

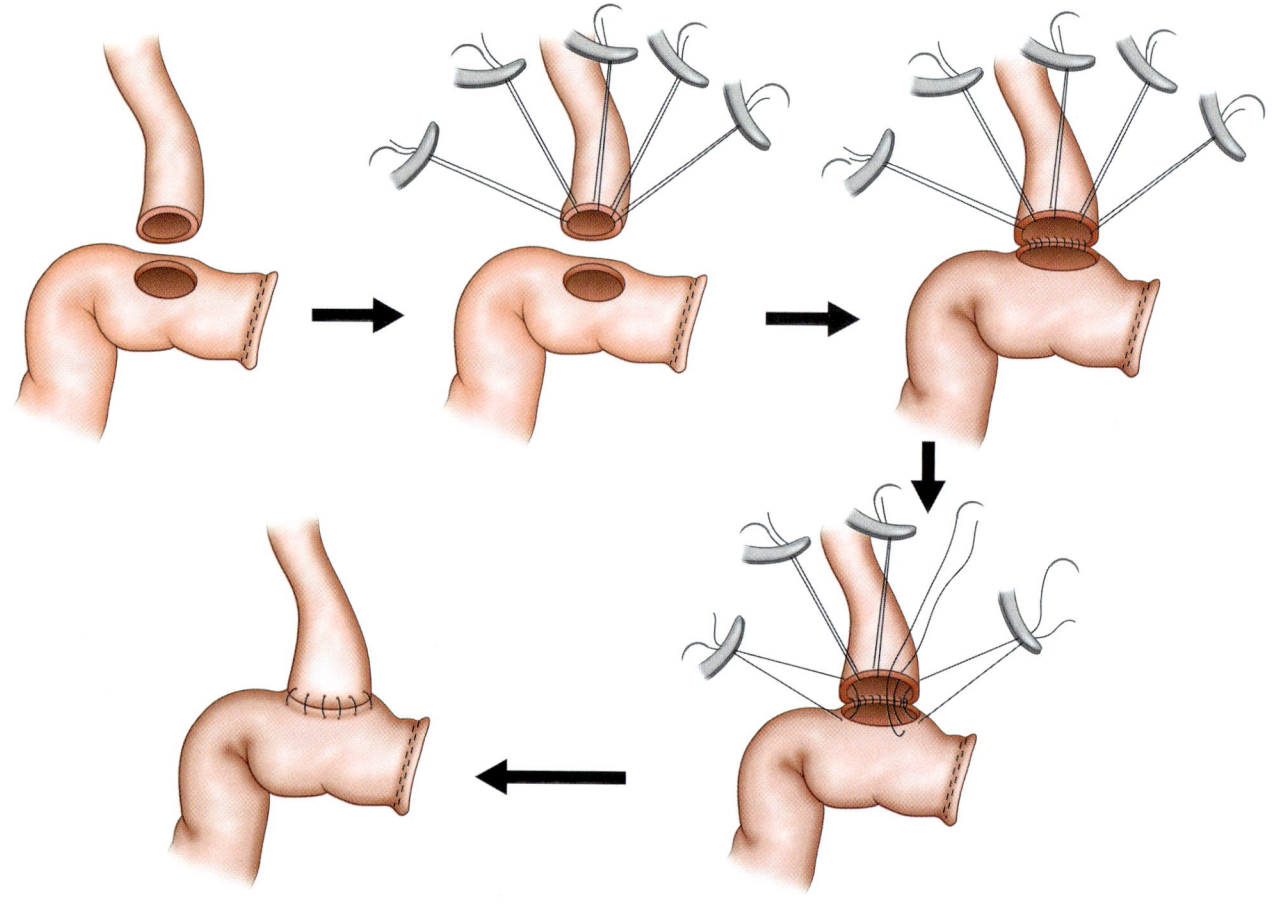

Steps of hepaticojejunostomy

apart. Throughout the anterior wall of both, ensuring that posterior wall anyway is not taken during the suturing of anterior wall.

Now, tying all sutures one by one and the knots of the anterior wall be on the outside. Lastly, cut both the corner sutures and the anastomosis is completed.

Step 6: Jejunojejunostomy: Now, the jejunojejunostomy is fashioned approximately 70 cm distal to the anastomosis. Jejunojejunostomy is made end-to-end or side-to-side either by stapler or hand swen in one layer. Lembert suture may be used.

Step 7: Closure of mesenteric gap: Using 4-0 silk or vicryl, close the mesenteric rent, intermittently and fix the entering jejunum with transverse mesocolon. Hemostasis is achieved completely. Clean the abdomen with normal saline. Place a drain in hepatorenal pouch. Abdomen is closed in layers.

Postoperative Care

- Nasogastric suction for 2 days minimum
- Inj. Pantoprazole 40 mg BD for 5–7 days
- Drain to be kept till the drainage has essentially ceased. Less than 30 ml.

People say, "never expect anything in return from anyone". But, the truth is, when we really love someone, we naturally expect a little care from them.

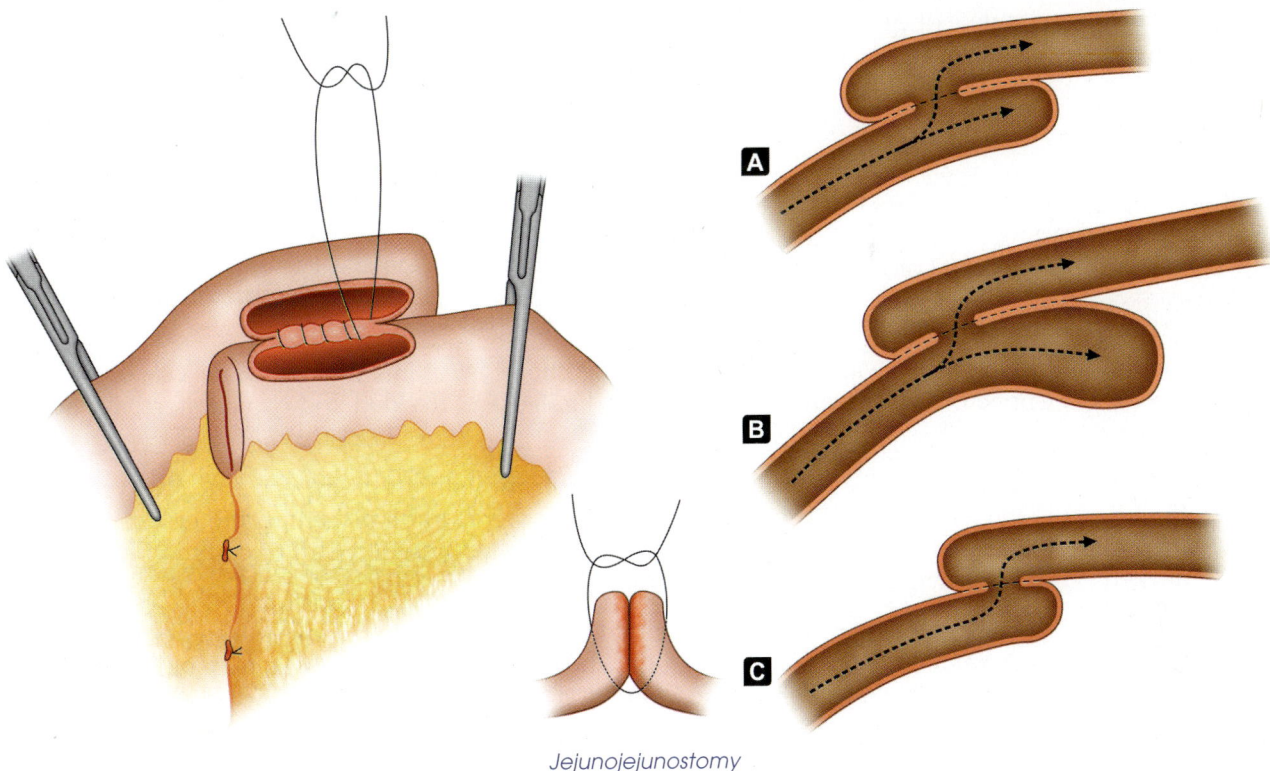

Jejunojejunostomy

Complications

i. *Bile leak:* Occasionally, the bile drainage persists more than 7 days, particularly after Roux-en-Y anastomosis. If it persists, potassium supplement is essential.

ii. *Postoperative duodenal ulcer:* As all the bile diverted into the Roux-en-Y hepaticojejunostomy, there is increased tendency of duodenal ulcer formation. So, continue proton pump inhibitor for a month or 2 months.

iii. Cholangitis: It is rare unless the anastomosis becomes stenotic.

iv. Stenosis of anastomosis: Cholangitis or jaundice may be the sign.
   So, patient is advised for periodic check up of liver function tests to detect the complications early. Transhepatic or endoscopic dilatation may be the relieving treatment modality.

v. Delayed gastric emptying: Following hepaticojejunostomy, with or without gastrojejunostomy, 10–15% patients develop delayed gastric emptying. So, we can use prokinetic drugs, like metoclopramide, itopride, etc.

6.6.4 CHOLEDOCHOLITHOTOMY

Indications

- Presence of palpable stone in CBD
- Endoscopic removal of stone is failed
- Dilated CBD (>10 mm)
- Multiple gallbladder stones

Change hurts and makes people insecure, confused and angry. People want things to be same to make life easier. If you are leader, you cannot let your people hang on to the past.

- History of recent jaundice or presence of jaundice
- Aspiration of lethogenic bile.

Procedures

1. General anesthesia
2. Supine position with a sand bag behind the right hypochondrium and epigastrium
3. Cleaning and draping
4. Incision: Kocher's subcostal or midline incision.

Step 1: Abdomen is opened. Palpate the gallbladder and CBD stone to confirm it.

Step 2: Hold the gallbladder with swab holding/Moynihan's cholecystectomy forceps. Dissect Calot's triangle, peritoneum to be stripped off. Cystic duct and artery are ligated and divided and cholecystectomy done as usual fashion.

Step 3: The bile duct is dissected by lifting the peritoneum from its anterior aspect. It is always better to confirm the bile duct by aspirating bile. Two stay suture, 3-0 vicryl to be placed on the either side of the dissected supraduodenal part of bile duct. Now, incise the elevated anterior wall of common bile duct by holding the stay suture to a length of maximum 1.5 cm.

Step 4: Removal of stone: Use a Desjardin's choledocholithotomy forceps to remove the stones from the bile duct (Choledochoscope may be introduced through the choledochotomy and stones may be retrieved by a Dormia basket catheter through choledochoscope.) Larger stones may be milking toward choledochotomy and remove.

Step 5: Irrigation of bile duct: After removal of stones at the level of satisfaction, irrigate the bile duct with normal saline to flush the small fragments or debris. (It is always better to do intraoperative cholangiogram to confirm the complete clearance of the stones.) If the stone is impacted in the ampulla, a papillotomy and the removal of stone is mandatory.

Step 6: Insert a "T" tube and close the common bile duct with 4-0 PDS/vicryl. Alternatively, a choledochoduodenostomy may be opted. "T" tube cholangiogram may be done to confirm the complete removal of stones. Then, the tube is taken out in the abdominal wall and fix it nicely.

Step 7: Hemostasis is secured: Clean the abdomen with normal saline. Place a drain at hepatorenal pouch. Close the abdomen in layers.

Problems and Management

1. Suppose after cholecystectomy and choledocholithotomy, "T" tube cholangiography shows a residual stone—how to manage it?

Answer: Only prevention of this situation is to do on table "T" tube cholangiogram to detect any residual stone. The numbers of ways to tackle such stones are:
   i. *Flushing:* If stone/stones is/are small, irrigate with normal saline. Otherwise it is better to irrigate with heparinized saline (250 mL NS + 2,500 IU heparin) through "T" tube for 5–7 days.
   ii. After 4–6 weeks when the "T" tube tract is matured, the "T" tube is removed and now the "T" tube tract is dilated under the control of fluoroscopy. With the help of Dormia basket catheter, the stone may be extracted. This technique is called Burrheme technique.
   iii. *Dissolution method:* Cholesterol stone may be dissolved by infusing cholesterol dissolving agents, like methyl tert-butyl ether via "T" tube, may resolve the stone.

The most beautiful thing in this world is to see your loved ones smiling and the next best thing is to know that you are the reason behind that smile.

iv. *Choledochoscopy:* Choledochoscope may be passed through the matured "T" tube and stones may be extracted with direct vision.

v. *Endoscopic method:* Endoscopic sphincterotomy and extraction of stones through a Dormia basket catheter.

vi. *ERCP stone retraction:* Up to 1.5 cm stones can be extracted by ERCP (endoscopic retrograde cholangio-pancreatography). But, the complications, like cholangitis, pancreatitis, bleeding, perforation, are common (5–10%) even mortality is 1–5%.

vii. Extracorporial shock wave lithotripsy (ESWL): A single stone, moderate in size 2 cm, ESWL is applied to remove the stone.

2. Other techniques include to remove these stones:
 i. Laparoscopic choledocholithotomy
 ii. Open choledocholithotomy.

3. Suppose the stone/stones are detected after removal of "T" tube—how to manage?

Answer:

 i. Endoscopic method: Endoscopic sphincterotomy and extraction of stones through a Dormia basket catheter.

 ii. ESWL: If the stone is too large, it may not be suitable and up to 50% cases, endoscopic procedure, stenting, biliary drainage, etc. may be required.

 iii. Percutaneous transhepatic: Pass a cholangioscope first, then Dormia basket catheter is introduced through the cholangioscope, and remove the stones.

 iv. Laparoscopic choledocholithotomy

 v. Open choledocholithotomy is the alternate technique.

6.6.5 RADICAL CHOLECYSTECTOMY

Indication

1. Operable carcinoma gallbladder
2. As a completion surgery for incidental carcinoma GB (when HPE after open/lap chole for presumed gallstone disease shown cancer invading muscularous or deeper).

Pitfalls

1. Hemorrhage during hepatic wedge resection
2. Bile duct injury, bile leak.

Procedure

1. Supine position with a sand bag at the right back to elevate the operating area
2. General anesthesia
3. Incision: Right subcostal extending toward the left subcostal region.

Step 1: Staging: Staging laparoscopy to rule out liver metastasis/peritoneal.

Step 2: Open the abdomen and assess the operability, i.e. exclude liver metastasis, infiltrating to surrounding structures, hepatic ducts, artery, lymphnodes (LNs), ascites or frozen porta.

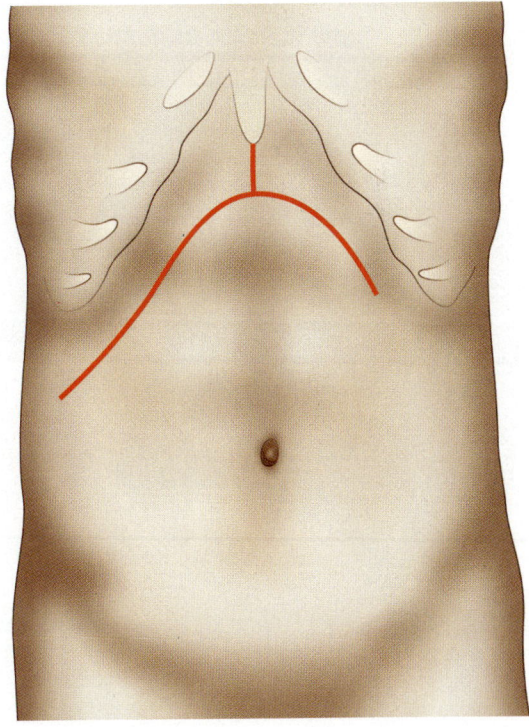

Kocher's right subcostal incision extending to left subcostal region

All our dreams can't be translated into reality, but they can act as a foundation stone for a glorious future.

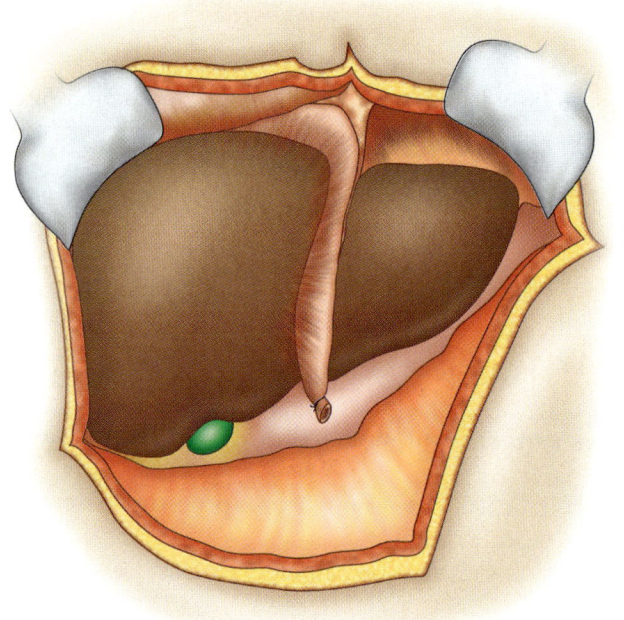

Division of falciform ligament

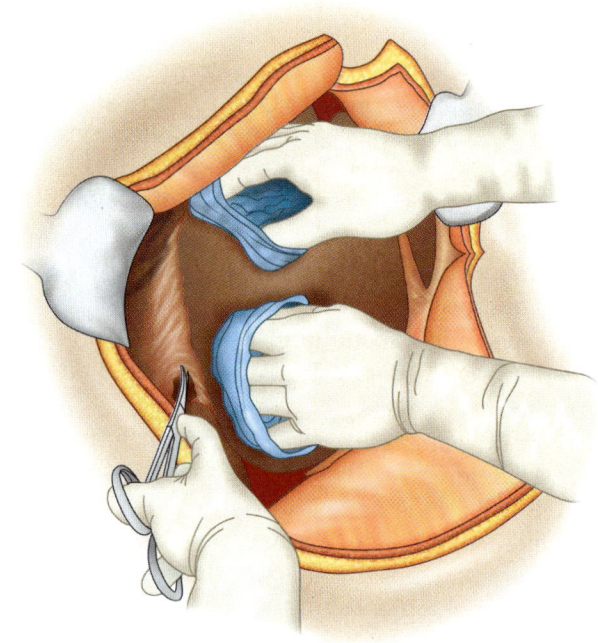

Division of triangular ligament to mobilize liver

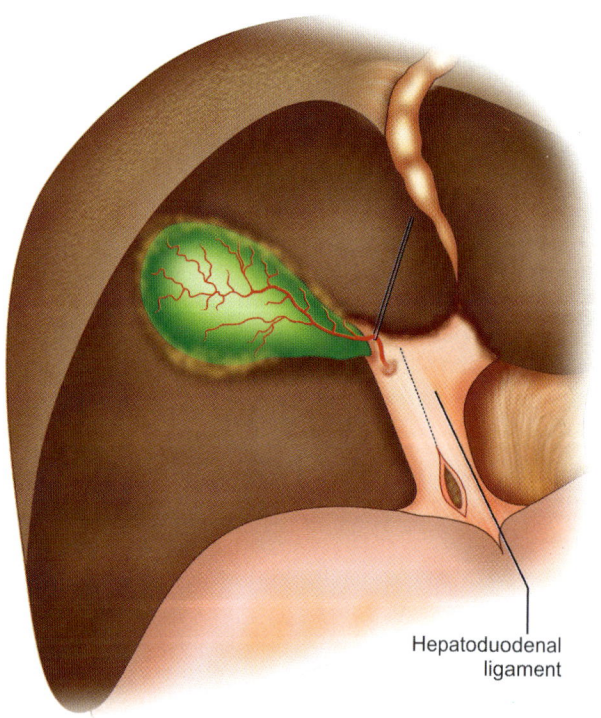

Hepatoduodenal
ligament

Right
hepatic
artery

Common
hepatic
duct

Proper
hepatic
artery

Common
bile duct

Cystic duct   Lymphatic
tissue

Dissection of porta hepatis

Always pray to have eyes that see the best in people, a heart that forgives the worst, a mind that forgets the bad and a soul that never loses faith in God.

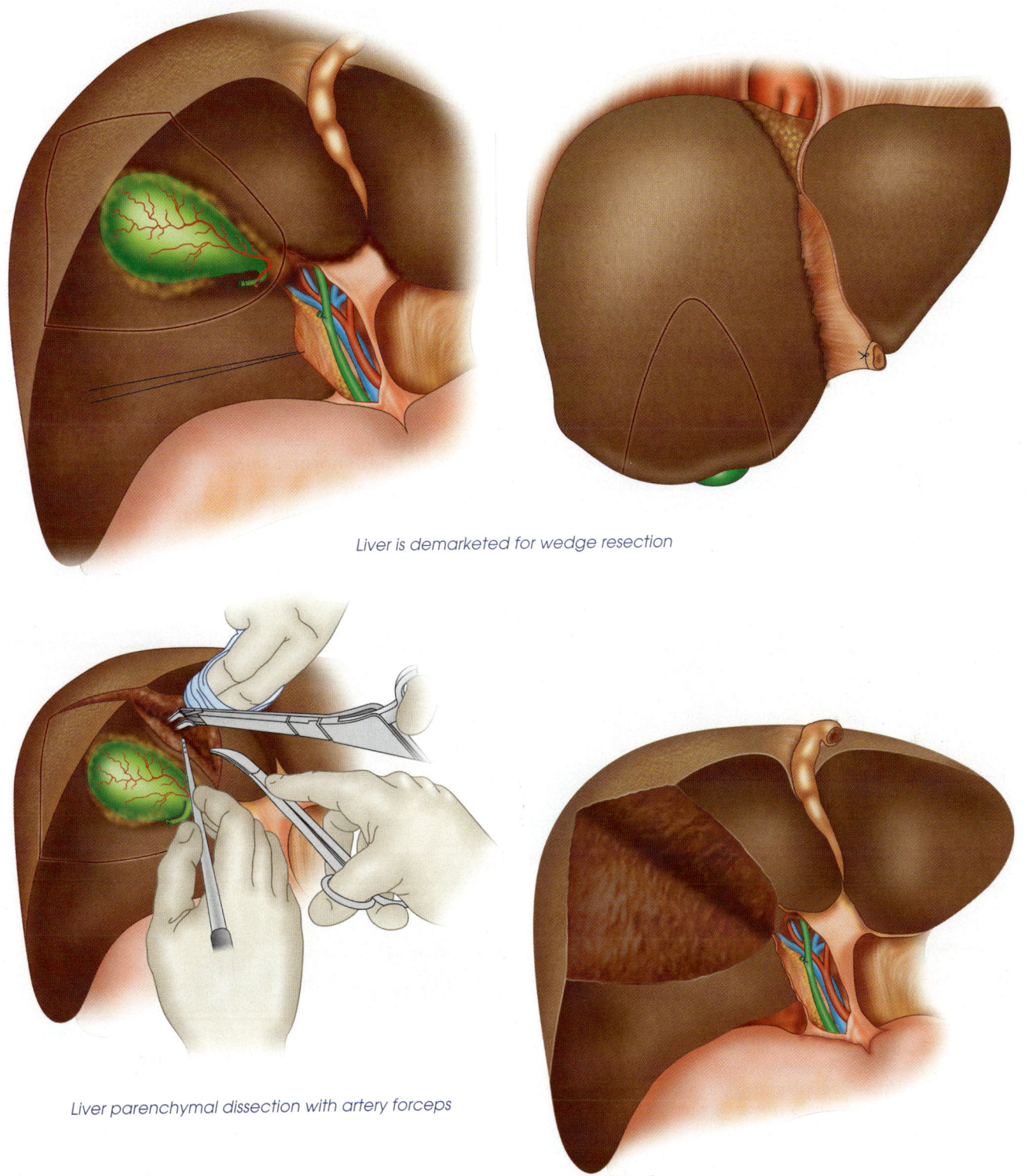

Liver is demarketed for wedge resection

Liver parenchymal dissection with artery forceps

Picture after radical cholecystectomy

I cried when I had no shoes. Suddenly, I stopped crying when I saw a man without leg. Life is full of blessings, sometime we do not understand.

If operable proceed further, divide the falciform ligament. Mobilize the right hepatic lobe by dettaching right triangular ligament, coronary ligament. (Few abdominal swab may be kept behind the liver to bring it further down.)

Step 3: Dissection of porta hepatis, and LNs strip of peritoneum and loose areolar tissue are stripped above downward. All nodal tissues are dissected off the cystic LN, common hepatic artery, bile duct and porta, i.e. station I LNs are to be removed.

Calot's triangle dissected, cystic duct, cystic artery are ligated and divided as close to the bile duct.

• Place feeding tube or vascular tape all around the bile duct and hepatic artery to clear off the duct and artery properly.

• The hepatoduodenal ligament is stripped below upward.

Some surgeons prefer to remove retropancreatic and retroduodenal LNs even retrocholedochal nodes after excising the bile duct (LNs dissection is essentially described by the author as below).

Step 4: Wedge resection of the liver: Define the margin, minimum 2 cm, of resection of the liver. Utilize sharp dissection, cautery clips to resect parenchyma of the liver. In segment IV and V or tissue clysis method, by artery forceps, tie the visible vessels and bile ductules one by one with 3-0 polypropylene.

Hemostasis to be achieved in every step. Few mattress suture may be used to close the defect of the liver.

Step 5: Hemostasis and closure: The operative area to be irrigated with normal saline and sucked it dry. All bleeding points are electrocoagulated. Hepatic area bleeding to be controlled by electrocoagulation or best way to control by argon beam spray coagulation. Place a subhepatic drain and abdomen is closed in usual fashion.

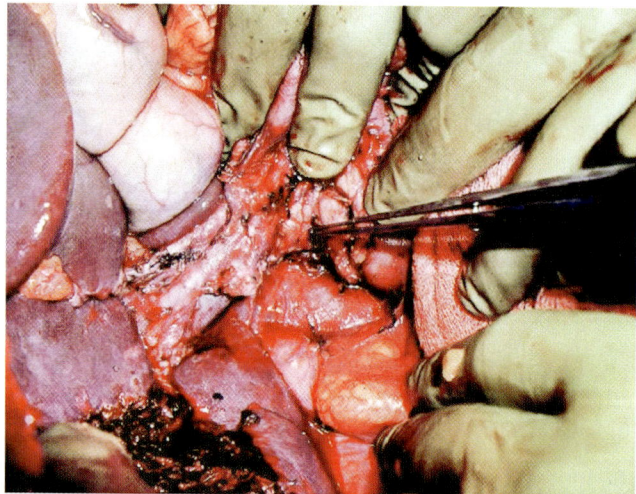

Dissection along the posterior surface of the pancreatic head and the duodenum. Forceps pointing to the exposed pancreatic head; the inferior vena cava can be seen behind. The dissection has proceeded cranially to expose the portal vein from behind (Courtesy: Dr Durgatosh Pandey)

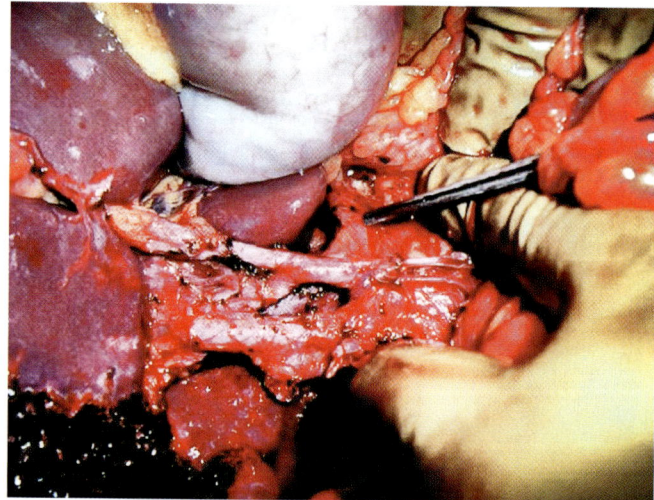

Forceps pointing to the common hepatic artery. The hepatic artery branches have been dissected. The common bile duct (CBD) is also dissected. The right hepatic artery is seen until it goes behind the common bile duct. The dissection in the triangle formed by the hepatic artery, CBD and the superior surface of the pancreas exposes the anterior surface of the portal vein (Courtesy: Dr Durgatosh Pandey)

People are not beautiful as they look, as they walk, as they wear. People are wonderful as they love, as they care and as they share.

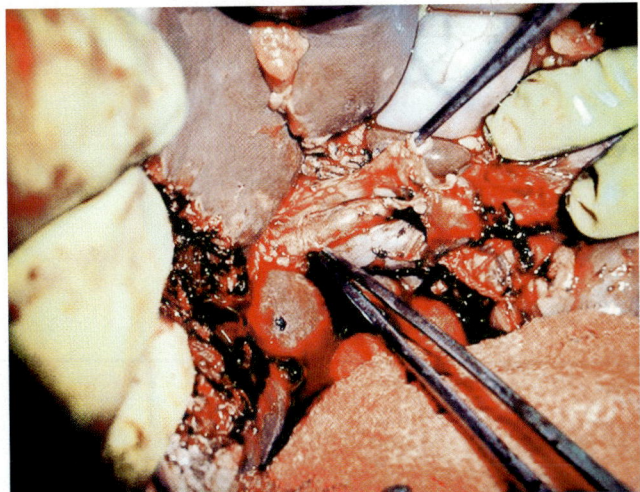

Complications

1. *Early:* Hemorrhage, reactionary biliary leakage
2. *Others:* Chest involvement, ileus, pancreatitis, surgical site infection, etc.
3. *Late:* Biliary stricture, recurrence.

Surgical Technique

Having excluded the presence of distant disease via a laparoscopy followed by a formal laparotomy, the following steps were undertaken.

Kocherization of the duodenum and dissection of the lymphnodes behind the pancreatic head and the duodenum is shown on page 129. The duodenum is kocherized to expose the inferior vena cava and aorta. Any aortocaval node, if enlarged, is sampled. The lymphnode dissection starts by removing the fibro-fatty tissue and nodes behind the head of pancreas and the duodenum and exposing the posterior surface of the pancreatic head. As the dissection proceeds cranially, the portal vein is exposed from behind. This retroportal dissection is continued as cranially as possible toward the hepatic hilum. There is no significant branch of the portal vein posteriorly and this part of the dissection is easily carried out. The superior pancreaticoduodenal vein that drains into the portal vein is usually protected by the uncinate process of the pancreas. In certain situations where this vein terminates into the portal vein at a level above the head of the pancreas, it can be easily identified and preserved. In about 20% of patients, an aberrant or accessory right hepatic artery arises from the superior mesenteric artery and courses along the portal vein. This is carefully identified and preserved, if present. Occasionally, some troublesome bleeding can be encountered while removing the lymphnodes behind the pancreas; this is controlled generally by pressure or cauterization.

Exposure of the common hepatic artery is shown on page 132 (right-sided figure). The gastrohepatic ligament is divided and the hepatoduodenal ligament is encircled to prepare for the pringle maneuver, if necessary. The dissection starts by exposing the superior border of the pancreas and this tissue is swept superiorly. This exposes the common hepatic artery and an LN dissection is performed along this artery and is extended to remove the celiac nodes as well. Small branches of the artery may be encountered and are dealt with either using electrocautery or surgical clips. Extending the dissection toward the liver exposes the gastroduodenal branch which is preserved, and the right gastric artery which is divided to facilitate easy retrieval of the LNs in this region. Division of the right gastric artery also aids the exposure and dissection of the anterior surface of the portal vein that is done as a later step.

Dissect along the hepatic artery branches is shown in below figure. The common hepatic artery is skeletonized and traced toward the liver. In the process, the tissue along the right and left hepatic artery is removed and these branches are skeletonized. The right hepatic artery would generally course posterior to the bile duct and further dissection along this is reserved for the next step. Often, a branch to segment 4 is seen separately; this is dissected and preserved. The left border of the portal vein is also exposed while dissecting the hepatic artery branches. The dissection is continued into the hepatic hilum.

Skeletonization of the common bile duct is shown on page 132 (right-sided figure). The pericholedochal tissue and nodes are dissected from below upward so that the bile duct is exposed. If the gallbladder is

CBD has been retracted anteriorly to dissect the right hepatic artery behind it until the hepatic hilum. Retroportal dissection is also completed

An arrow can be shot only by pulling it backward, so when life is dragging you back with difficulties, it means that it is going to launch you into something great.

intact, the cystic artery is divided flush with the right hepatic artery, and the cystic duct is identified and divided flush with the common bile duct. If a revisional surgery is being performed, the cystic duct stump is identified and resected at its junction with the common bile duct. The dissection proceeds cranially until the hepatic hilum; in the process, bifurcation of the right and left hepatic ducts is often exposed. The right hepatic artery is now dissected from behind the bile duct and this dissection proceeds until the hepatic hilum. If the cystic duct margin is involved grossly or by frozen section, the bile duct is resected and a Roux-en-Y hepaticojejunostomy performed at the end of the surgery.

Dissection of the anterior surface of the portal vein is shown on page 133. Attention is now paid to the triangle formed by the superior border of pancreas below, common bile duct on the right, and hepatic artery-gastroduodenal artery on the left with the artery and duct meeting superiorly at the apex of the triangle. The fibro-fatty tissue and LNs in this triangle are dissected; this exposes the anterior surface of the portal vein. The bile duct is gently retracted to the left and the tissue along the anterior surface of the portal vein is dissected to skeletonize the portal vein until the hepatic hilum. This completes the regional lymphadenectomy for gallbladder cancer.

This is followed by removal of the gallbladder and an appropriate liver resection, tailored to the degree of liver invasion.

Genitourinary

7.1 NEPHRECTOMY

7.1.1 PARTIAL NEPHRECTOMY

Indications

1. Solitary kidney with pathology
2. Pathology in bilateral kidneys
3. Small kidney tumor ≤4 cm
4. Stone in nonduplex kidney/stone is located at one pole of the kidney/stone located in lower most calyx.
5. Traumatic polar rupture of kidney

Procedures

1. General anesthesia
2. Kidney position/supine
3. Incision: Loin (lumbar) incision/midline (transperitoneal) [Two main indications of transperitoneal approach are (1) ruptured kidney and (2) small renal cell carcinoma (RCC) in one pole.]

Step 1: Mobilize the kidney: As described in radical nephrectomy.

Step 2: Cross clamp the vascular pedicle: The renal artery and vein are isolated and taped first. Then apply a soft cross clamp to occlude the renal vessels to reduce blood loss during dissection. The occlusion should not be more than 15 minutes at a time to avoid temporary damage as damage occurs after 15 minutes of warm ischemia.

Remember: Permanent loss of function of the kidney may occur, if the occlusion persists 30 minutes or more. Usually, to increase parenchymal tolerance of ischemia, sterile ice pack is placed around the cross clamped.

Step 3: The capsule of the kidney is incised in the coronal plane and reflected as an anterior and posterior flaps.

Step 4: Now, the parenchyma has been divided as two flaps and all visible parenchymal vessels have to be ligated prior to release of the clamp.

Step 5: Open calyces are closed with a continuous absorbable suture first followed by closure of parenchymal flaps with absorbable suture. The capsular flaps are now folded back over the raw surface and suture it loosely.

Never try to go back and repair the past, that is impossible but be prepared to construct the future which is predictable.

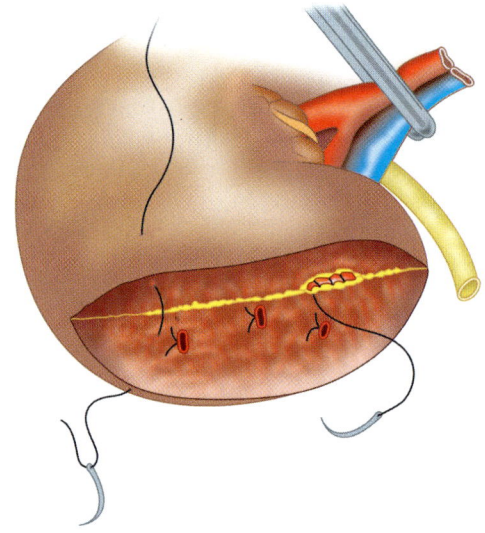

Partial nephrectomy

Step 6: Closure of the abdomen: Hemostasis to be achieved completely. Abdomen is now closed in usual fashion.

7.1.2 RADICAL NEPHRECTOMY

Anatomy of Kidney

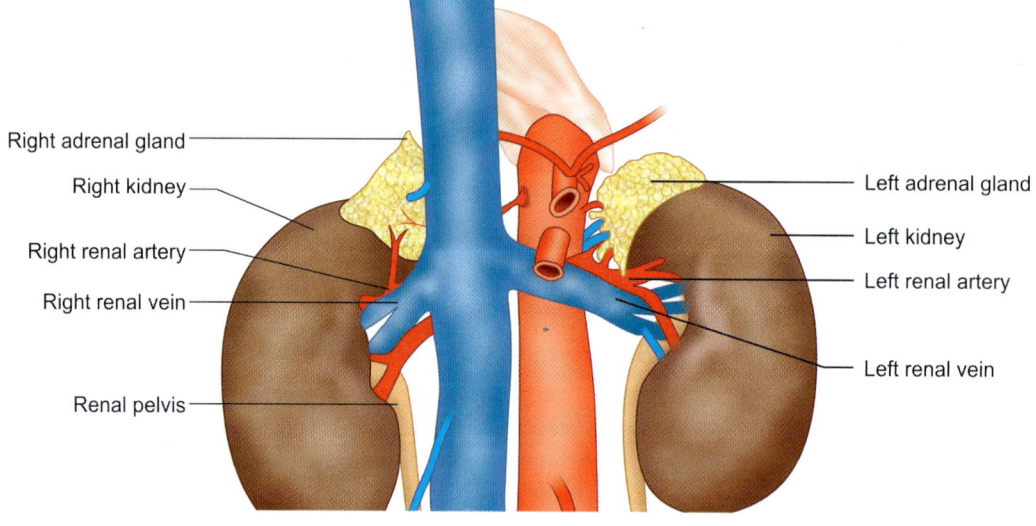

Location and vascular relation of kidney

Indications

Radical Nephrectomy

1. Renal cell carcinoma (RCC), if not suitable for partial nephrectomy (>4 cm tumor)
2. Transitional cell carcinoma (TCC) pelvis or ureter.

Our greatest weakness lies in giving up. The most certain way to succeed is always to try just one more time.

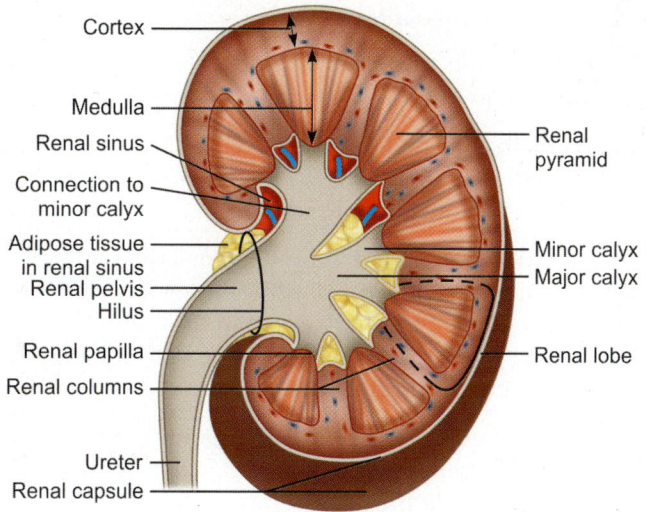

Anatomy of kidney on cross-section

Other Indications for Nephrectomy

1. Ruptured kidney, severe renal injury with avulsion of renal pedicle
2. Renal calculus with gross destruction of kidney
3. Hydronephrosis with non-functioning kidney
4. Chronic pyelonephritis, pyonephrosis
5. Donor nephrectomy for kidney transplant

Procedure for Transperitoneal Radical Nephrectomy

1. General anesthesia
2. Supine position for transperitoneal approach
3. Incision: Conventional midline incision.

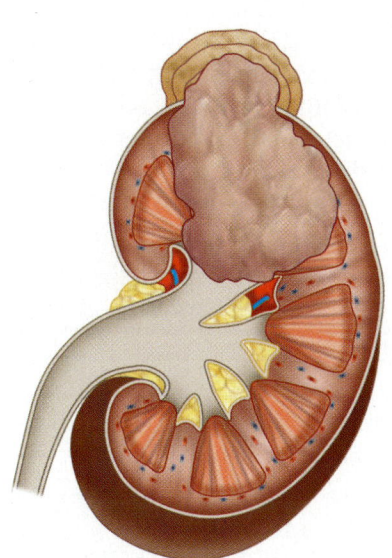

Tumor at upper pole of kidney

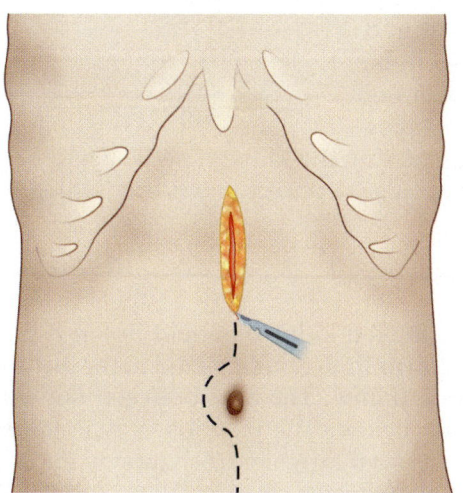

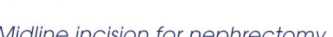

Midline incision for nephrectomy

Love starts from your house, to your neighborhood, to your community, to your nation and to the whole world. Spread love to all those you meet.

Description of Transperitoneal Radical Nephrectomy

Step 1: Abdomen is opened and assess the tumor, liver metastases, distant metastases, ascites, etc. Small bowel is to be packed opposite side or toward pelvis.

Step 2: Peritoneum to be incised on the right side lateral aspect of ascending colon, hepatic flexure and second part of duodenum. On the left side, descending colon, splenic flexure and the transverse colon are mobilized and brought medially to expose the kidney and renal vessels.

Step 3: Mobilization and vascular control of diseased kidney: Plane is just outside the perinephric fat. (Adrenal can be spared. It is not necessary to remove, if it is free of tumor invasion.) Early control of renal vessels before full mobilization of kidney. Look for renal helium. In the renal hilum, the structures from anterior to posterior are vein, artery and pelvis (VAP). Dissect at renal hilum and tape both the vessels. (If you ligate the vein first, the kidney will be enlarged due to intact arterial flow and chance of hemorrhage is more.)

Step 4: Ligation and division of renal vessels: Ligate and divide the artery first. (In case of large right renal tumor, it is better to ligate the artery in between aorta and IVC.) Double ligation or transfixation is advisable for additional security. Now ligate and divide the vein.

Step 5: Mobilization of whole kidney: After vessels control and division, mobilize the kidney all around and detach from all the surrounding structure including adrenal gland. Be careful to keep the fascia gerota intact. Next, the ureter is ligated and divided as lower as possible and kidney with tumor to be removed along with intact fascia of Gerota, lymphnodes, part of ureter with or without adrenal gland.

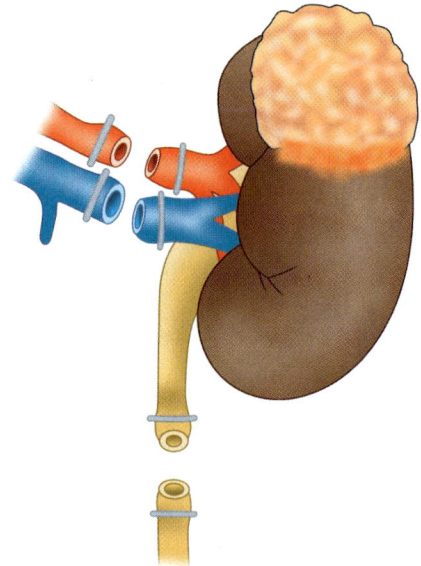

Remember: Where the adrenal gland is required to be removed; it is very important to secure adrenal vessels. It is difficult to secure right adrenal vein as it lies very high in the triangle between IVC and liver and open into IVC.

Step 6: Hemostasis to be achieved completely. Repair the underline muscles, if required. Then, drain is placed at the kidney bed and abdomen is closed in usual fashion.

Note: When the tumor thrombus is inside the renal vein (particularly in right side as it is very short), Satinsky clamp to apply laterally on the IVC where the renal vein enters, is divided and the rent of IVC is sutured with 5-0 prolene. In large tumor, additional feeding vessels also to be ligated and divided. When there is a dense adhesion and pedicle not separated or not well visualized, the assumed pedicle can be clamped en

Tumor at upper pole of the kidney

masse and the kidney to be removed keeping the clamp. After removing the kidney, pedicle will be ligated and transfixed with vicryl. When all planes are obliterated, subcapsular nephrectomy is advisable.

Description of Retroperitoneal Radical Nephrectomy

1. General anesthesia
2. Kidney position for retroperitoneal approach: For approach to the left kidney, patient lies in right lateral position. The upper arm is supported on an arm rest. The right lower limb is kept flexed at the hip and knee to 90° and the left lower limb is kept extended supported on a pillow. The area between the left costal margin and the iliac crest is widened by placing the sand bag below. The position is maintained by a leather strap or a broad band of adhesive strap fixing the iliac crest and the greater trochanter to the operation table. The left shoulder is also anchored to the operation table by adhesive strap.
3. Cleaning and draping.

A knowledgeable person makes you realize how wonderful the world is; but it is only a loving person who makes you realize how wonderful you are in the world.

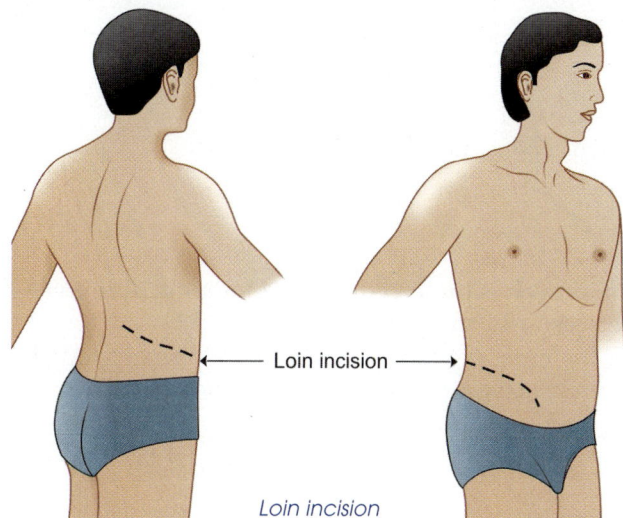

Loin incision →

← Loin incision

Loin incision

Incision

Loin incision: An oblique incision starting just above the renal angle (junction of 12th ribs and lateral border of erector spinae). And the incision is being continued downward and forward toward the anterior superior iliac spine 2 cm below the costal margin and ends 3–5 cm above and anterior to the anterior superior iliac spine (ASIS) to lateral border of rectus sheath.

Step 1: Division of the superficial muscles: The subcutaneous tissue is incised in the same line. Latissimus dorsi posteriorly and anteriorly the external oblique muscles are divided.

Then, the serratus posterior and the internal oblique muscles are incised in the same line.

Step 2: Division of thoracolumbar fascia: With the blunt and sharp dissection, the parietal peritoneum is stripped off from the transversus abdominis muscles. The thoracolumbar fascia is to be divided up to the lateral border of erector spinae muscle and the transversus abdominis muscle is divided.

Step 3: Dissection at perinephric space: The cut margin of thoracolumbar fascia is retracted and the parietal peritoneum is stripped off further medially and the perinephric space is exposed. Now dissect around the fascia of Gerota.

(In case of benign disease, fascia of Gerota is incised and kidney is exposed to mobilize along with the perinephric fat which looks pale yellow in color. But in malignancy, you have to remove the kidney along with fascia of Gerota).

Step 4: Mobilization of the kidney: In case of malignancy incised, the kidney is mobilized all around along with fascia of Gerota, but in benign disease fascia of Gerota incised and the perinephric space reached. With blunt dissection, the kidney is mobilized from the lower pole, posterior surface all around. The accessory vein and artery, mainly observed at the lower pole, are to be ligated and divided. At the upper pole, the kidney is to be separated from adrenal gland by blunt dissection. (Even in case of malignancy, adrenal gland may be spared, if it is not invaded.)

Step 5: Ligation and division of renal vessels: In this approach, renal artery lies posterior to the renal vein. So, it is easier to tackle the artery first. The renal artery is ligated, transfixed and divided. Then, the renal vein is to be doubly ligated and divided. Now, the proximal ureter is identified, dissected, ligated and divided. Now, the kidney is removed.

Step 6: Hemostasis and closure: Complete hemostasis to be achieved. Place a drain in the renal fossa. Abdomen is closed in layers.

Which is the longest word in English? "SMILES" because there is a "MILE" gap between S and S. So, let's keep smiling.

7.1.3 PYELOLITHOTOMY

Indications

i. Stone lies within the pelvis.
ii. Dislodgement of stone from calyces to pelvis.

Procedures

1. General anesthesia
2. Kidney position (Lumbar approach is preferred most of the time as it gives direct access to the kidney but it is a fixed space, in between rib, and iliac crest.
3. Left/right lateral position: The inner leg (knee) is flexed and the hip too. And upper leg will be extended fully. Place pillow in between two legs and the sand bag below the loin with a wide strapping to prevent the patient from rolling over.
4. The right upper limb is supported on an arm rest and left upper limb is kept forward, so that the patient's weight should not be over it.
5. Incision: An oblique incision starting just above the renal angle (junction of 12th rib and lateral border of erector spinae).

And the incision is being continued downward and forward toward the anterior superior iliac spine 2 cm below the costal margin and ends 3–5 cm above and anterior to the ASIS to lateral border of rectus sheath. Expose the kidney layer by layer.

Step 1: Divide the superficial fascia: The skin, and subcutaneous tissue are incised. The lower fibers of latissimus dorsi are incised along the line of incision. When the incision is extended forward it cuts external oblique, and its aponeurosis. On deepening the incision at its highest part incising serratus posterior inferior, quadratus lumborum with lumbar, fascia is exposed. At the anterior part of the incision, the internal oblique is incised at the same line.

Step 2: Divide thoracolumbar fascia: Thoracolumbar fascia is incised, taking care the subcostal nerve. The incision is extended backward up to the erector spinae. Now, the parietal peritoneum is stripped off from the transversus abdominis muscle and thetransversus abdominis muscle is divided.

Step 3: Expose the perinephric space: On retracting the lumbar fascia, the peritoneum is further stripped off medially, and the perinephric space is exposed.

Step 4: Incise fascia of Gerota and expose the kidney: At the lateral aspect, incise the fascia and extend it to expose the perirenal fat deep to which the kidney lies.

Step 5: Mobilize the kidney: Now, the kidney is mobilized all around by sharp and blunt dissection. The lower pole, anterior surface and posterior surface are well exposed.

Step 6: Dissection of pelvis of the kidney: The posterior surface of the pelvis is dissected from the surrounding fat. The kidney is held by left hand such a way that the tips of index finger and middle finger lie beneath the pelvis and thereby thumb above it which can prevent the slippage of stone.

Step 7: Open the renal pelvis: Make a semilunar incision over the stone in the extrarenal pelvis and remove the stone/stones from the pelvis or from accessible calyx. In case of intrarenal pelvis, a plane to be developed between the intrarenal pelvis and the overlying parenchyma, retract both the sides and remove the stone, ensuring that no fragments are left behind. (The term extended pyelolithotomy is used when the incision is extended into the neck of the calyces to remove Staghorn calculus.)

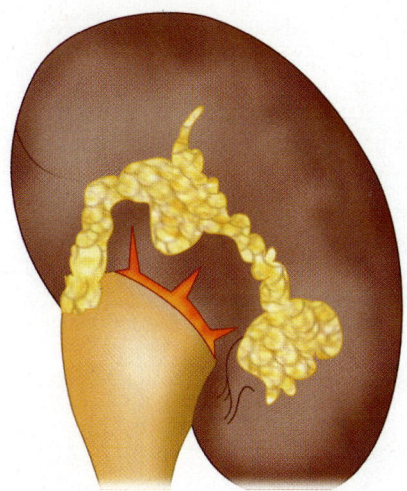

The semilunar incision to open the pelvis

Step 8: Close the incision: The incision is closed with vicryl 3-0 (absorbable sutures) and a ureteric stent is left in situ for 4–6 weeks. Hemostasis to be achieved in every step. The abdomen is closed with or without a drain.

Remember: Open pyelolithotomy is rarely done today. Lithotripsy or percutaneous pyelolithotomy is the procedure of choice.

7.1.4 PYELOPLASTY

Indications

i. Idiopathic congenital pelviureteric junction (PUJ) obstruction causing hydronephrosis.
ii. Hydronephrosis due to PUJ obstruction where adequate renal function is preserved and reasonable thickness of functioning parenchyma is intact.

Procedure

1. General anesthesia
2. Kidney position
3. Cleaning and draping
4. Lumbar/loin incision as described above.

Step 1: Exposure of kidney: As above.

Step 2: Dissection at pelvis and pelviureteric junction: Renal pelvis and upper part of ureter are dissected and mobilized. The excess renal pelvic tissue and pelviureteric junction is excised.

Step 3: Pelviureteric anastomosis: Now spatulate the ureter and pelvis as shown in the photograph. Insert a double "J" stent and ureter is anastomosed with pelvis, using 3-0 polyglactin suture. For better drainage, well-dependent pelviureteric junction is to be made.

Step 4: Closure of the wound: Hemostasis to be achieved completely.
- Wound is closed as above.
- Abdomen is closed in an usual fashion. (Endoscopic balloon dilatation of narrowed pelviureteric junction is called pyelolysis is gaining popularity day by day though the results are not convincing till date.)

You have not lived today until you have done something for someone who can never repay you.

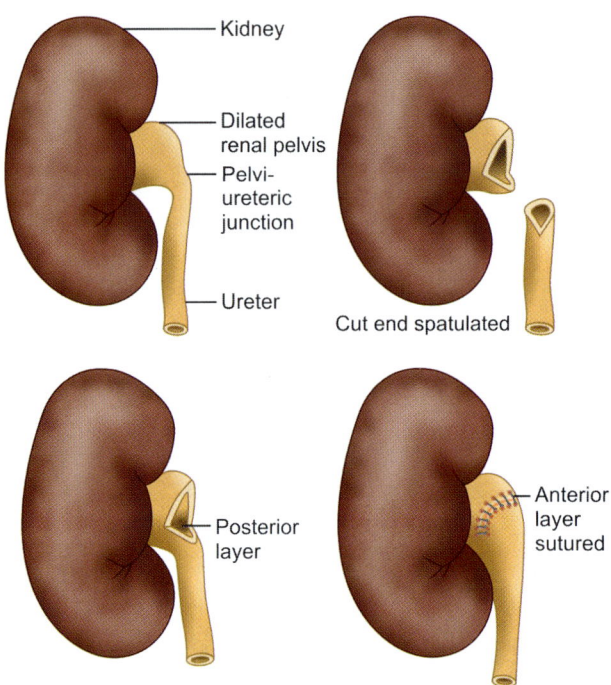

Anderson-Hynes pyeloplasty

7.1.5 ILIOINGUINAL BLOCK DISSECTION (IIBD)

Indications

Metastatic inguinal lymphnodes in:
1. Both male and female genitalial and anorectal cancers
2. Skin cancers below umbilicus, i.e. lower abdomen, perineal and groin and both lower limbs, like skin adnexal tumor, squamous cell carcinoma (SCC), melanoma, etc.
3. Lower extremity soft tissue sarcomas with involvement of inguinal nodes (rare)

Important Points to be Noted

1. High chance of skin flap necrosis (up to 62% worldwide)
2. Injury to femoral vessels and nerve
3. Subcuticular lymph collection
4. Late lymphatic edema.

Preoperative Special Care

1. Arrange elastic stocking for the patient
2. From toes to upper thigh, evaluate the extent of disease, i.e. involvement of femoral vessels particularly femoral vein. Be ready for vascular reconstruction, if required.
3. Be ready for flap reconstruction with tensor fascia lata, flap (preferred by most of the surgeons) or transverse rectus abdominis myocutaneous (TRAM) flap.

Do not give way, hold tight. It is when everything seems lost that all is saved.

Surgical Anatomy

Boundary of inguinal lymphnode dissection: Inguinal node is located in the femoral triangle based on inguinal ligament. So, the boundary of femoral triangle is above by inguinal ligament, laterally by medial border of sartorius, medially by lateral border of adductor longus and below the apex of the triangle is formed by the crossing of adductor longus and the sartorius muscles. The boundary of pelvic dissection is:

1. Above, by the apex of the triangular area formed by the bifurcation of the common iliac artery
2. Laterally, the genital branch of genitofemoral nerve
3. Medially, the bladder wall
4. Posteriorly, obturator nerve
5. Below, the fascia covering the obturator internus and levator ani.

Inguinal Lymphnodes

There are two sets of inguinal nodes on each side. The superficial nodes below inguinal ligament form a horizontal group and the deep inguinal nodes along the upper 7 cm of great saphenous vein form the vertical group. The deep inguinal nodes form a chain along the upper part of femoral vein and in the femoral canal. Superficial nodes drain the superficial part of lower abdominal wall, perineum and lower limb. The deep nodes (usually 3, 4 nodes) drain deeper tissues of both lower abdomen and lower limb. Both superficial and deep nodes drain into external iliac group of nodes.

Operative Procedure

1. Position—lower limb to be kept in mildly abducted, flexed as well as externally rotated.
2. Incision—may be
   • Oblique incision
   • Curved (lazys) incision
   • Vertical incision.

Note: Although the exposure is more in vertical incision but skin flap necrosis is very common (7.5–65%). In lazys incision, exposure is better and skin necrosis is relatively less in comparison to vertical incision. In oblique incision, chance of necrosis is lowest but exposure is little difficult.

Remember: It is not truly required to dissect skin flaps beyond the confines of the femoral triangle as it has no therapeutic value and it may impair blood supply to the skin.

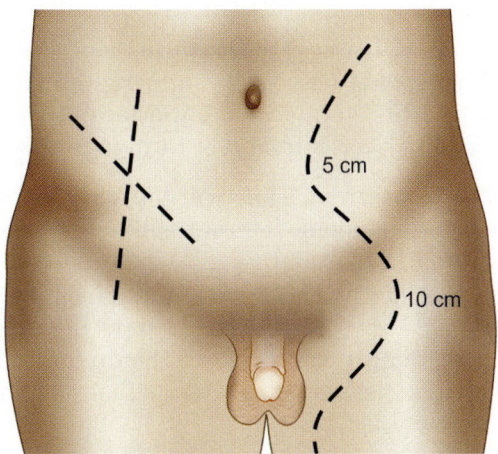

Different conventional incisions for groin dissection

Step 1: *Raise the skin flaps:* Skin flap in raised in between fascia of Camper (fatty layer) and fascia of Scarpa that leaves 4.5 mm of subcutaneous fat on the skin 5 cm cephalad above the inguinal crease and 6–8 cm caudal is the limit for raising the skin flap. Take stays suture on the flap to avoid shearing effect.

Step 2: *Femoral triangle dissection:* The upper limit of this dissection is 5 cm above the inguinal ligament where a transverse incision is made through the fat to expose the external oblique aponeurosis. Then all tissues, fatty fascia and nodes, are stripped off the aponeurosis down to the level of the inguinal ligament. All efforts made to secure the superficial vessels crossing the field. In walls, spermatic cord to be identified and preserved carefully. Expose the medial border of sartorius muscle and lateral border of adductor longus. Continue the dissection removing all fatty tissue lymphnodes, and fascia, in between two muscles and from lateral to medial direction and then toward the apex of femoral triangle. At the apex, great saphenous vein to identify and then ligate and divide at its junction with femoral vein. (Some surgeons preserve the vein to reduce the lymph edema of lower limb.)

Step 3: *Dissection of femoral artery, vein and nerve:*
It is easier to identify the femoral artery and vein near the apex of femoral triangle. Elevate the areolar tissue and fat from anterior surface of femoral vessels proceeding toward inguinal ligament. Now dissect the specimen from the medial border of the femoral triangle toward the lateral border and expose the medial aspect of femoral vein. (Medial aspect of the vein is usually struck to enlarged nodes. So, careful dissection is required to separate the vein. If it is not possible to take the segment of vein, plan for reconstruction. The segment loss is less than 2 cm, end to end anastomosis is possible, otherwise vein graft repair is essential). Remember, there are no branches on the medial aspect of the vein. Now, pectineus muscle, and femoral canal are exposed. Remove all lymphnodes of this canal as well as the

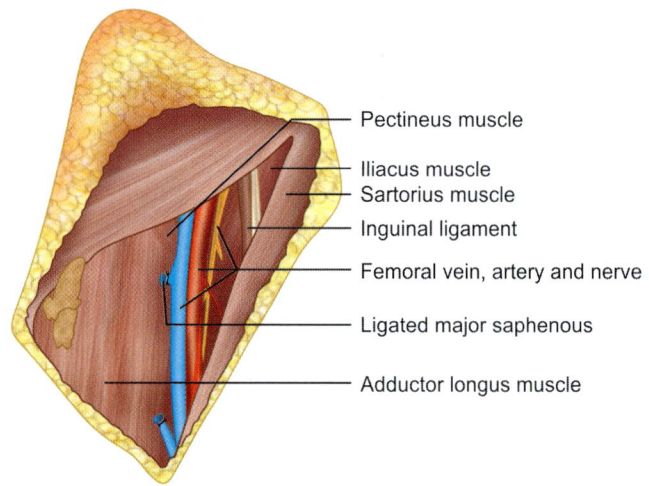

- Pectineus muscle
- Iliacus muscle
- Sartorius muscle
- Inguinal ligament
- Femoral vein, artery and nerve
- Ligated major saphenous
- Adductor longus muscle

After dissection of inguinal region

triangle. Bare the whole length of femoral vein and artery in the triangle. Small branches going to the specimen are to be ligated and divided. Femoral vein lies lateral to femoral artery covered with thin femoral sheath. Expose the nerve by incising the sheath just below inguinal ligament and preserve all branches of femoral nerve. Now, detach the specimen. Irrigate operative field and achieve complete hemostasis.

Step 4: *Transposition of sartorius muscle:* Transect the sartorius muscle at its insertion and separate proximal 6–7 cm of the muscle and cover the femoral vessels by suturing the cut end of the muscle to the inguinal ligament with 20 absorbable sutures. This step is very important to protect femoral vessels from the consequences of a possible necrosis which is very common to form in inguinal dissection.

Step 5: *Pelvic lymphnode dissection:* Make an incision over the external oblique aponeurosis in the direction of its fibers, 3–4 cm above the inguinal ligament. Internal oblique muscle to be divided then incision to be carried through the transversalis muscle and underlying fascia not through peritoneum.

Deep inferior epigastric vessels identified just above the inguinal ligament arising from external iliac artery and vein, are to be ligated and divided. Now, use the gauge dissection to sweep the peritoneum in cephalad direction and hold it with a retractor. Identify and preserve the ureter which usually remains adhered to the peritoneal layer. The area to be dissected between the external iliac and the internal iliac vessels down to the obturator fascia overlying obturator foramen.

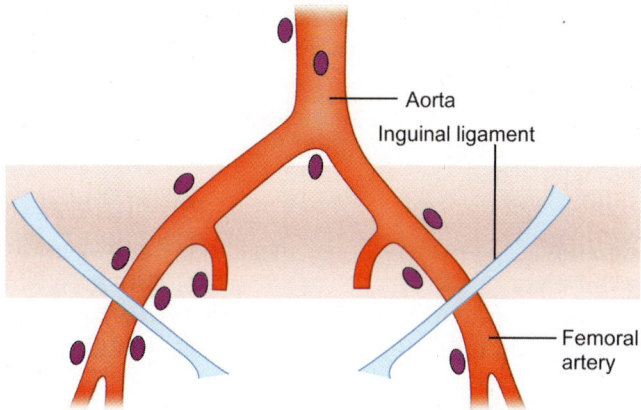

Location of pelvic lymphnodes

First dissect the fat and lymphnode overlying the external iliac artery and vein beginning at the level of inguinal ligament and proceed in a cephalad direction to the junction with the internal iliac vessels.

Remember: Iliac vein is very fragile. Small laceration of the vein may produce considerable bleeding and that is difficult to control. So be careful dissecting over and around the iliac vein.

Now, sweep the fat and lymphatic from the apex of the triangle, i.e. the bifurcation of common iliac artery in a downward direction. Identify and preserve the obturator artery and vein and nerve. Dissect all fatty tissue and lymphnodes off the obturator vessels and nerve posteriorly and remove the specimen. Hemostasis to be achieved in every step of dissection and the end meticulously. Close the incision of lower abdomen in layers with 2-0 nonabsorbale suture. Fascia transversalis, overlying aponeurosis, to be closed. Next close the defect in femoral canal by suturing the inguinal ligament down to Cooper's ligament or the pectineal fascia from below.

Usually, drain is not required in the pelvis.

Step 6: Transposition of sartorius muscle: Transect the sartorius muscle at its insertion. Free the proximal 5–7 cm from the attachments and transpose it over the femoral vessels. Suture the cut end to the inguinal ligament using interrupted 3-0 vicryl.

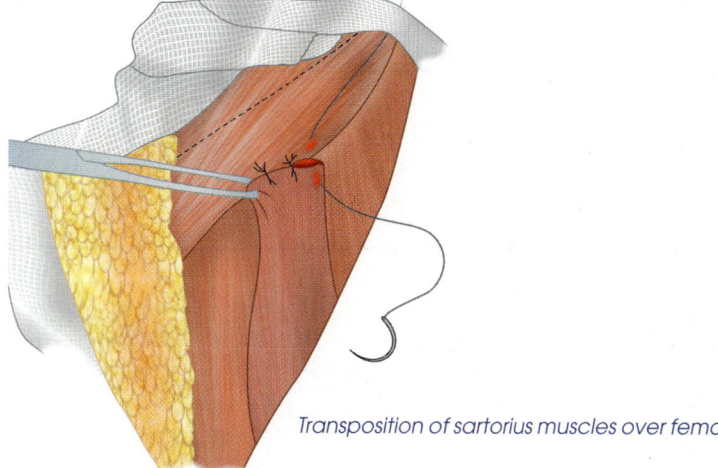

Transposition of sartorius muscles over femoral vessels

Truth and trust are two pillars of strong relationship. If you do not trust a person, you won't say truth and if you do not say truth, the person won't trust you.

Step 7: Drainage and closure: Close suction drain to be placed at the femoral triangle above the sartorius muscle after irrigation of the operative field. Trim away the part of skin flap that seems to be devitalized to close the skin with 3-0 nylon.

Author has designed his own technique by the name, Ray's "river flow" Incisional Technique. With his technique, he has done around 65 cases of ilioinguinal block dissection (IIBD) but there is no single flap necrosis. The technique is described as below.

1. *Ray's "river flow" incision (two parallel curvilinear incisions—inguinal and iliac)*

    Inguinal incision: Approximately, 5–7 cm curvilinear incision is made 4 cm below and parallel to inguinal ligament.

    Iliac incision: Approximately, 5–7 cm curvilinear incision is made 4 cm above and parallel to inguinal ligament. The curves of each incision indicate medial and lateral limits of both the dissections.

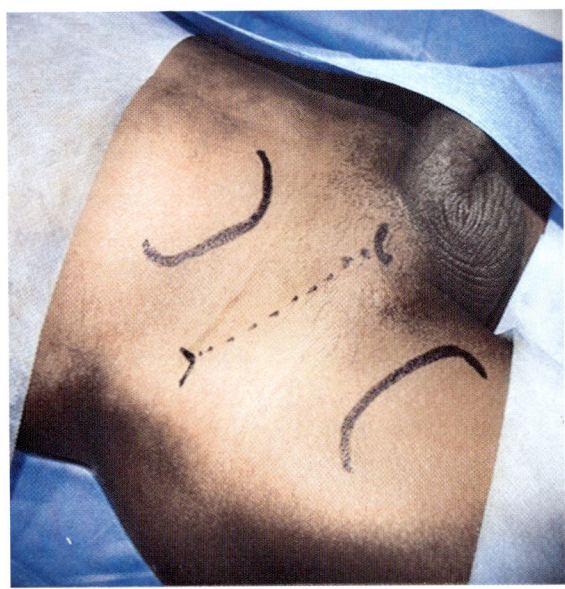

Ray's river flow incision (two parallel curvilinear incisions)

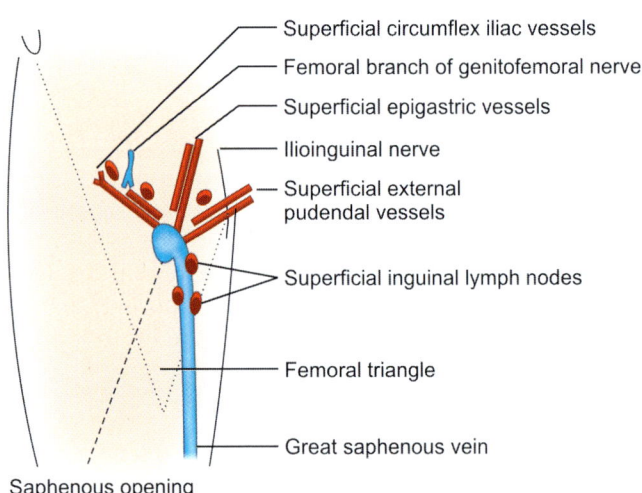

- Superficial circumflex iliac vessels
- Femoral branch of genitofemoral nerve
- Superficial epigastric vessels
- Ilioinguinal nerve
- Superficial external pudendal vessels
- Superficial inguinal lymph nodes
- Femoral triangle
- Great saphenous vein

Saphenous opening

Anatomical consideration of blood supply in the groin

2. *Flap is raised just below the fascia of Scarpa*

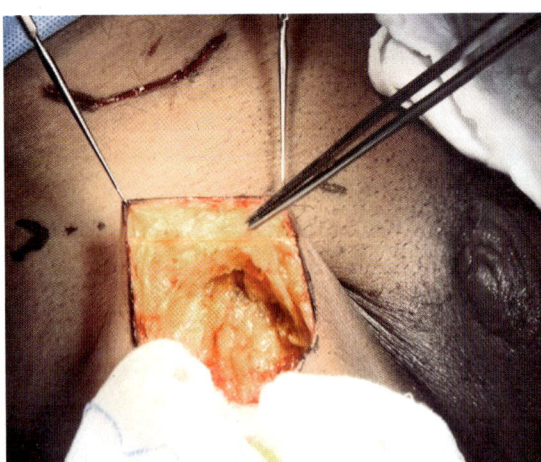

Raise the flap just below the membranous layer (fascia of Scarpa)

Higher, always higher! Let us never be satisfied with what is accomplished.

3. *The boundary of inguinal dissection*
   - Upper limit: 3 cm above the inguinal ligament, i.e. external oblique aponeurosis and spermatic cord.
   - The lateral limit of dissection is kept up to the medial border of sartorius, not beyond.
   - The medial limit is kept up to the lateral border of adductor longus, not beyond.
   - Lower limit: Apex of the femoral triangle.

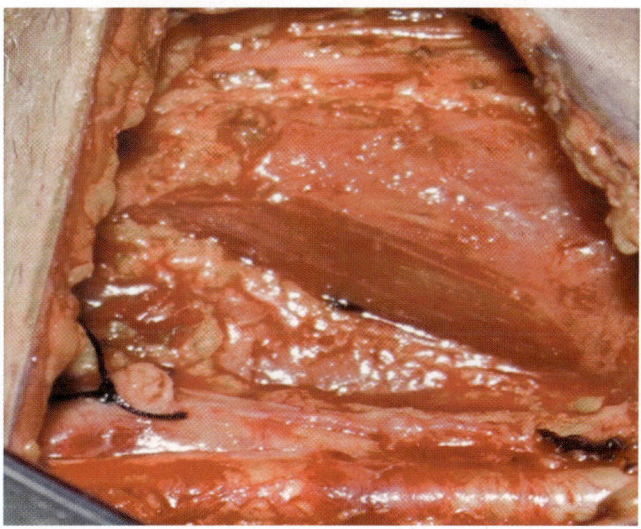

Boundary of inguinal dissection

4. *Technique of iliac dissection:* The external oblique muscle is divided along the skin incision. The internal oblique and transversus abdominis muscles are split along the muscle fibers. Then, we enter into the retroperitoneal space. Lymphnode dissection in the iliac territories is performed with standard technique.
5. *Boundary of standard iliac dissection*
   - Above: Up to common iliac bifurcation
   - Below: Pelvic diaphragm, i.e. up to levator ani and obturator internus muscles

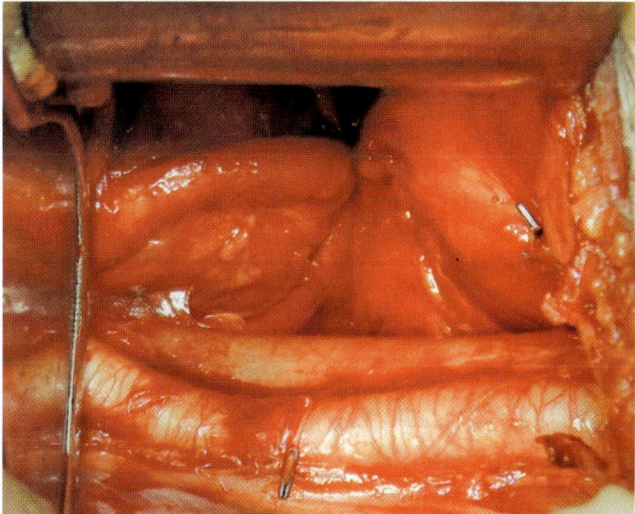

Picture after iliac dissection

There is great beauty in simplicity.

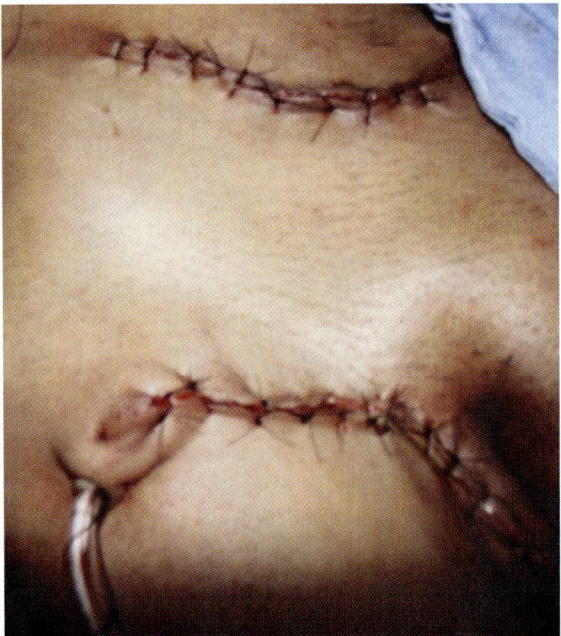

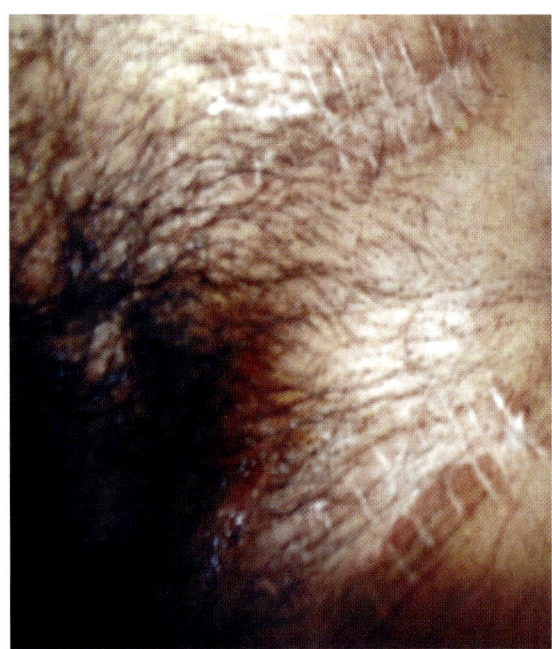

Picture just after closure of the river flow incision   *On follow-up, the picture of wound healing*

- Laterally: Genital branch of genitofemoral nerve
- Medially: Up to bladder wall and obturator nerve posteriorly

The advantages of the incision are:

i. Medially, it spare fossa ovalis owing to its curve, thereby sparing the emerging part of the superficial vessels, namely superficial circumflex iliac, superficial epigastric and superficial external pudendal, supplying the superficial fascia of the thigh.

ii. Both the curves define the lateral and medial limits of the boundary. One should not dissect beyond these limits.

iii. Due to these curves, surgeons can go down easily up to the apex of femoral triangle which is the lower limit of the dissection, without much more stretching by the retractor.

We raise the flap just below the membranous layer of the superficial fascia and did the stand inguinal dissection, i.e. medially up to the lateral border of adductor longus, laterally the medial border of the sartorius, superiorly 3 cm above the inguinal ligament, i.e. the external oblique aponeurosis and spermatic cord/round ligament and inferiorly the apex of the femoral triangle.

Postoperative Advice

Apart from routine fluids, antibiotics, etc., following points to be noted:

1. Apply elastic stocking to fit the operated lower limb from the proximal part of toes to the upper thigh
2. Keep the patient at bedrest and elevate the limb for 3 days. There after patient is permitted to walk and short time sitting in a chair
3. Ask the patient to move the limb while lying on the bed
4. Drain to be removed when the volume is 40 mL or less
5. Elastic stocking to be worn for latest 6 months
6. Ask the patient to elevate the limb thrice a day for 1 hour each time for 2 months (6–8 weeks) to prevent permanent lymph edema of the limb.

At the hour of danger, a perfect quietness is required.

7.1.6 HIGH INGUINAL ORCHIDECTOMY

Indication

Carcinoma testis.

Procedure

1. Spinal anesthesia
2. Supine position
3. Cleaning and draping
4. *Incision:* An inguinal incision is made 2 cm above and parallel to the medial two-thirds of inguinal ligament.

Step 1: The skin, and superficial fascia are incised in the line of incision. One or more superficial epigastric veins cross the line are to be cauterized or ligate.

Step 2: External oblique aponeurosis identified, the fascia covering it (Gallaudet's fascia) to be incised along with the aponeurosis in the direction of its fibers. Preserve ilioinguinal nerve.

Step 3: Take the cord out by putting two index fingers at the level of pubic tubercle from both sides. Now, encircle the cord and its posterior mesentery containing genitofemoral nerve with a tape. Dissect the cord adequately to encircle all around.

Step 4: Division of spermatic cord: Apply a non-crushing clamp across the cord at the deep ring. Transfix it with 2-0 vicryl or 2-0 prolene and keep 3–4 cm long nonabsorbable suture (for future identification of the stump during pelvic lymphnodes, dissection, if indicated) and divide the cord and the proximal stump with long nonabsorbable suture is to put inside the abdominal cavity.

Step 5: Mobilization of the testis: The diseased testis is then mobilized all around through the superficial inguinal ring and delivered through it and remove the whole specimen.

Remember: When the preoperative diagnosis is doubtful, i.e. the tumor markers are marginally elevated and ultrasonography (USG) suggestive of malignancy the procedure should be like this. Soft clamp is placed across the cord at the level deep ring do not transfix, and divide it, before this you deliver the testis, inspect and palpate it. If any doubt of malignancy do an open biopsy (Chevassu's maneuver) and send for frozen section. If it confirms malignancy, follow the above steps of high inguinal orchidectomy otherwise remove the clamp, reconstitute the testis, place the testis into the scrotum and fix it at least three points (orchiopexy) of the tunica albuginea to the tunica vaginalis with 3-0/4-0 prolene suture.

Step 6: Hemostasis to be achieved completely. Place a suction drain to prevent scrotal hematoma. External oblique is closed with 2-0 vicryl and skin is closed in usual fashion.

7.1.7 RETROPERITONEAL LYMPHNODE DISSECTION (RPLND)

Surgical Anatomy

Roberts reported first RPLND in 1902 through transperitoneal approach. But, the patient died because of peritonitis.

Indications

A. Primary (Upfront RPLND)

Seminoma: Primarily treated with chemotherapy (CT)/radiotherapy (RT). Upfront RPLND is not indicated.

Live within; be not shaken by outward happenings.

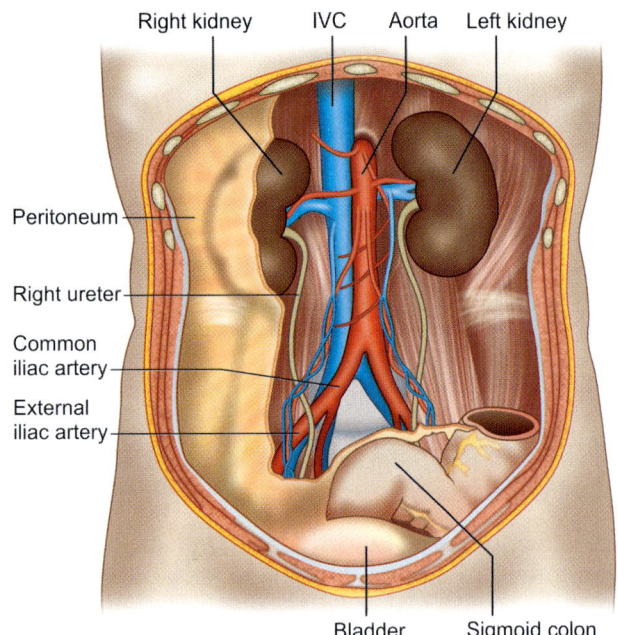

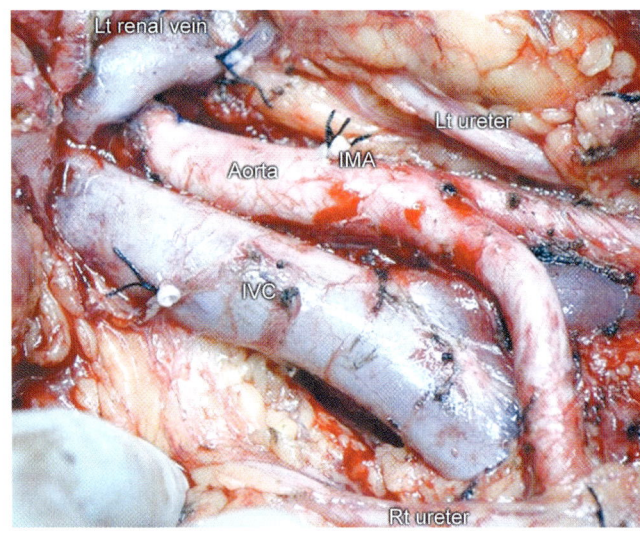

Surgical anatomy of RPLND (Courtesy: Dr Durgatosh Pandey)

Remember: In seminoma stage II disease (low tumor load), if the retroperitoneal node is less than 5 cm, RT is the treatment of choice. But in high tumor load stage II and stage III, patients with bulky retroperitoneal nodes (lymphnode size more than 5 cm) chemotherapy is the treatment of choice.

Nonseminomatous germ cell tumor (NSGCT)
- Stage I (tumor limited to testis) NSGCT - 30% cases, pathological involvement of peritoneal lymphnodes is obvious. RPLND is curative in this category but in many institutions CT is the preferred treatment option.
- Stage II (low tumor barden) where the retroperitoneal nodes are less than 3 cm. The options are RPLND followed by CT followed by RPLND, if required. (Stage III and high tumor load stage II where the RPLNs are more than 3 cm, CT is the treatment of choice.)

B. Secondary (Post-CT/RT) RPLND

1. *Seminoma:* Post-CT more than 3 cm residual retroperitoneal mass mandates RPLND.
2. *NSGCT:* Post-CT, residual retroperitoneal mass just larger than 1 cm at the site of disease is considered malignant component and bilateral RPLND is recommended.

C. Basic Concept of RPLND

Template RPLND is recommended only for upfront surgery. Post-CT, RPLND should be completed, no template dissection is mandatory. Classical RPLND: Bilateral classical RPLND comprising of removal of all lymphnodes along with lymphatic tissues from the boundary as follow.

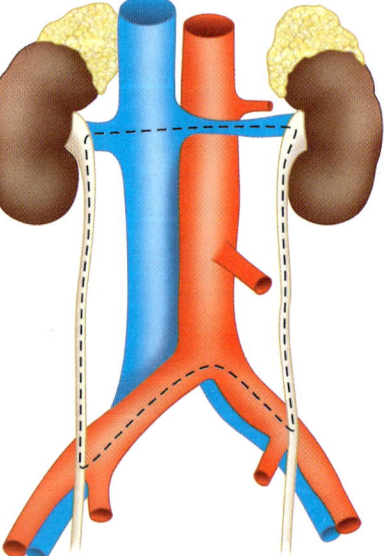

Standard boundary of RPLND

- Above the renal vessels both the sides
- Laterally ureter in each sides
- Below up to the level where ureter crossing the iliac vessels both the sides.

So the nodes are removed, namely, precaval, paracaval, retrocaval, intraortocaval, preaortic, para-aortic and both common iliac group of nodes.

D. Nerve Sparing RPLND

For left-sided testicular tumor: The dissection is usually limited to the ipsilateral retroperitoneal lymphnodes as we know very rarely the left-sided primary spreads to the contralateral side, i.e. to the right retroperitoneal nodes.

So, the boundary of the dissection is like the left-sided classical RPLND as above as the right-sided sympathetic nerve chain will be intact to preserve fertility.

In case of right-sided testicular tumor, bilateral RPLND is recommended as more than 50% cases, the left retroperitoneal lymphnodes are involved. So in right side, complete RPLND, like classical RPLND, but in the left side, the lower limit of the dissection should be up to "inferior mesenteric artery".

So that hypogastric plexus will be intact to preserve fertility.

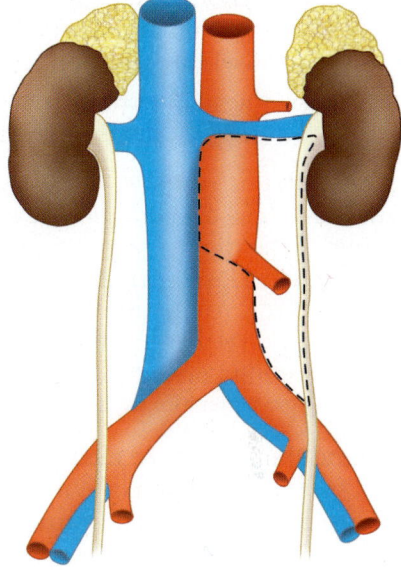

Boundary of RPLND for left-sided testicular tumor

Pitfalls

1. Great vessels injury
2. Ureteric injury
3. Prolong ilius
4. Respiratory complications.

Preoperative Preparation

1. Incentive spirometry for respiratory exercise.
2. Bowel preparation, the day before operation.

Approaches

There are two approaches:
a. Abdominal approach
b. Thoracoabdominal approach (when the bulky nodes are around or above the renal hilum).

Procedure

1. General anesthesia
2. Position: Very very important: In abdominal approach, the position is supine. And in thoracoabdominal approach, the position is described below. The same sided shoulder is to be kept at 45° angle by placing sand bag or sheet root under the back and the arm is to place over the arm rest. The pelvis is nearly supine. The OT table would be flexible so that there will be a wide separation of the costal cartilage and the anterior superior iliac spine (ASIS). Both lower limbs will be straight.

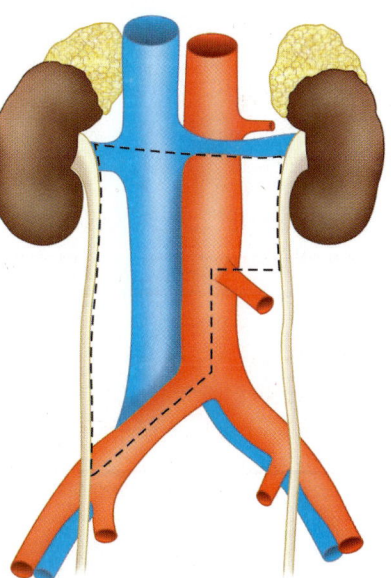

Boundary of RPLND for right-sided testicular tumor

3. Cleaning and draping
   - Incision: For abdominal approach (when the bulky nodes above the level of renal hilum)
   - Midline incision from xiphisternum to symphysis pubis
   - For thoracoabdominal approach
   - The incision begins over the 9th rib in the midaxillary line, extends across the costochondral junction up to epigastrium, then usual midline incision just below xiphisternum to symphysis pubis
   - The muscle and the periosteum are incised and subperiosteal resection of the ribs is done
   - Now the abdomen is opened in the midline in usual fashion.
     (Here only the steps of RPLND abdominal approach are described).

Step 1: Mobilization of peritoneum: The peritoneal mobilization is to start superiorly where the peritoneum attaches to the diaphragm. The superior extension of Gerota's fascia and the thin layer of fibroareolar tissue between the diaphragm and the Gerota's fascia to be identified. This is an avascular plane. Three vessels penetrate the fascia of Gerota, namely, celiac artery, superior mesenteric artery (SMA) and inferior mesenteric artery (IMA). Anatomically, SMA is medial to the junction, where superior mesenteric vein and splenic vein form the portal vein, and passes directly over the left renal vein. It is to be preserved anyway. Next, the IMA to be identified near the duodenojejunal flexure.

Step 2: Mobilization of gut: The small intestine, and ascending colon (duodenum, pancreas–when nodes are around the hilum) are mobilized by incising the posterior mesenteric attachments, from the level of cecum and from the foramen of Winslow to the ligament of Treitz. The inferior mesenteric vein may be ligated and divided near its insertion into splenic vein, if required. The inferior mesenteric artery may be ligated in young but in elderly people try to preserve it. The intestine can then be mobilized more and elevate the pancreas to expose the renal hilum. Next, along the line of Toldt, incise the peritoneum to mobilize the whole right colon.

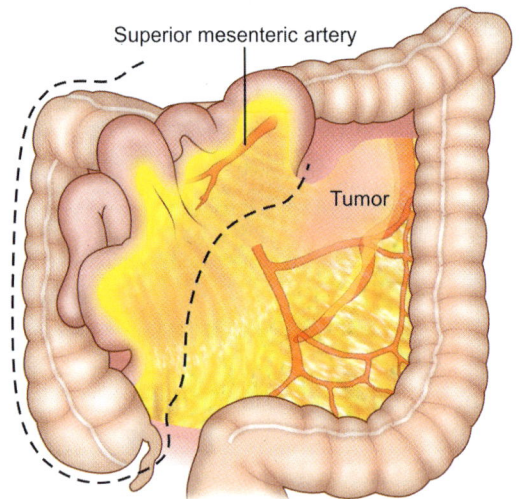

Superior mesenteric artery

Tumor

The mobilization of small intestine, ascending colon and duodenum by incising the posterior parietal peritoneum

Now, whole small intestine and the right colon to be packed inside the wet warm OT towel and to be kept over the chest wall (all the time of dissection be careful of any injury to SMA).

Step 3: The nodal tissue dissection: The nodal tissue over the aorta and IVC is divided along the line of vessels, creating three pockets:
   i. Right of the vena cava

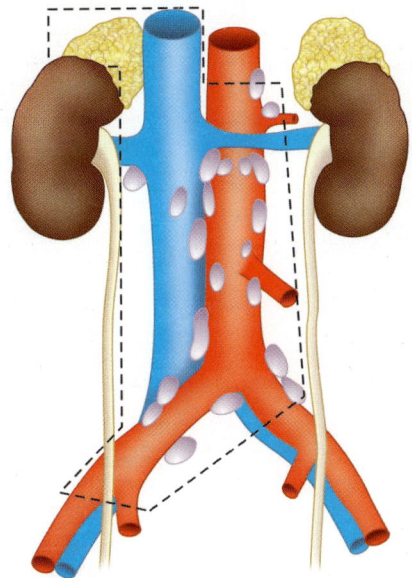

Lymphnodes involvement in right-sided testicular tumor

ii. In between aorta and IVC

iii. Left to the aorta.

Dissect all the nodes and tissues off the vessels. Split and roll techniques are useful for this. In this technique, split the peritoneum over the IVC and aorta and remove all lymphnodes lymphatics from three compartments, i.e. (i) compartment between right ureter and IVC, (ii) between IVC and aorta and no (iii) between aorta and left ureter.

Step 4: The boundary of the dissection is to be determined first. The dorsal limit of the dissection is the anterior spinous ligament. (The nerve sparing RPLND depends upon the extent of the disease and the patient's status and usually it is done in upfront surgery.)

Step 5: In the left-sided nerve sparing technique: The ureter is reflected laterally which is the lateral limit of the dissection. Sympathetic fibers are to identify either where they cross the left common iliac artery or by reflecting the lymphatic tissue medially off the psoas. The sympathetic fibers are then dissected free. The lymphatic tissue is split over the aorta. The lumbar arteries, distal to renal hium are ligated and divided by retracting the aorta with a vessel retractor. These are paired arteries. The lumbar veins are to be ligated and divided in the same manner. All the posterior attachments are divided and the specimen to be separated from the anterior spinous ligament. Thus, the aorta is completely mobilized. Remove all the nodal tissue behind the aorta and the

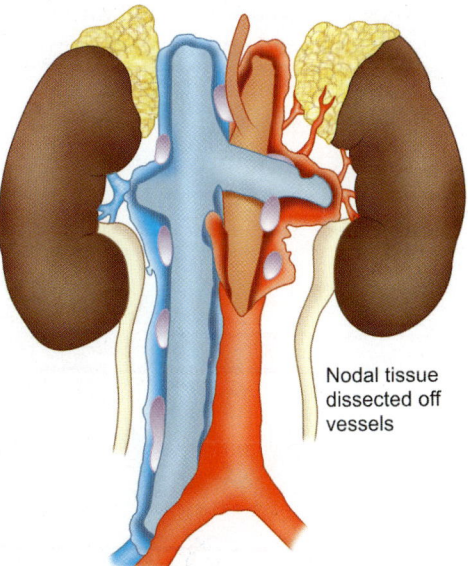

Nodal tissue dissected off vessels

Nodal dissections in three compartments by split and roll technique

IVC. The gonadal and posterior ascending lumbar veins are ligated and divided. The renal artery to be dissected from the aorta origin to the site where it crosses the cruss of the diaphragm. All the lymphatic tissues are snept medially and inferiorly, over the anterior vertebral ligaments to the opposite side.

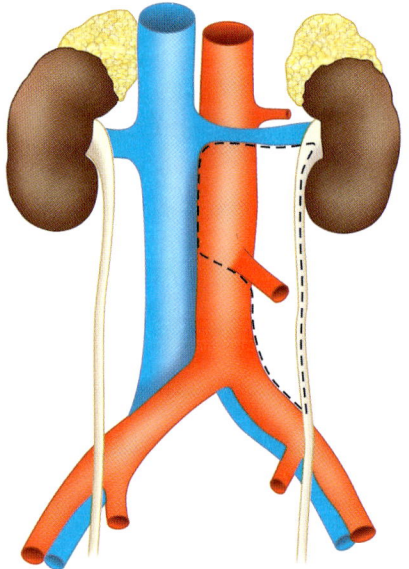

Boundary for nerve sparing RPLND for left-sided testicular tumor

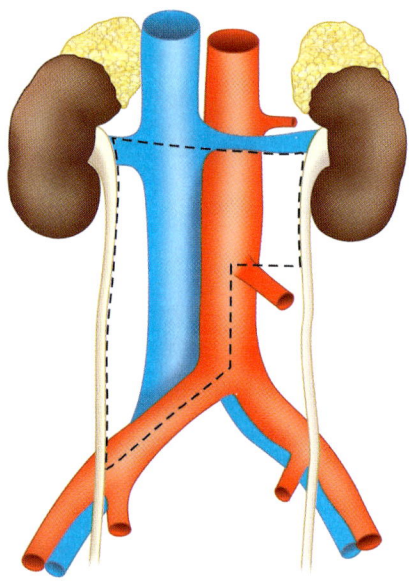

Boundary for nerve sparing RPLND for right-sided testicular tumor

Step 6: *The right-sided nerve sparing technique:* After mobilization of peritoneum, the lymphatic tissue is to split along the aorta and then along the IVC. The interaorta caval tissue is then rolled to the right (left to the patient) and the efferent sympathetic fibers are identified which is to be preserved. Lumbar arteries and veins are to be ligated and divided and the renal hilum to be dissected.

Now, the total specimen of lymphnodes and lymphatic tissue is to be dissected off the anterior spinous ligament and remove it. All the time of dissection, care to be taken for ureter and sympathetic fibers.

Step 7: *Meticulus hemostasis to be achieved.* Clean the retroperitoneal area thoroughly with normal saline. Place a drain. Reapproximate the cut opened peritoneum and close the abdomen in usual fashion.

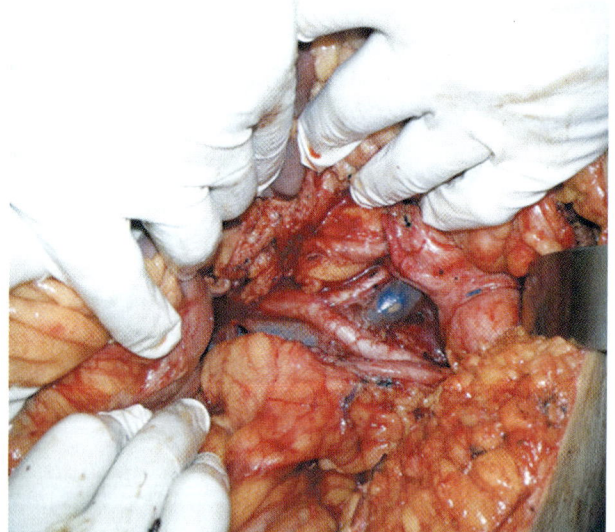
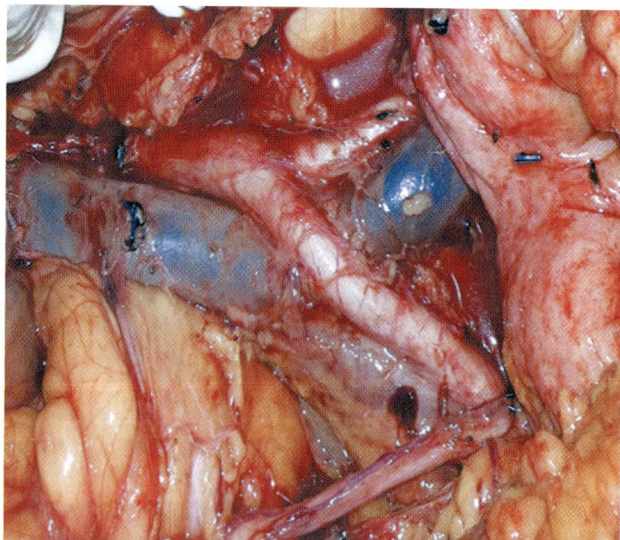

Post-RPLND picture

A person changes his house, changes his clothes, changes his relations, changes his friends, but is still unhappy? Because he never changes himself.

Complications

1. Hemorrhage and hematoma. Injury to the great vessels
2. Surgical site infection
3. Prolonged ileus
4. Enterocutaneous fistula
5. Aorta enteric fistula
6. Pancreatitis
7. Lymphocele, chylous ascites are important complications.
8. Injury to ureters
9. Inability to ejaculate, retrograde ejaculation, etc.

7.1.8 TOTAL PENECTOMY

Anatomy of Penis

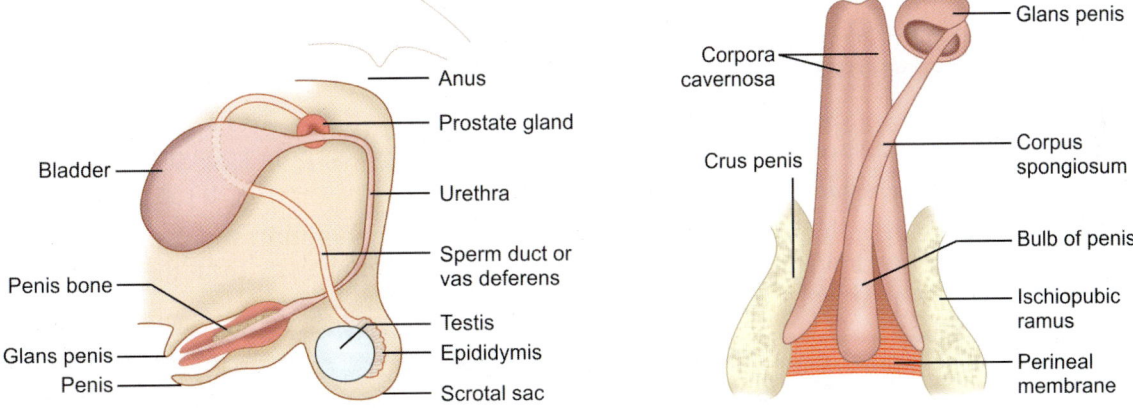

Anatomy of penis

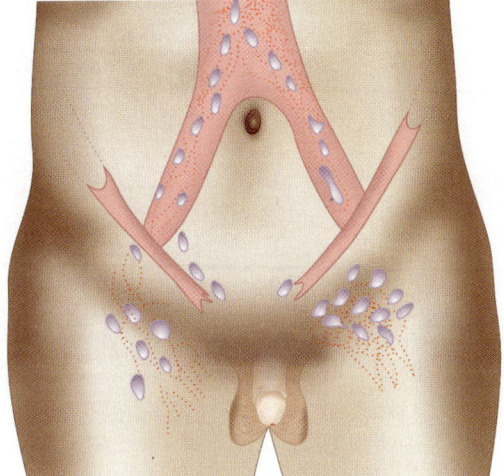
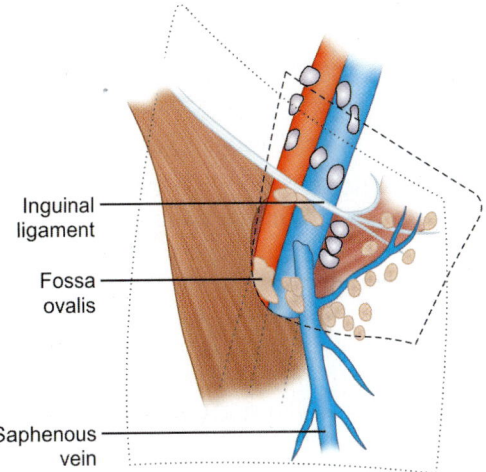

Lymphatic drainage in penile growth

It is not that people stop smiling when they grow old. The fact is, people look old when they stop smiling. Donate a smile everyday.

Indications

The growth involves the long segment of the shaft of the penis where 2 cm proximal margin is not effectively achievable.

Procedures

1. Spinal/penile block
2. Supine position
3. Cleaning and draping
4. Tourniquet may be used at the root of penis leep max for 20 minutes, release for 2 minutes and use monopolar cautery. Not bipolar to preserve the blood supply.
5. Incision: A circumferential incision around the root of the penis with a 2 cm long extension toward the symphysis pubis.

Step 1: Deepen the incision and ligate dorsal vein, artery, then deep dorsal vein and artery of the penis at the midline one by one and divide.

Step 2: Resection of corpora cavernosa and ischiocavernosus muscle: The two corpora cavernosa with ischio-cavernosus muscle is excised from their origin of the ischiopubic rami, over running with 3-0 vicryl suture to prevent bleeding.

Step 3: Resection of corpora spongiosum with urethra: The separated corpora spongiosum is to cut along with the proximal urethra 2 cm from the root of the penis.

Step 4: Make an opening in perineum, at a suitable distance behind the scrotum and the urethral opening is brought out through the opening. Spatulate it and suture with skin 2 mm away from the margin to prevent retraction, using 3-0 nylon. Thereby a new perineal urethrostomy is created.

Step 5: Bilateral orchidectomy: Bilateral orchidectomy is usually done along with total penectomy. (In view of preventing psychosexual abnormality and avoiding overhanging testes over the perineal urethrostomy to pass urine easily.) Place an arterial clamp over each spermatic cord beyond the testis and divide it and over-run with vicryl 3-0 suture. Excise the extrascrotal skin and suture the edges both the sides with 3-0 nylon.

Step 6: Hemostasis to be achieved. Put a Foley's catheter and keep it for 10 days. Dressing is done.

Remember: In carcinoma penis, ilioinguinal lymphnode dissection is considered, if the malignant lymphnode is suspicious or fine-needle aspiration cytology (FNAC) proven and in opposite site if suspicious node or FNAC proven malignant node, do ilioinguinal dissection, otherwise only inguinal dissection although prophylactic inguinal lymphadenectomy is still controversial. [Groin dissection related to carcinoma penis described in ilioinguinal block dissection (IIBD).]

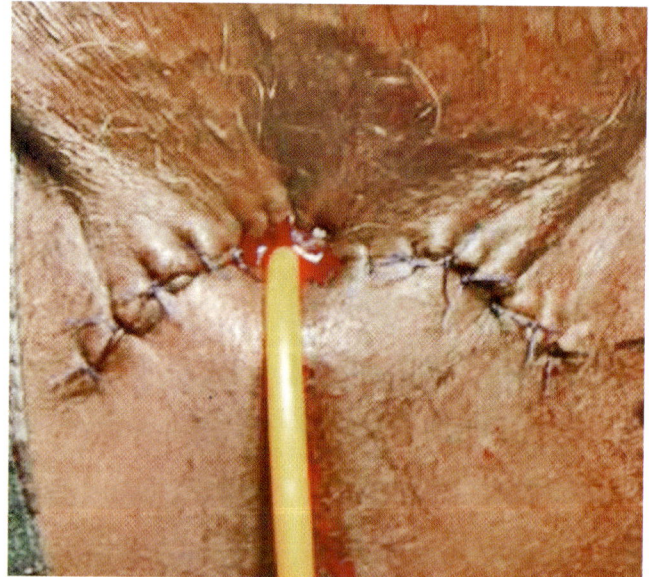

Perineal urethrostomy

Life has so many great options but you do not have to pick what seems to be the best. Just pick what makes you happy and it will be the best.

7.1.9 PARTIAL PENECTOMY

Anatomy of Penis

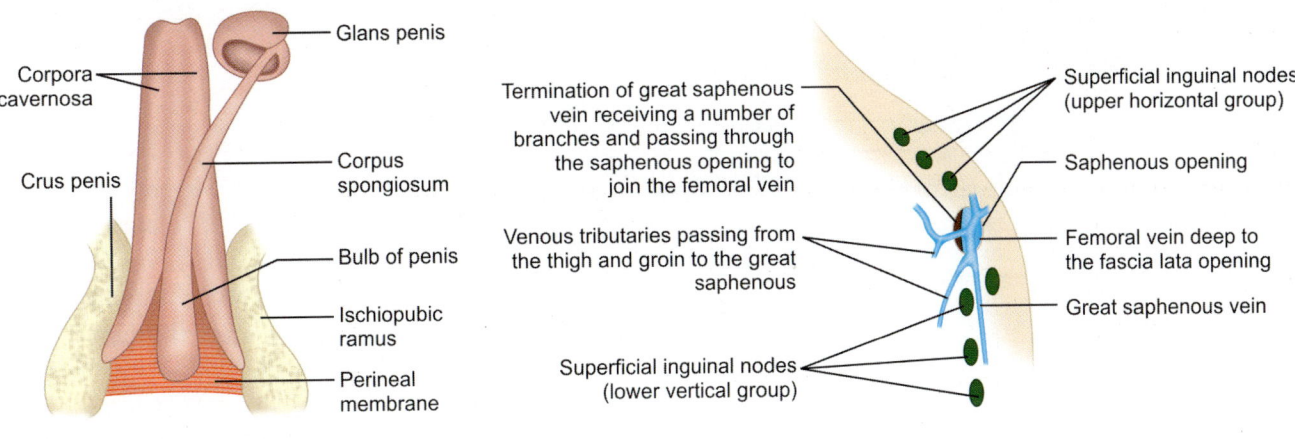

Anatomy of Penis

Anatomy of lymphatic drainage at groin

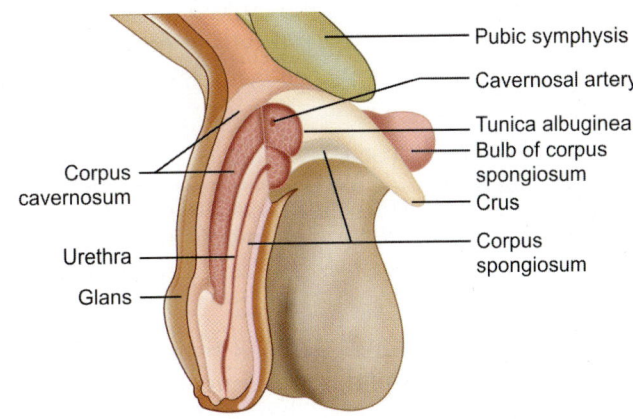

Anatomy of penis

Indications

Penile cancer where 2 cm clear proximal margin is obtainable, i.e. tumor is in the preruce, glans or distal shaft. Other tumors involving distal shaft or glans of the penis or both, like

- Condyloma acuminata
- Buschke-Lowenstein tumor
- Balanitis xerotica obliterans, etc.

Procedures

- Spinal/penile block
- Supine position
- Cleaning and draping

Life is an echo; all comes back, the good, the bad, the false and the true. So, give the world the best you have and the best will come back to you.

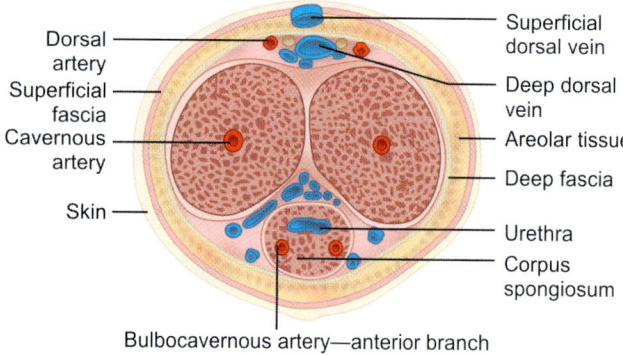

Penile anatomy on cross-section

- Tourniquate may be used at the root of penis leep max for 20 minutes, release for 2 minutes and use monopolar cautery. Not bipolar to preserve the blood supply.
- Incision: Mark the incision first with gention violet. It is 2 cm proximal to the proximal margin of the tumor and put half of the circumference on dorsal aspect. On the ventral aspect, longer flap is marked.

Step 1: Dorsal flap and longer ventral flap are raised.

Step 2: The corpora cavernosa is divided completely. Apply a hemostatic artery forceps to prevent bleeding. Now overrun both the corpora with 3-0 vicryl suture, removing the hemostatic artery forceps gradually.

Step 3: Corpora spongiosum along with the urethra is divided 1 cm distal to the division of corpora cavernosa, i.e. keep it slightly longer.

Step 4: Make a nick on the ventral skin and urethra along with spongiosa is to be brought out through the opening of the ventral skin flap. The opening of the corpus spongiosum may be enlarged by small cuts both the sides. Now, the mucous membrane of the urethra is sutured with the skin 2 mm away from the margin to prevent unwanted retraction. Thus, a new urethral orifice is created at the ventral aspect of the penis.

Step 5: Hemostasis to be achieved completely. Now, both the edges of the two flaps are approximated with 3-0/4-0 nylon. Put a Foley's catheter (keep it for 10 days) and keep the penis straight with the help of dressing [groin dissection related to carcinoma penis described in ilioinguinal block dissection (IIBD)].

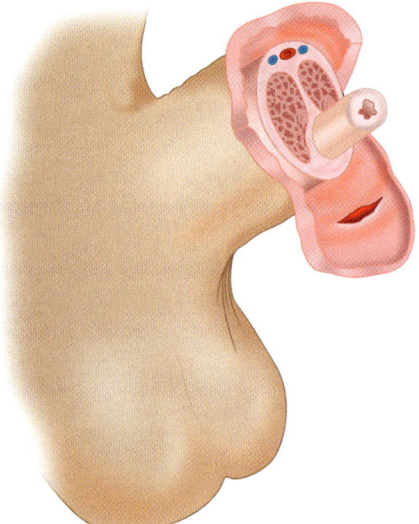

Partial penectomy

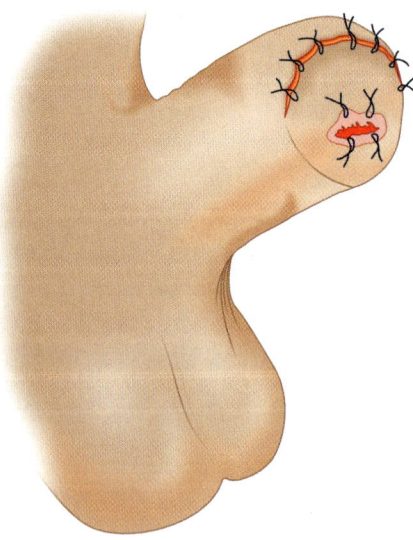

Closure after partial penectomy

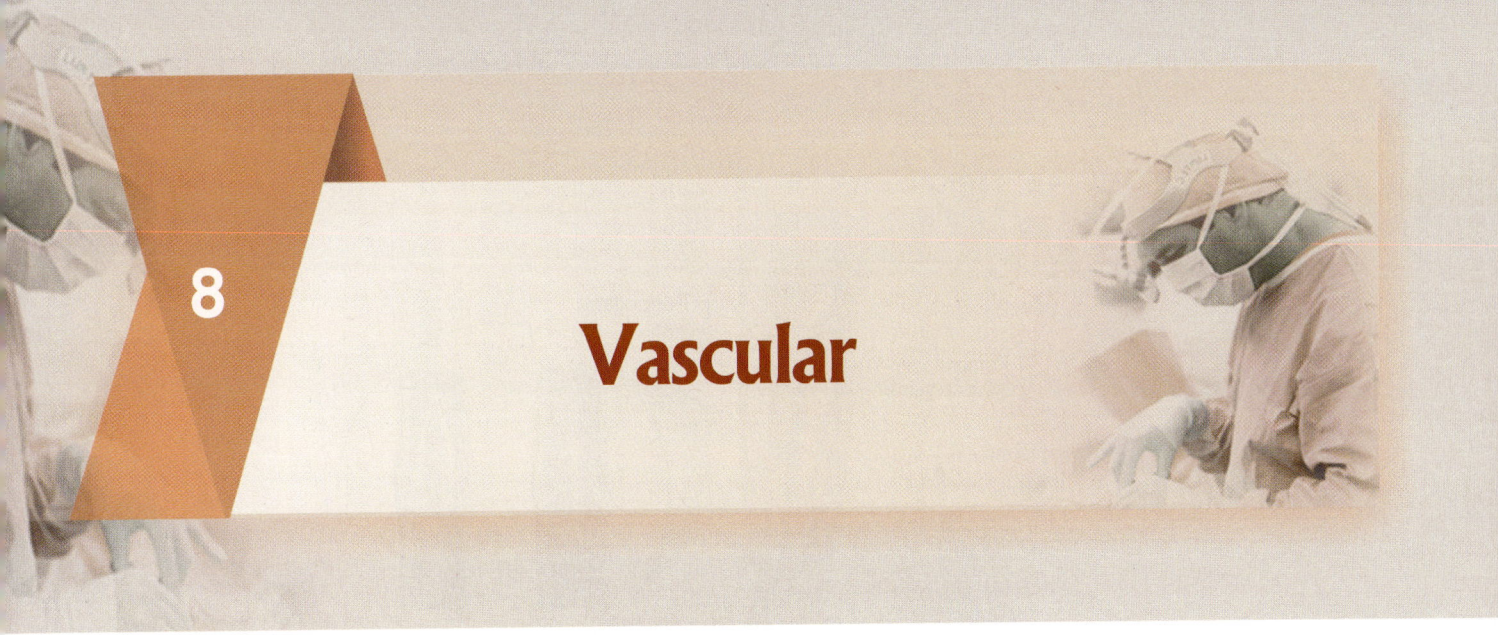

Vascular

8

8.1 TRENDELENBURG'S OPERATION (SAPHENOFEMORAL LIGATION)

Anatomy

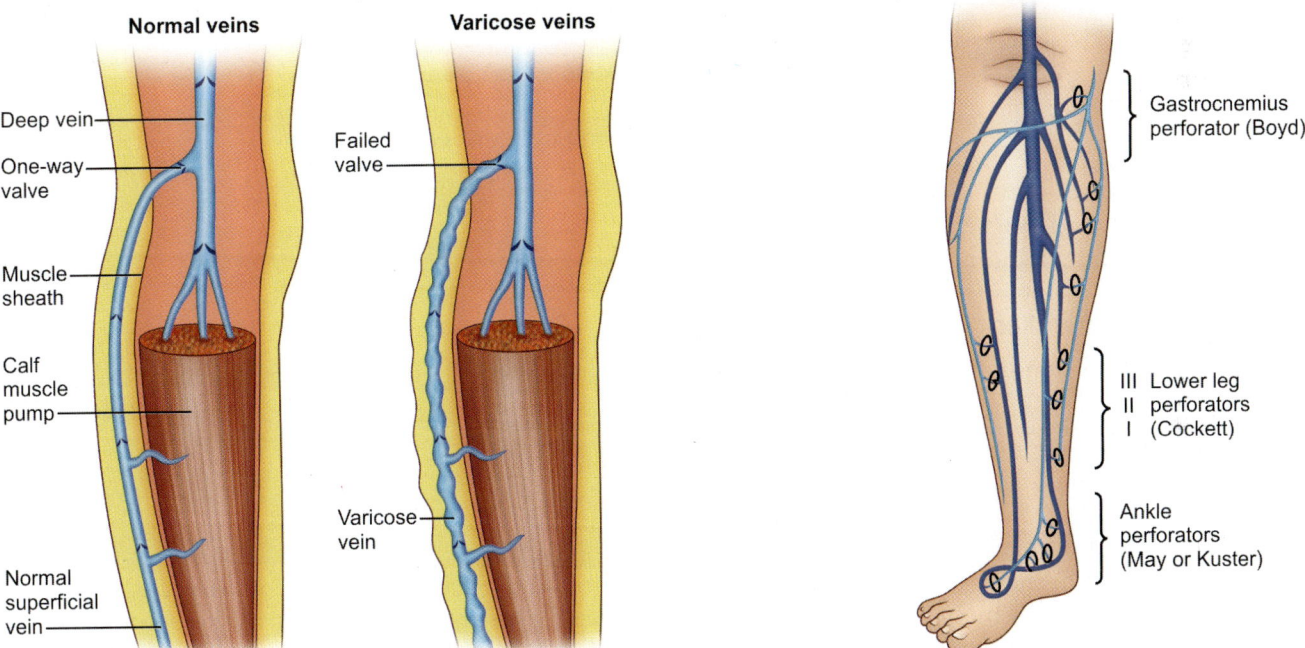

Anatomy of great saphenous vein and lower limb perforators

Indications

- Symptomatic varicose veins
- Grade IV varicose veins
- Varicose veins with complications.

Pitfalls

- Hemorrhage
- DVT

Not dreams, but night changes. Not destiny, but path changes. Always keep your hope alive, luck may or may not change, but time definitely will change.

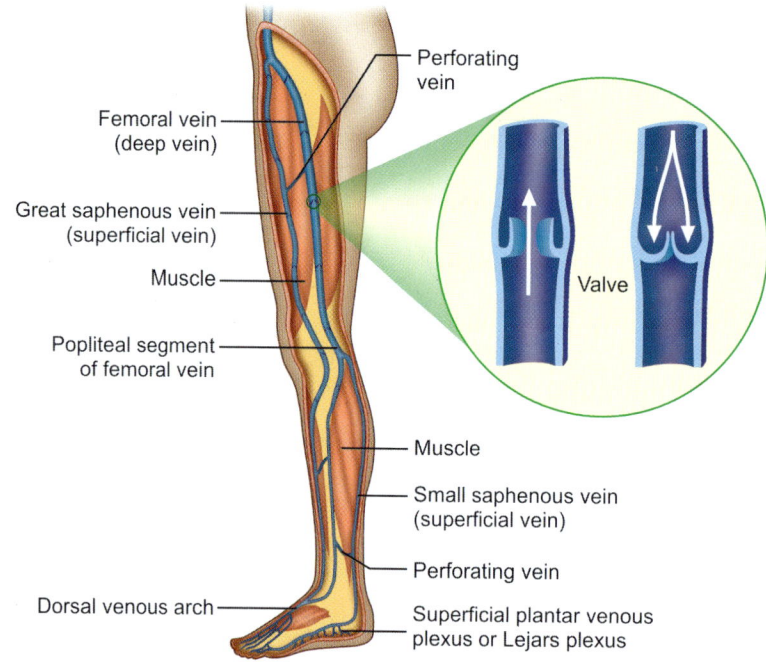

Femoral vein (deep vein)

Great saphenous vein (superficial vein)

Muscle

Popliteal segment of femoral vein

Perforating vein

Valve

Muscle

Small saphenous vein (superficial vein)

Perforating vein

Dorsal venous arch

Superficial plantar venous plexus or Lejars plexus

Anatomy of great saphenous vein and lower limb perforators

- Recurrence of varicose vein
- Injury to common femoral vein

Preoperative Preparation

Vein is marked on standing position and the area of perforators incompetence is encircled.

Procedures

1. Spinal anesthesia
2. Supine position
3. Cleaning and draping
4. *Incision:* A 6–8 cm incision, 2–3 cm below and parallel to the inguinal ligament from the site of femoral artery pulsation to the medial border of adductor magnus. (Few surgeons make a groin crease incision for better cosmetic results but it is more often affected by intertrigo and more prone to develop infection.)

Step 1: The incision is deepened through the subcutaneous fat and through the fascia of Scarpa. The great saphenous vein lies in the fat just below this layer, at the fossa ovalis. Dissect the vein both proximally and distally. Ligate and divide all four named tributaries (superficial circumflex, superficial epigastric, superficial pudendal and deep external pudendal) and unnamed tributaries draining into the femoral vein just above and below the saphenofemoral junction.

Step 2: Ligation of saphenofemoral junction: The saphenous vein must not be divided until it has been undoubtfully indentified. It is always better to identify the common femoral vein to continue both proximally and distally to the saphenofemoral junction.

Accepting many WRONG persons may not affect your life, but rejecting one right person will leave you something missing throughout your life.

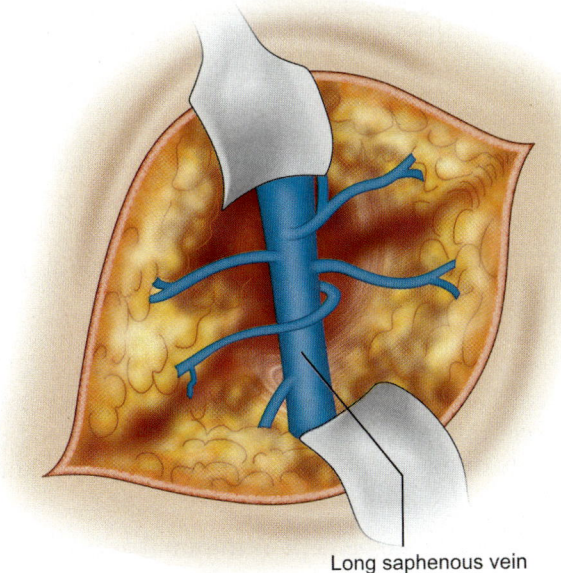

Long saphenous vein

Long saphenous vein and its tributaries

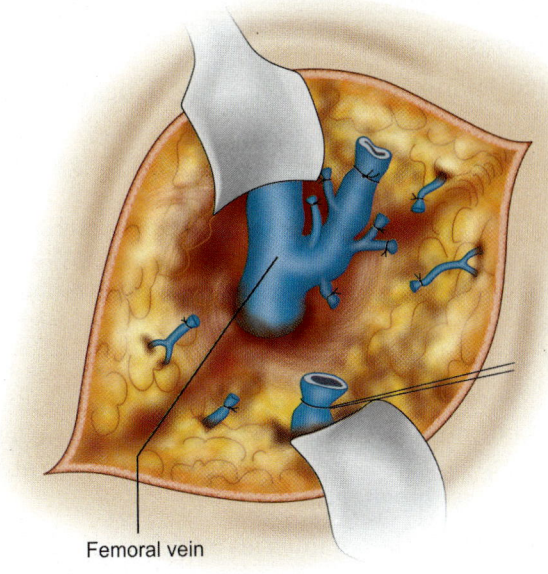

Femoral vein

Transfixation at saphenofemoral junction

Remember: The color of LSV is different from CFV. Dissect both medial and lateral aspects of common femoral vein. Then, the LSV is ligated flush at the saphenofemoral junction or just close to the saphenofemoral junction with 2-0 silk/vicryl. Now, take one transfixation suture and divide the vein in such a way that there will be no deformity of common femoral vein.

Remember
1. Biting the common femoral vein with a stitch and leaving a long stump of LSV are the main causes of development of DVT.
2. If at any stage major bleeding occurs, do not apply any artery forceps blindly. Just do two things—apply firm pressure with a gauze swab and elevate the foot end of the table to reduce the venous pressure and wait for 5 minutes and then reassess the damage and ligate or repair the vein as required.

Step 3: Stripping of the LSV: Now, insert the Mayo's stripper into the saphenous vein at the groin and pass it through the vein up to just below knee. Make an incision over the tip of the stripper and take it out. Apply a suitable metal cap at the tip and give a traction of the stripper from above, the vein will come out. [If the stripper is extended much below the knee, there is a fair chance to damage the saphenous nerve as it runs side by side to the GSV (great saphenous vein).]

Step 4: Stripping of leg varicosities: Make small incisions over the marked varicosities and sip the veins with the help of two artery forceps at the leg and apply a good pressure on the lower limb along the vein.

Step 5: After achieving good hemostasis, close the groin wounds and all wounds in the limb with 3-0 nylon. After sterile dressing, apply pressure bandage (crepe bandage)/stocking starting from foot to groin and keep it for 5–7 days.

Note on short saphenous vein (SSV) surgery:
• Prone position
• Open popliteal fossa. Identify SSV, ligate it carefully close its junction with popliteal vein.
• No need to strip SSV, like LSV. Make multiple incisions and remove the varicose vein in the limb.
• Save the sural nerve during the procedure.

Thinking that we are perfect and that others need to be corrected is just like cleaning the mirror instead of cleaning of our face.

8.2 AMPUTATION

Indications

The limb/limbs which are either dead, deadly or deadloss.
a. Dead—dry gangrane
b. Deadly (dying)—diabetic foot, wet or gas gangrene, spreading cellulitis, severe sepsis, melanoma, osteosarcoma.
c. Dead loss (devitalized)—crush injury, congenital anomaly, severe rest pain, paralysis, etc.

Below knee amputation (Burgess amputation) points to remember: Ideal length of tibia for below knee amputation is 15 cm from knee and minimum length is 8 cm.

Steps of Incision

Step 1: Burgess posterior longer flap technique is well accepted. The long posterior flap is marked out and it should be one and half times the diameter of the leg and width is half time the circumference of the leg at the site of amputation. Anterior flap is to cut down at the level of the division of the bone 15 cm below the knee, i.e. from tibial tuberosity.

Step 2: Anterior flap of muscles and skin is off form, underlying bone is to be kept as minimal as possible—1 cm is adequate.

Step 3: The anterior incision is deepened up to tibia. The tibia is divided 1 cm proximally and beveled anteriorly. The fibula is divided 1 cm more proximally.

Step 4: The posterior flap will retain deep fascia and muscles throughout of its length to maintain skin perfusion. The muscle bulk is to be reduced to make a rounded stump.

Step 5: All arteries and veins are ligated as they are encountered and nerves are divided too. Anterior tibial vessels and nerves are divided first, on deepening gradually, laterally the peroneal vessels to be encountered. On medial side, the long saphenous vein is ligated and divided.

Step 6: In between solius and tibialis posterior, the posterior tibialis vessels and nerve are to be ligated and divided.

Step 7: The posterior muscles are divided obliquely thereby deep muscles are mostly removed but a part of superficial gastrocnemius bellies and soleus remain.

Step 8: The posterior surface is now freed from all attachments. Now, the tibia is divided 1 cm to be proximally and beveled. The fibula is divided 1 cm more proximally.

Step 9: The posterior muscle mass is sutured over the bone to deep fascia and few stitches with the periosteum of the bone. The skin of both flaps is closed over a suction drain after ensuring hemostasis. The stump bandage will be light to maintain the circulation to the flaps.

Variations

1. For young active person who does not have peripheral vascular disease is suitable for two musculocutaneous flaps. Equal lengths of these flaps have the advantage that the suture line will be away from the stump.
2. Skew flap technique (skew means skin) and muscle flaps are fashioned separately. Skin flaps are based on the blood supply of the skin and venous drainage is related to both long and short saphenous veins and a single posterior muscle flap relies on collateral vessels.

All birds find shelter during a rain. But, an eagle avoids rain by flying above the clouds. Problems are common. But, attitude makes the difference.

Above Knee Amputation

Points to remember: The site of selection for above knee amputation is 25–30 cm from the tip of greater trochanter. Ischemia and trauma are two main indications.

Steps

1. The incision is made either equal anterior and posterior myocutaneous flaps or a longer anterior flap. Author prefers the equal flaps.
2. The vertical part is extended over the subsartorial canal to the femoral vessels.
3. The incision is deepened through subcutaneous tissue fascia lata. Gradually, anteriorly the lower end of quadriceps muscles, medially the adductors, gracilis sartorius and poteriorly the hamstring are divided.
4. Periosteum is elevate, femur is divided and beveled.
5. The quadriceps muscles are sutured to hamstring muscles and adductors are sutured to the iliotibial tract to maintain the balanced muscle action of the stump.
6. The fascia lata is repaired.
7. Hemostasis is to be achieved.
8. Skin is closed placing a suction drainage.

8.3 LUMBAR SYMPATHECTOMY

Surgical Anatomy

There is a lumbar sympathetic trunk on each side of the vertebral body. The trunk lies retroperitoneally on the anterolateral surface of the bodies of lumbar vertebrae in the paravertebral gutter.

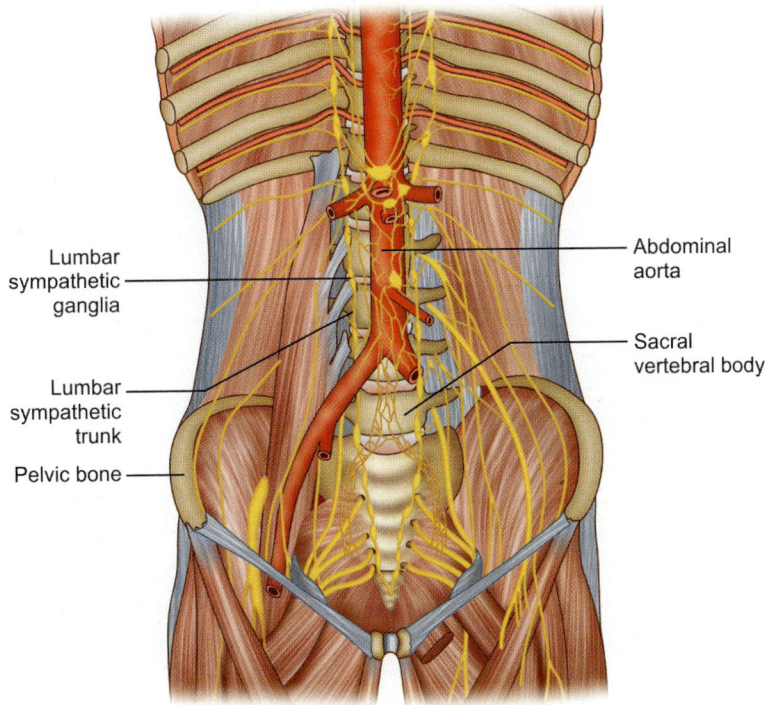

Surgical anatomy of lumbar sympathetic trunk

Everyday do something that will inch you closer to a better tomorrow.

The Lumbar Sympathetic Trunk

The preganglionic sympathetic fiber for the lower limbs, arising from lower T4, T5 and L1 segments via the gray rami communicantes, the preganglionic fibers reach the corresponding sympathetic ganglia from spinal cord and through the white rami communicantes postganglionic fibers connect sympathetic ganglia to the peripheral nerves.

On the left side, it lies in between the psoas and the aorta on right side. It is in between the psoas muscle and the IVC. The IVC may overlap slightly the right sympathetic trunk.

Sympathetic trunk to be differentiated from lymphatics. Sympathetic trunk has rami communicantes and ganglia. Below the first lumbar segment, only white rami communicantes are there. The genitofemoral nerve lies on the anterior aspect of psoas muscle, whereas sympathetic trunk runs medial to the muscle. And there is no ganglia or rami communicantes in the genitofemoral nerve.

Rami communicantes, both gray and white, connect sympathetic trunk with spinal cord and peripheral nerves. Gray rami communicantes carry the preganglionic sympathetic fibers from spinal cord to sympathetic ganglia. The white rami communicantes carry postganglionic fibers from sympathetic ganglia to the peripheral nerves.

In Lumbar Sympathectomy

L1, L2, L3 and L4 ganglia need to be removed for sympathetic denervation of lower limb.

But in case of bilateral lumbar sympathectomy, one-sided L1 ganglia has to be preserved to prevent impotence. L1 ganglion lies under the crus of diaphragm.

In chemical sympathectomy, though very specific expert centers have been doing, the lumbar sympathetic trunk is blocked under fluoroscopic control by injecting 5 mL phenol in water (1:15) into the lumbar sympathetic trunk. Injection to be applied just by the side of 2nd, 3rd, 4th lumbar vertical bodies.

Pitfalls

- Fail to increase skin perfusion in an ischemic lower limb
- Only temporary relief of rest pain.

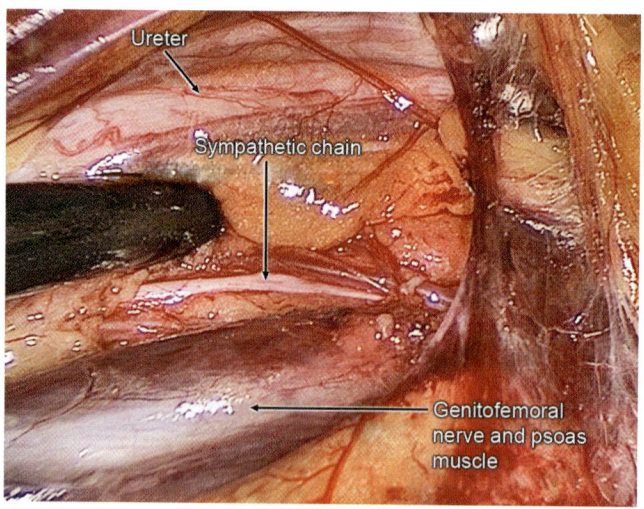

Identification of sympathetic chain medial to psoas muscle

Always pray to have eyes that see the best in people, a heart that forgives the worst, a mind that forgets the bad and a soul that never loses faith in God.

Procedure

1. General anesthesia
2. Supine position with slight elevation of the flank on the side of operation
3. Cleaning and draping
4. Incision for retroperitoneal approach
   - An oblique loin incision from anterior axillary line/lateral border of erector spinae to lateral border of rectus sheath.
   - A transverse incision: Starts from a point below the tip of 12th rib to the lateral border of rectus sheath at the level of umbilicus.

Step 1: The skin and subcutaneous tissue is incised in the line of incision.

Step 2: Division of muscles and aponeurosis: In oblique incision, the external oblique muscles and aponeurosis, internal oblique, transversus abdominis are splited along the direction of fibers (in transverse incision, all muscles are incised along the line of incision.)

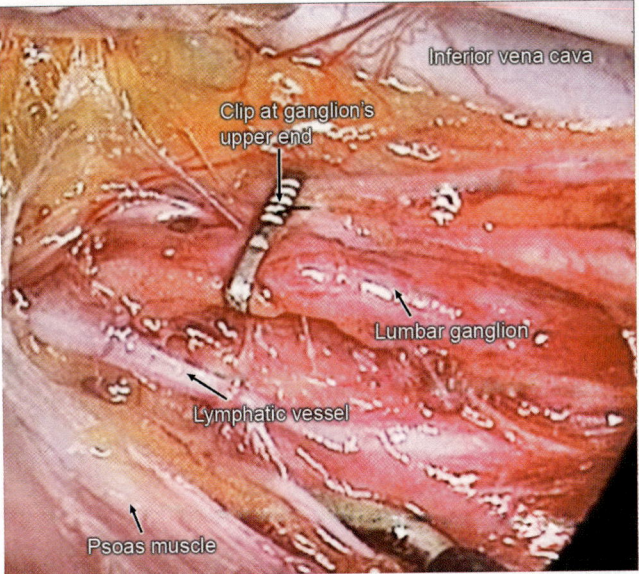

Clip or ligate at ganglion's upper end

Step 3: Stripping of peritoneum: While the flat muscles are divided, the peritoneum is exposed along with extraperitoneal fatty tissue. Now, the peritoneum is stripped medially and forward from the side of abdominal wall, till the inner border of the psoas major is exposed. The gonadal vessel and the ureter to be identified and displaced from peritoneal surface.

Step 4: Identification of sympathetic chain: It lies in the paravertebral gutter, i.e. lateral to the body of lumbar vertebrae and medial to psoas muscle. (In the right side, it may be overlapped by the IVC and left by aorta.) The sympathetic chain is identified by its ganglia and rami communicantes.

Remember: 3G (1) paravertebral gutter, (2) gray rami communicantes and (3) ganglion to identify the sympathetic chain.

The first lumbar ganglion is located high up under the cover of crus of diaphragm, just above the renal vessels. For complete, sympathetic denervation of the lower limb, 1st to 4th lumbar ganglia are to be removed. In case of bilateral sympathectomy, one side L1 ganglia to be preserved to prevent impotence and ejaculatory dysfunction.

Step 5: Dissection of sympathetic chain: The first lumbar ganglion is identified under the retraction of the crus, dissect it, ligate and divide. Tackle the lumbar vessels on the way. The sympathetic chain is dissected downwards up to 4th lumbar ganglia lying behind the common iliac vessels. All ganglia are dissected ligated and divided more than a centimetre apart.

Step 6: Hemostasis to be achieved. See the increased skin temperature of the limbs. Abdomen is closed in layers.

The happiest people on earth are not those who live on their own terms. But those who change their terms for the ones whom they Love and care.

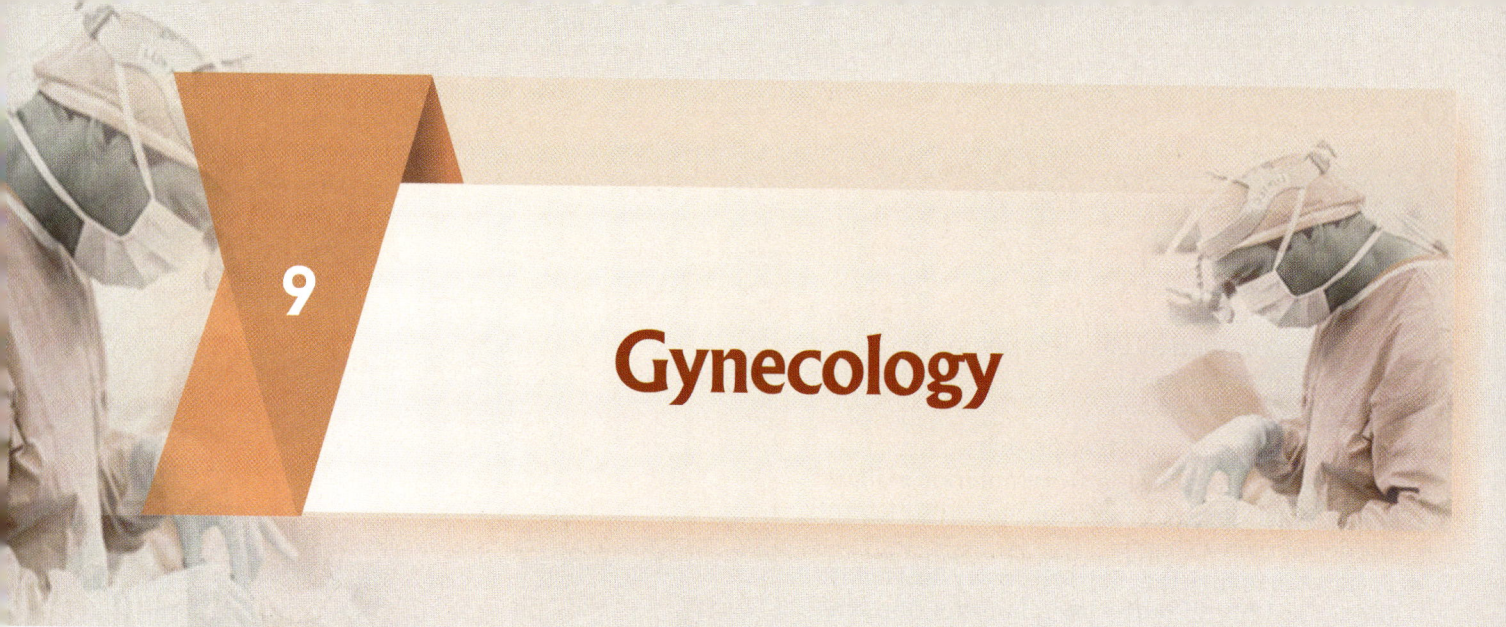

Gynecology

9

9.1 ABDOMINAL HYSTERECTOMY

Surgical Anatomy of Pelvis and Female Genital Tract

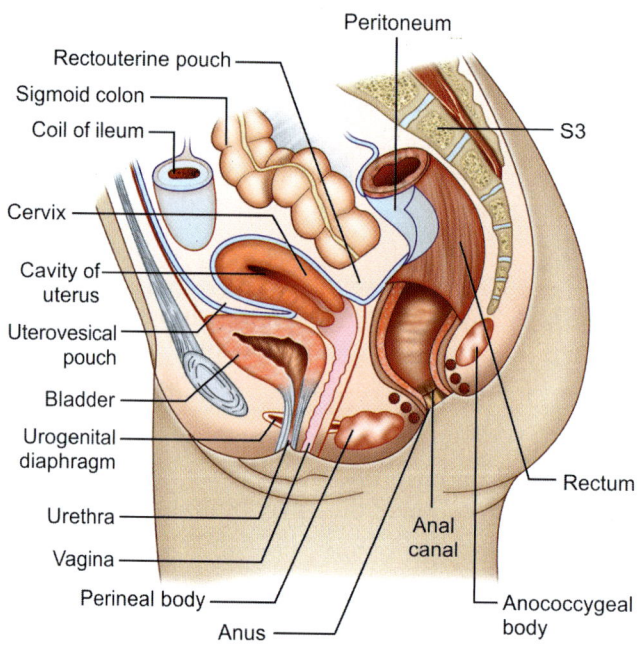

Anatomy of female pelvis in sagittal section

Indications

1. Large symptomatic fibroid: Type I
2. Dysfunctional uterine bleeding (DUB): Type I
3. Carcinoma
   - Cervix: Radical hysterectomy (Type III)
   - Endometrium: Type II

Success is not only a goal, it is a journey, when you commit yourself to the journey, and the goal is surely there to be attained.

- Fallopian tube: Type II
- Ovary: Type II.

Pitfalls of the Surgery

- Ureteral injury: Most formidable
- Pitfalls others: Bladder, bowel injury, hemorrhage, etc.

Types of Hysterectomy

Type I: Extrafascial: Vagina minimal tissue removed, bladder partially mobilized, ureter not mobilized, uterine artery ligated at uterus, parametria resected at uterus and uterosacral ligament transected at uterus.

Type II: Modified radical: Vagina upper 1–2 cm removed, bladder partially mobilized, ureter unroofed in parametrial tunnel, uterine artery ligated medial to ureter, parametria resected medial to ureter and uterosacral ligament transected at midpoint of ligament.

Type III: Radical: Vagina upper one-third to half removed, bladder completely mobilized, ureter completely dissected until entry into bladder, uterine artery ligated at origin from hypogastric artery, parametria resected at pelvic side wall, uterosacral ligament transected at distal attachment.

Type IV: Extended radical: Vagina same as class III, bladder completely mobilized but not resected, ureter all periureteral tissue removed, uterine artery ligation at origin and ligation of superior vesical artery, parametria same as class III, uterosacral ligament same as class III.

Type V: Partial exenteration: Vagina same as class III, portion of bladder resected, distal ureter removed, uterine artery same as class IV, parametria same as class III, uterosacral ligament same as class III.

Procedures

1. Spinal/general anesthesia
2. Supine position, pelvic examination and catheterization
3. Cleaning and draping
4. Incision depends on simplicity, expected exposure, need for extension of the incision, previous surgical scar and cosmesis. Usually, lower midline from umbilicus to symphysis pubis or Pfannenstiel incision.

Step 1: Abdomen is opened in usual fashion. Assessment of pelvis and whole abdominal cavity including liver, kidney, peritoneal cavity. Keep the patient's head down, push the intestinal coil upward with the help of a wet op towel and place the self-retaining retractor.

Step 2: Elevation of uterus: Take a "figure 8" deep bite suture at the fundus of the uterus for the purpose of elevation and traction of the uterus. Otherwise, place a broad ligament clamp at each cornu so that it crosses the round ligament. The tip of the clamp may be placed close to the internal OS. It is useful for uterine traction and to prevent back bleeding.

Step 3: Entering the retroperitoneal spaces: The actual procedure starts by entering the retroperitoneal space. The

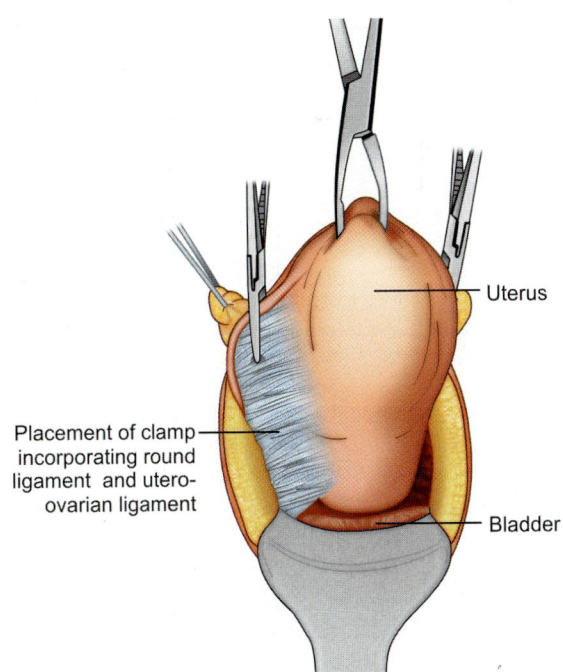

Uterus

Placement of clamp incorporating round ligament and utero-ovarian ligament

Bladder

Traction of uterus and placement of clamp

There is no need to be perfect to inspire others. Let others get inspired by how we deal with our imperfections.

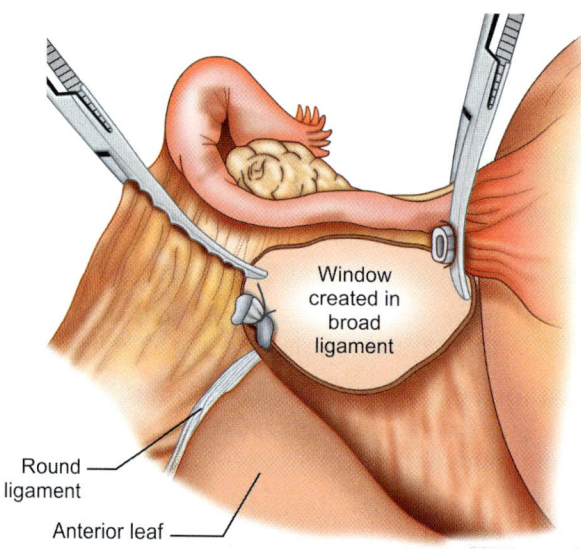

Ligation and division of infundibulopelvic ligament

round ligament is dissected, ligated and divided close to the pelvic side wall. The peritoneum incised and exposing the retroperitoneal space.

At this time, salpingo-oophorectomy may be performed (although salpingo-oophorectomy is not the integral part of hysterectomy but it is done usually) when required. Before ligating ovarian vessels, identify the ureter as the saying is "water (ureter) under the bridge (gonadal vessels)." Now, the paravesical and pararectal spaces are developed. The anterior leaf of broad ligament is incised along the vesicouterine fold and separate the peritoneal reflection of the bladder from the lower uterine segment.

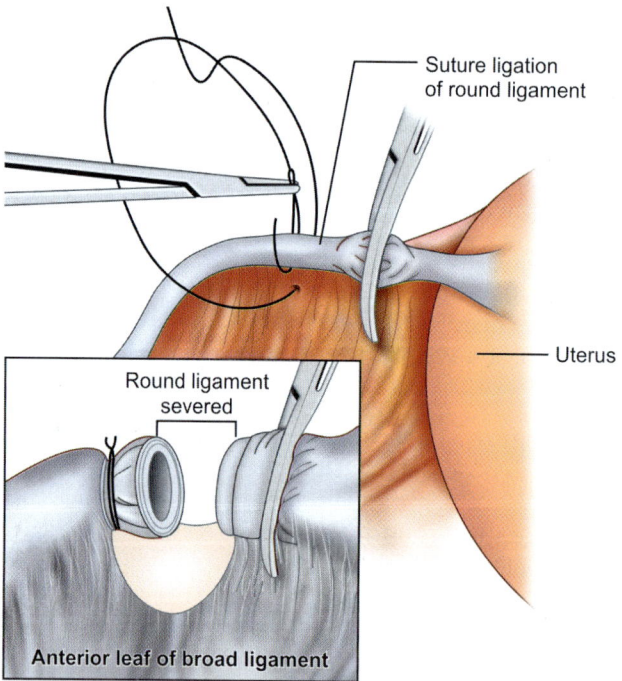

Ligation and division of round ligament and opening of broad ligament

The boundary of paravesical space is:
   i. Bladder and obliterated umbilical artery medially
   ii. The external iliac vessels laterally
  iii. Posteriorly the cardinal ligament
  iv. The obturator fossa and obturator internus muscle inferiorly. The pararectal space is bounded medially by rectum, ureter; laterally pelvic wall, internal iliac vessels; anteriorly cardinal ligament and posteriorly by sacrum.

Step 4: Identification of ureter and safeguard: Enter the retroperitoneum by incising the posterior leaf of broad ligament. Remain lateral to both infundibulopelvic ligament and iliac vessel. The ureter is identified crossing the common iliac artery or down below it is usually below the gonadal vessel [water (ureter) under the bridge]. The ureter to be kept attached to the medial leaf of the broad ligament to maintain its blood supply.

The same way identify the ureter of another side and loop both with vascular tape.

Now, ligate infundibulopelvic (utero-ovarian) ligament. The peritoneal opening is gradually enlarged and extended cephalad to infundibulopelvic ligament and caudal to uterine artery. This opening allows proper exposure of ureter, and infundibulopelvic ligament. Ureter is to be separated from the close proximity of uterine artery and infundibulopelvic ligament.

Step 5: Mobilization of bladder and ligation of uterine vessels: Identify the peritoneal reflection over the cervix and lower uterine segment. For the bladder mobilization, enter the avascular plane between the lower uterine segment and the bladder. Give a good countertraction of the bladder, holding Foley's bulb or placing retractor. On the bladder edge, expose the cervix and upper third of anterior vaginal wall.

Now, uterus is to retracted, cephalad and deviated one side. Uterine vessels are to be skeletonized and placed a curved clamp perpendicular to uterine artery at the junction of the body and cervix, caring the ureter laterally. The vessels are cut and ligated properly. The same procedure to be repeated opposite side.

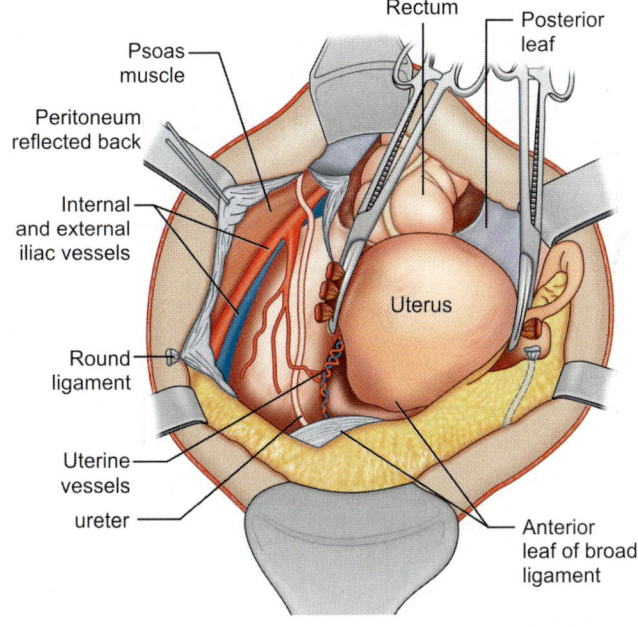

Identification of ureter at the medial leaf of broad ligament

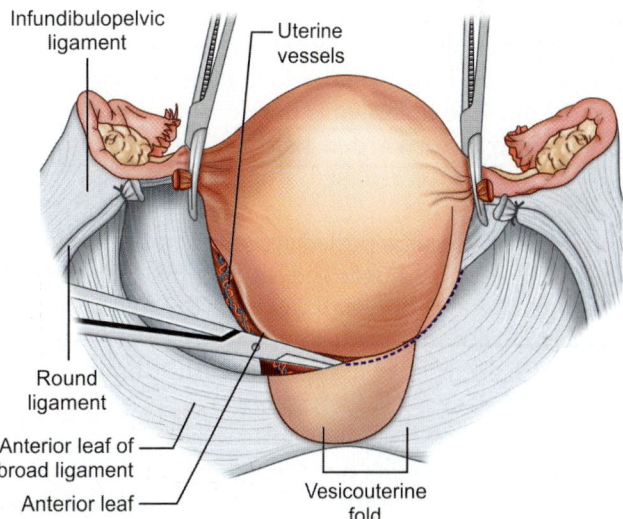

Broad ligament is detached from the bladder at the vesicouterine fold

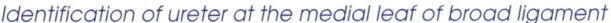

A good plan for today is better than a great plan for tomorrow. Look backward with satisfaction and look forward with confidence.

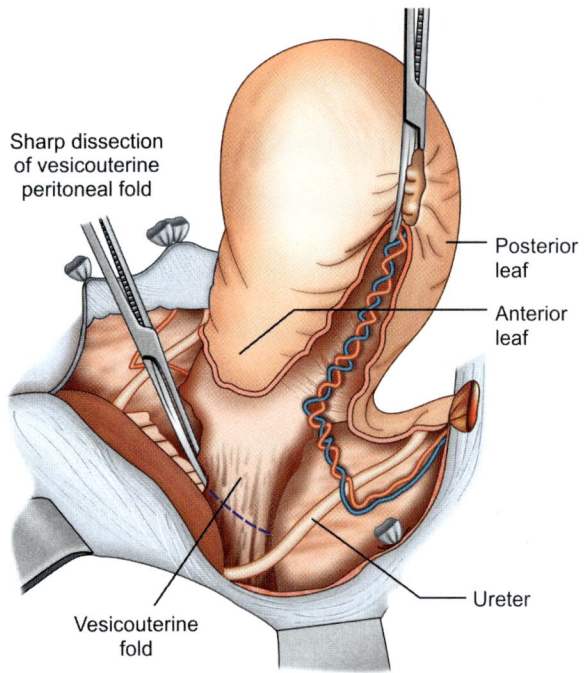

Sharp dissection
of vesicouterine
peritoneal fold

Posterior
leaf

Anterior
leaf

Ureter

Vesicouterine
fold

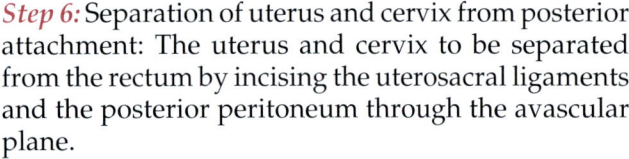

Mobilization of bladder at vesicouterine plane

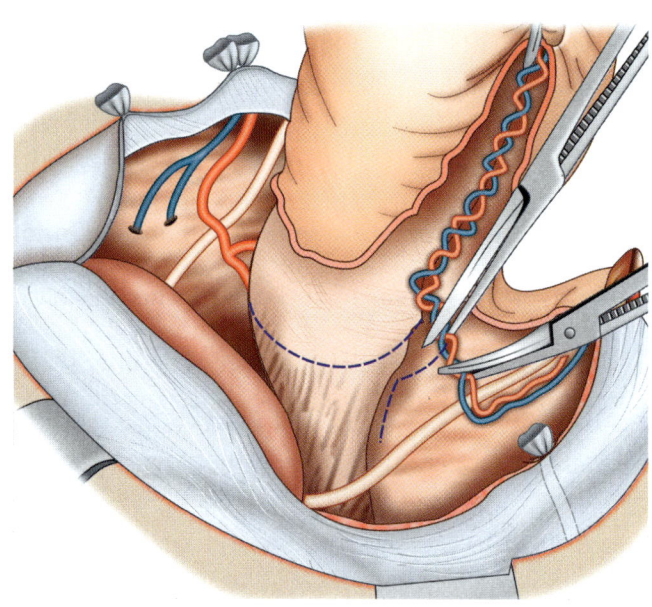

Ligation and division of uterine artery

Step 6: Separation of uterus and cervix from posterior attachment: The uterus and cervix to be separated from the rectum by incising the uterosacral ligaments and the posterior peritoneum through the avascular plane.

Step 7: Division of cardinal ligament and removal of uterus: Cardinal ligament is divided by placing two straight clamps medial to the uterine vessel pedicle, 2–2.5 cm apart for a distance of 3 cm and parallel to the uterus. The ligament is then divided and ligated. The clamp is forwarded below till the junction of cervix and vagina reached. Repeat the same step for the opposite side.

Now, the uterus is pulled cephalad and the external os is to palpate. Enter the vagina on the midline through the anterior wall (leaving the desire length in case of modified radical or radical hysterectomy) and cut it all around avoiding foreshortening of the vagina. The uterus is then removed.

Now, close the vaginal cuff with 1-0 vicryl with reverse cutting needle. A running locked suture is used for hemostasis along the cuff edge. The both edges of vaginal cuff may be fixed with remaining round ligament both the sides to prevent vault prolapse.

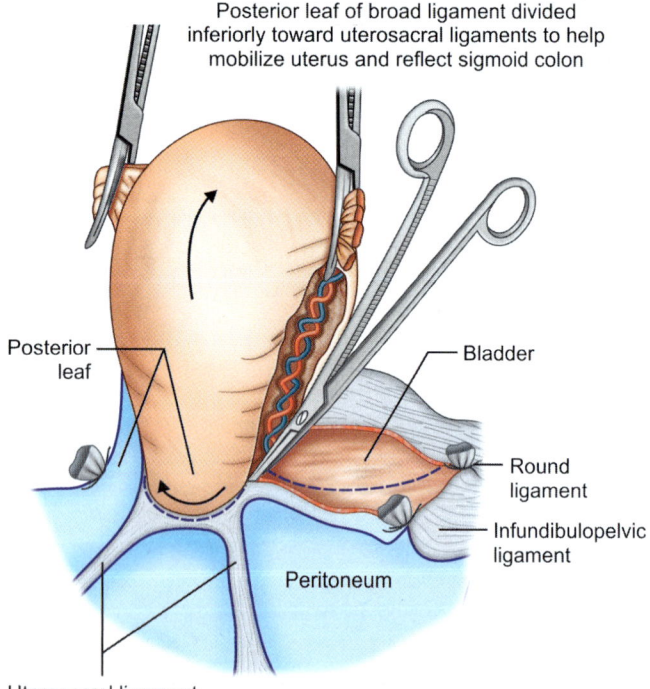

Posterior leaf of broad ligament divided
inferiorly toward uterosacral ligaments to help
mobilize uterus and reflect sigmoid colon

Posterior
leaf

Bladder

Round
ligament

Infundibulopelvic
ligament

Peritoneum

Uterosacral ligament

Uterus is detached from rectum posteriorly by incising uterosacral ligament

Don't feel bad that people remember you only when they need you. Feel privileged that you are like a candle which comes to mind when there is darkness in their lives.

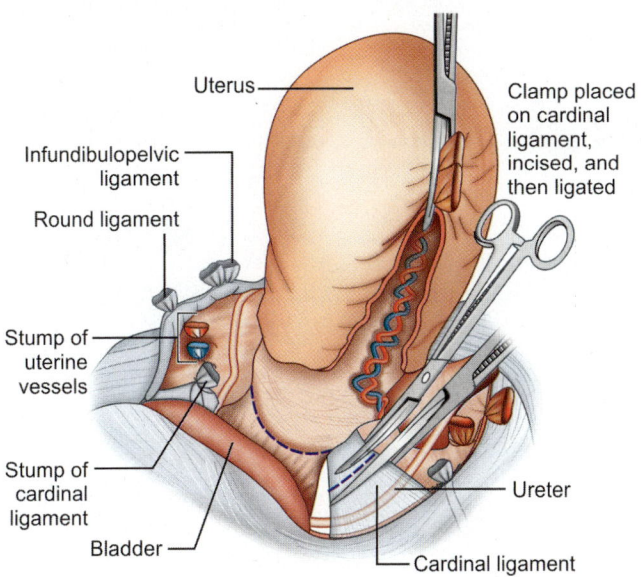

Ligation and division of cardinal ligament

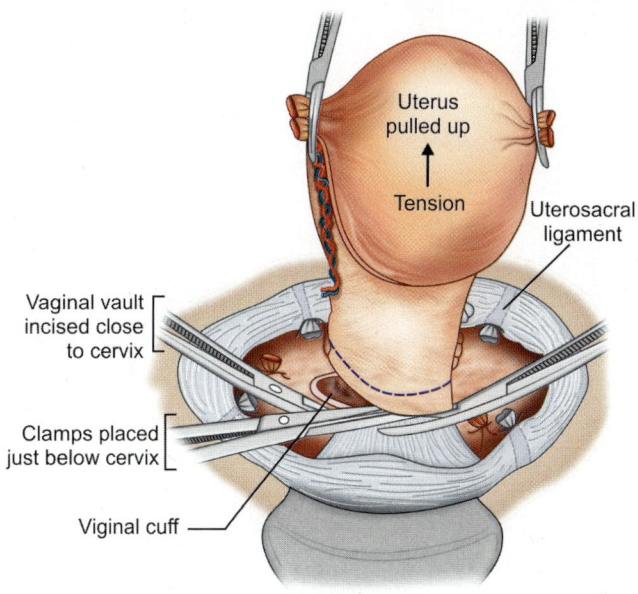

Transaction of vaginal wall all around

Step 8: Hemostasis and peritoneal closure: The pelvis is to be irrigated thoroughly with normal saline and complete hemotasis to be achieved throughout the pelvis.

Ureteral position and integrity to be checked to ensure that they are intact as before and do not seem to be dilated.

The approximation of pelvic peritoneum is not required to avoid adhesion, but fascia can be closed with an interrupted monofilament suture. Place a pelvic drain and abdomen is closed in usual fashion.

Complications

1. *Ureteral injury:* The most formidable complication because of the risk of renal impairment. Most ureteral injury can be avoided by the opening of retroperitoneum, proper exposure of ureter and by direct identification of the ureter.
2. *Bladder injury:* Very common due to close proximity of lower uterine segment, cervix and upper vagina. If injured, close it in two layers with 3-0 vicryl and keep the drain for 4–5 days.
3. *Bowel injury:* If any injury, the defect should be closed in perpendicular to the lumen.
4. *Hemorrhage:* Bleeding may occur from the uterine or ovarian vessels near the insertion of infundibulopelvic ligaments. The pressure pack is the easy way to control and identify the bleeding points. Ligate the vessels properly. Mass ligature should be avoided.
5. Others, like surgical site infection, wound dehiscence, etc., are not uncommon.

Vaginal cuff is closed with 1-0 vicryl and peritoneum is closed over the cuff

Don't decrease your goal to the extent of your ability. Increase your ability to the extent of your goal. That is the way to succeed in Life.

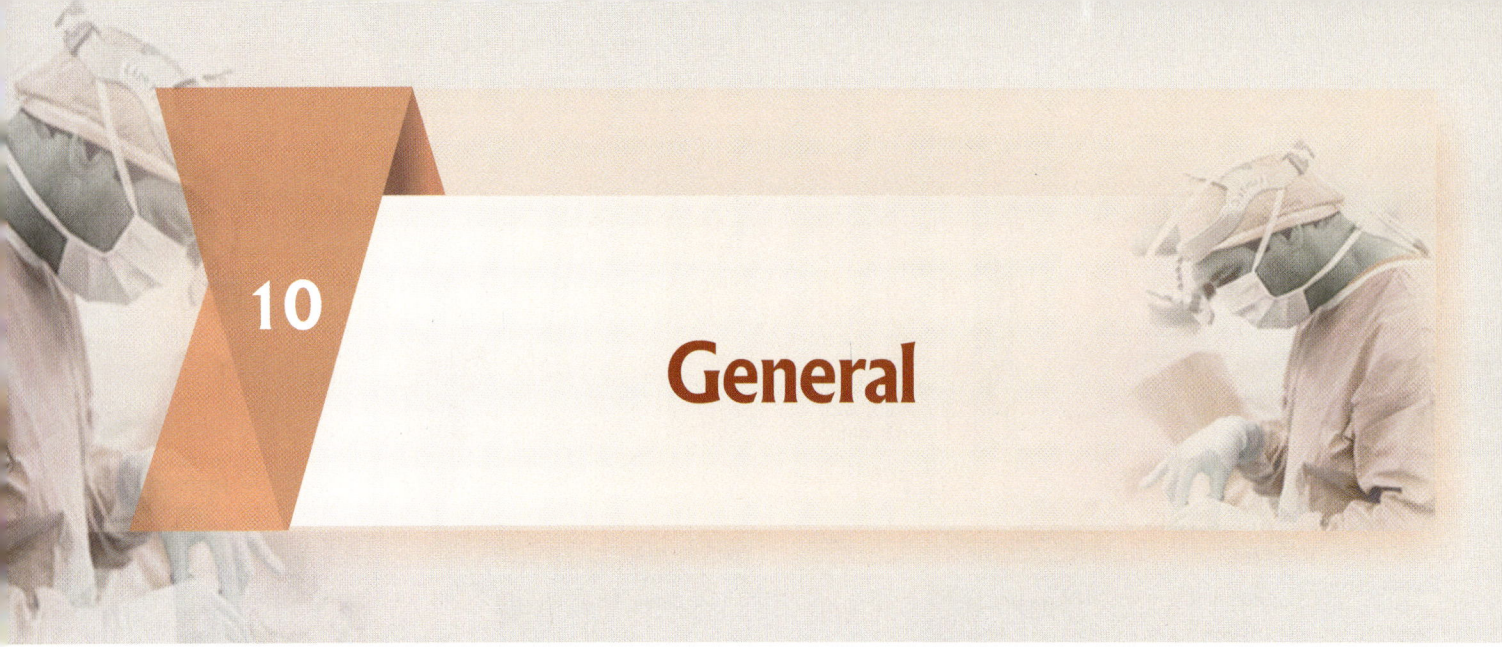

General

Surgical Anatomy

10.1.1 MESH REPAIR OF INGUINAL HERNIA

Indications

1. Presently, mesh-plasty for all symptomatic direct or indirect inguinal hernias.
2. Recurrent inguinal hernia
3. Where the fascia transversalis and adjacent structures are of insufficient quantity for anatomical repair.

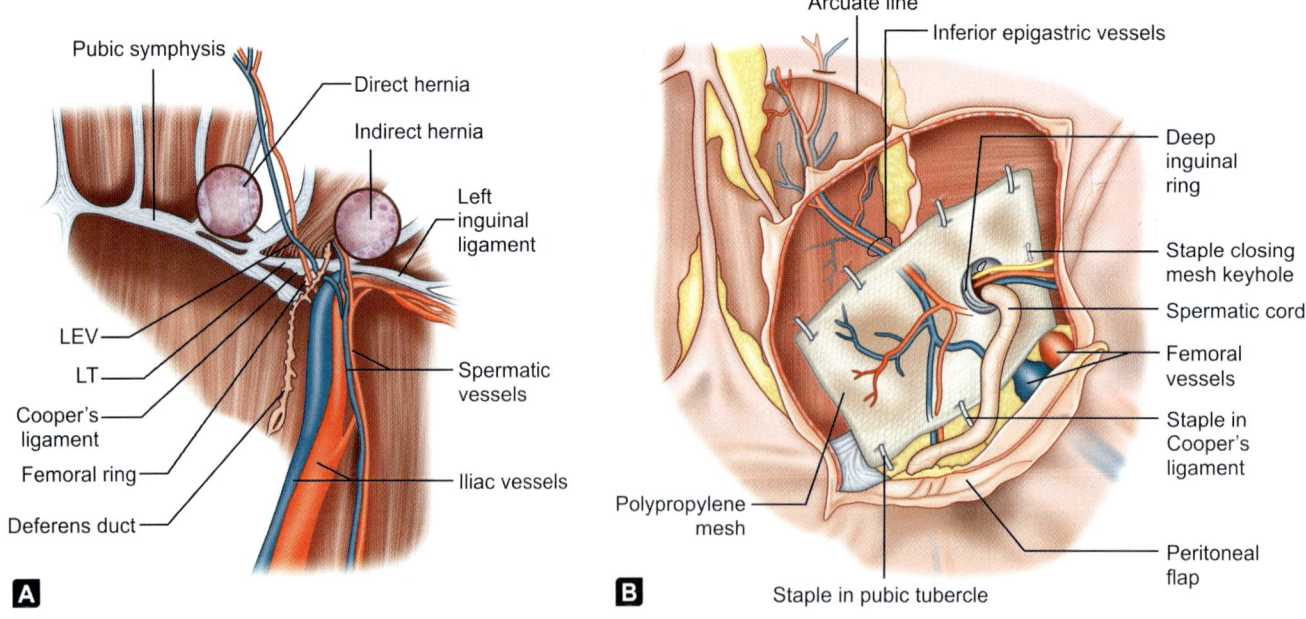

Anatomy of hernioplasty

Out of all relations, friends hold the best place—no commitments, no ego, no frustration, no break-ups. Just sharing the best and the worst.

Pitfalls

1. A missed indirect sac which may cause recurrence.
2. Mesh migration or curling may cause failure of hernia repair.
3. Technical failure causes immediate recurrence and tissue failure causes late recurrence.
4. Injury to spermatic cord and its contents, ilioinguinal nerve, etc.
5. Chance of infection in the mesh.

Preoperative Preparation

1. Advice for weight reduction
2. Correct constipation
3. Correct the underlying causes of strain, like chronic cough, benign prostatic hyperplasia (BPH), urethral stricture.
4. Avoid vigorous exercise, etc.

Procedures

1. *Anesthesia:* Spinal/regional block/field block
2. *Position:* Supine
3. *Incision:* The incision is made 2.5 cm above and parallel to the medial two-thirds of the inguinal ligament.

Remember: More horizontally placed skin crease incision will give a more cosmetic scar mark.

Step 1: The skin and superficial fascia are incised in the line of incision. One or more superficial epigastric veins cross the line are to be cauterized or ligated.

Step 2: External oblique aponeurosis identified the fascia covering it. "Gallaudet's fascia" to be incised along with the aponeurosis in the direction of its fibers. Preserve ilioinguinal nerve.

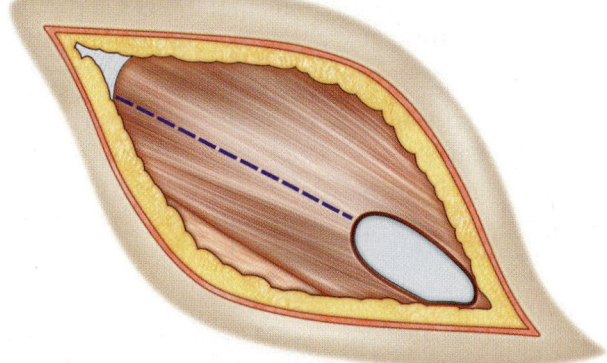

Step 3: Take the cord out by putting two index fingers at the level of pubic tubercle from both sides. Now, encircle the cord and its posterior mesentery containing genitofemoral nerve with a tape. Dissect the cord adequately to encircle all around.

Step 4: Identification of sac: Simply incise the cremester muscle (do not divide) in the direction of its fibers (longitudinally) to see the cord structure clearly. An indirect sac, if present, is found anteromedial to the

External oblique aponeurosis is to cut in the direction of its fibers

cord. It appears as a pearly white structure. The cord structures are then separated from the sac as far as the neck. Care to be taken to save the testicular vessels and the vas anyway. (The vas is very vulnerable to injury as it lies separate from other cord structures and closely applied to the sac.) Continue the dissection till the neck of the sac is exposed. Visualization of preperitoneal lappet, a cresentic thickening of peritoneum, is the limit of adequate dissection.

Step 5: Reduction of the content of the sac: The fundus of the sac is held with two artery forceps and opened. Put your finger inside the sac and adhered content to be separated and reduced inside the abdominal cavity.

Look for any thickening at medial and lateral wall to exclude additional sliding component to the hernia.

We never know which step will bring turning point in our life. So, keep working without expecting anything. Because happiness comes when it is most unexpected.

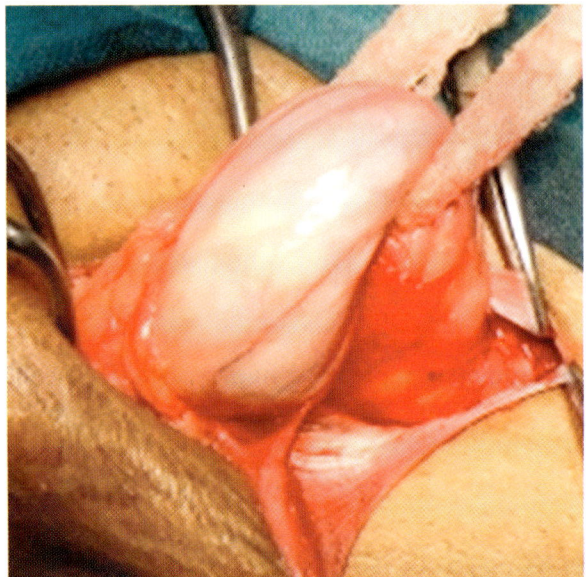
Separation of spermatic cord

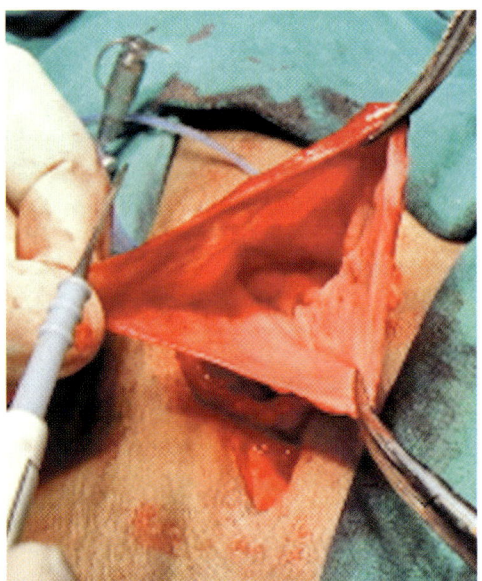
Content of the sac is reduced

Step 6: Transfixation at the neck and excise the sac: Now transfix at the or just above the neck, caring that underlying bowel is not in the transfixation suture and excise the sac.

Step 7: Look for the internal ring: If it is too patulous or wide 2 cm or more, do Lytle's repair, i.e. anatomical repair by plicating fascia transversalis to tightening the ring to its normal diameter.

Step 8: Look for the weakness of the floor by palpation, assess the weakness of the floor of inguinal canal. If direct hernial defect is present, reduce the content of the hernia with attached part of the sac into the preperitoneal space. Take a purse string suture with 3-0 prolene or PDS at the base of the unopened sac and tie the suture to close the defect. Or do an anatomical repair with the surrounding fascias to close the defect. (Many old surgeons prefer it but with the placement of mesh—practically it is not mandatory to close the defect anatomically.)

Step 9: Mesh repair (described by Lichtenstein): A mesh (usually prolene mesh) 8 × 6 cm is divided at lateral one-third and medial two-thirds approximately 4 cm to take the cord out. The cut edge, i.e. the split arch, will be placed toward the deep ring. The first suture (1-0 prolene) to take at pubic tubercle, keeping minimum 2 cm mesh ahead proximally to cover the myopectineal orifice of Fruchaud to prevent the recurrence.

The lateral edge of the mesh will be sutured with lower edge of pubic tubercle, lacunar ligament and the inguinal ligament, intermittently or continuously, with 3-0 polypropylene (prolene) beyond the deep ring. So that it covers the deep ring. The medial edge is sutured with conjoint tendon intermittently. Now, two split arches of the mesh are crossed over each

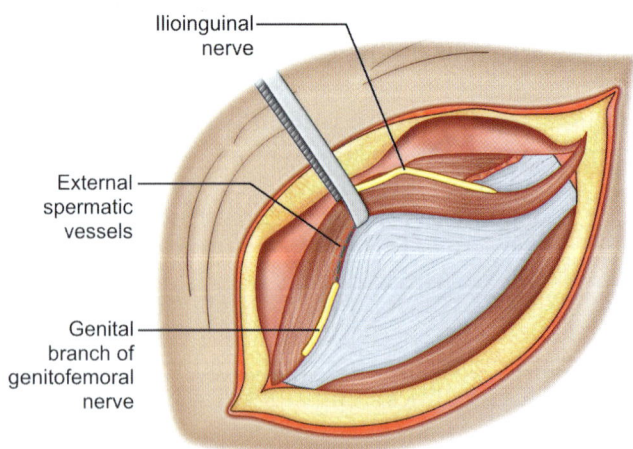

Ilioinguinal nerve

External spermatic vessels

Genital branch of genitofemoral nerve

Lichtenstein tension free mesh repair

other, creating a new deep ring through which the spermatic cord comes out, and suture it and fix it then. The mesh is placed the way that it is totally tension free. So, it is named as Lichtenstein tension-free mesh reapir.

Step 10: Hemostasis to be achieved completely. (Usually drain is not routinely required unless extensive dissection is there or trainee perfomed the surgery in his initial stage.) External oblique is closed with 3-0 vicryl. (Prolene can be used too, where more strength is required.) Subcutaneous layer to be closed with 3-0 vicryl and skin with 3-0 prolene, silk, nylon or stapler.

Complications

i. Chance of infection although rate is low in the present era of antibiotics.
ii. Mesh migration, though rare, into femoral vein, spermatic cord, has been reported.
iii. Recurrence rate is 1–5% till now with an expert hand too.

10.2 LAPAROSCOPIC INGUINAL HERNIA REPAIR

i. TEP (total extraperitoneal) repair
ii. TAPP (transabdominal preperitoneal) repair

10.2.1 TOTAL EXTRAPERITONEAL (TEP) MESH REPAIR

Anatomy for TEP

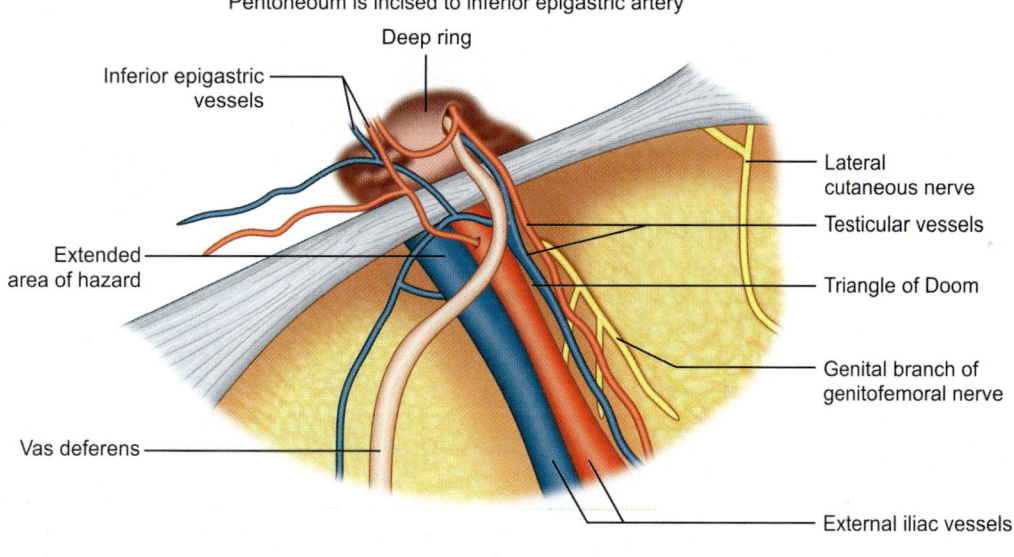

Basic anatomy for TEP

Indications

1. Bilateral inguinal hernia
2. Recurrent hernia has two noncontroversial indications for laparoscopic repair. (Bilateral hernias—they can be repaired simultaneously without additional incisions or trocar site. And in recurrent hernia—laparoscopic repair is the choice because it avoids the previous surgical field and repair can be done through healthy tissues and thereby the results are better.)

Life is like a cotton. Do not make it heavier by dipping in water of sorrow. But, make it lighter by blowing in joy of air. Enjoy every moment of life.

Pitfalls

1. Injury to inferior epigastric artery, external iliac vessels, obturator nerve, genitofemoral nerve, bladder, vas, etc.
2. Hernia may be missed, thereby, recurs immediately.
3. Inadequate fixation of mesh and failure of repair.

Preoperative Preparation

1. Insert Foley's catheter to decompress the bladder just prior to operation.
2. Injectable antibiotics at induction.

Procedure for TEP

1. General anesthesia
2. *Position:* Supine and arms to be kept on arm rest both sides.
3. Trendelenburg position allows the bowel to keep away from pelvis. Single video monitor at the foot of the table.
4. The surgeon stands opposite side of the operating hernia.
5. Cleaning and draping
   [TEP is now the standard technique and has virtually replaced the transabdominal preperitoneal (TAPP)].

Procedures

Step 1: Make the skin incision 10–12 mm just below the umbilicus. Open anterior rectus sheath ipsilateral side and retract the muscle laterally to expose posterior rectus sheath and with the same retraction, sufflate the preperitoneal space. Put your index finger over the posterior rectus sheath and gently develop a space.

Step 2: Insert a transparent balloon-tipped trocar (Usually, surgeons make this balloon-tipped trocar with two fingers of a glove.) into the space toward the symphysis pubis. Place the laparoscope in this trocar. Under direct vision, inflat the balloon with 150 mL of normal saline and keep it for a minute to create an extraperitoneal space and remove the balloon after removing the normal saline first.

Step 3: Two additional trocar to be placed. One 5 mm just above the symphysis pubis and another 5 mm in between the two. Place these trocars after initial dissection and under direct vision.

Step 4: Camera is being used through the umbilical trocar and laparoscopic dissecting and retracting instruments through the two 5 mm trocars. And, preperitoneal space to be dissected carefully.

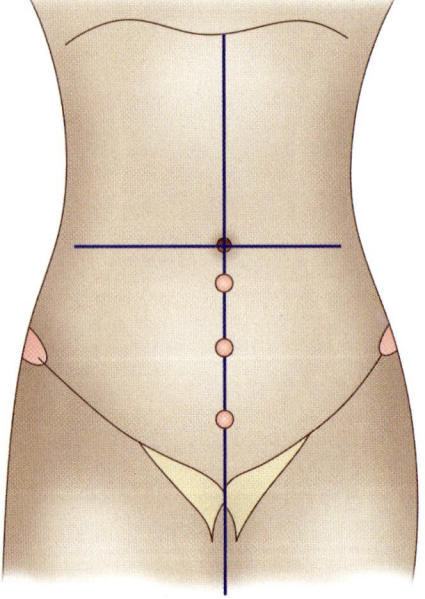

Ports placement for TEP

Step 5: Expose the Cooper's ligament from the symphysis pubis to just medial to the iliac vessels. This will expose the Hesselbach triangle posteriorly. During this dissection, hernial sac will be identified and reduced, taking care the aberrant obturator artery which usually crosses the Cooper's ligament near the femoral canal. Dissect the preperitoneal space all aspects, by pushing peritoneum and detach it from ventrolateral abdominal wall.

Step 6: Identify all the vital structures: "Triangle of Doom", and its contents, myopectineal orifice of Fruchaud, gonadal vessels, vas deferens, epigastric vessels, internal ring, all are to be saved during dissection. Look for

---

A generous heart will quickly become a precious heart.

complete reduction of the content of hernia sac. If it is not done easily, neck of the sac can be divided. Peel the peritoneum off the cord structures to complete the dissection of myopectineal orifice.

Step 7: A prolene mesh/double mesh (vicryl + prolene)/three-dimension (3D) mesh measuring 10 × 15 cm is rolled and placed through 10 mm camera trocar. Now, the mesh is unrolled and spread over the myopectineal orifice. Fix the mesh with tacker at Cooper's ligament and at ventral and lateral abdominal wall (do not put any tacks dorsal to iliopubic track laterally to avoid multiple nerve injury).

Step 8: Achieve complete hemostasis. Clean the preperitoneal space and mesh with normal saline. Remove all the trocars and desufflate the preperitoneal space. Close anterior rectus sheath with vicryl (2-0). Close the skin with 3-0 nylon or 2-0 silk.

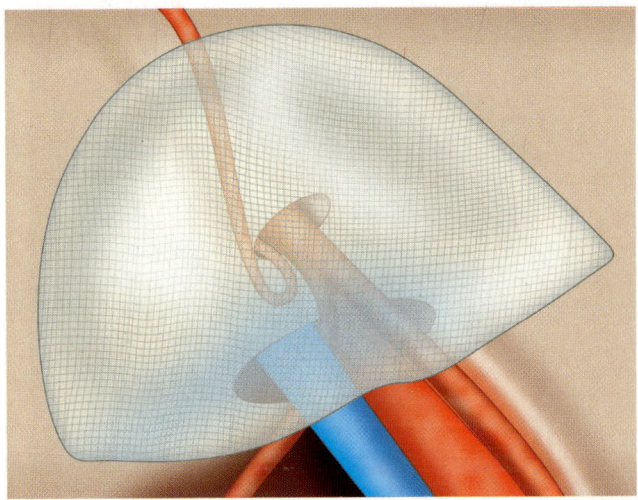

Placement of 3D mesh

10.2.2 TRANSABDOMINAL PREPERITONEAL (TAPP) MESH REPAIR

Procedures

1. General anesthesia
2. Position: Supine and arms to be kept on arm rest both sides
3. Trendelenburg position allows the bowel to keep away from pelvis. Single video monitor at the foot of the table
4. The surgeon stands opposite side of the operating hernia
5. Cleaning and draping.

Step 1: First trocar 10–12 mm is to place just below umbilicus. Laparoscope is inserted through the umbilical trocar and creates pneumoperitoneum. Make two additional ports 10 mm each on either side at the level of umbilicus, lateral to the rectus sheath under direct vision.

Step 2: Next, inspect both inguinal regions, identify the medial and median umbilical ligaments, the lateral umbilical fold. Median umbilical ligament (remnant of Urachus) may be divided for better exposure. The hernia is visible as an out pouching of the peritoneum.

Step 3: Incise the peritoneum along a line 2.5 cm above the superior edge of the hernial defect, from anterosuperior iliac spine to median umbilical ligament. Mobilize the peritoneal flap inferiorly and superiorly.

Step 4: Identifying the vital structures: Identify epigastric vessels, lower part of rectus abdominis muscle, symphysis pubis, Cooper's ligament, iliopubic tract. Dissect inferiorly caring femoral branch of genitofemoral nerve and lateral femoral cutaneous nerve. Now, skeletonize the cord

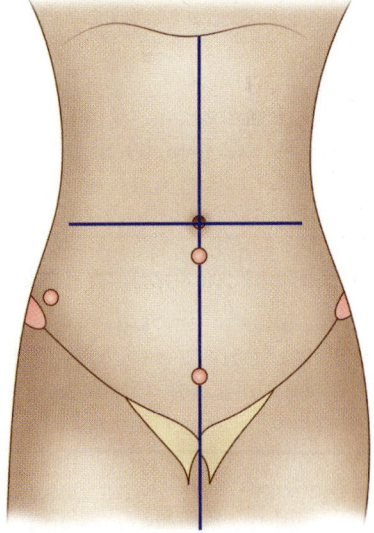

Ports placement for TAAP

structure too. Indirect hernia sac to be mobilized from the cord structure. If it is not separated easily, just divide the sac just distal to the deep ring, leaving the distal sac in situ. By gentle traction, direct sac is reduced easily along with preperitoneal fat from the hernial orifice.

If you win something without any trouble that's just a victory but if you win it through lot of troubles and hassles, it can create a history.

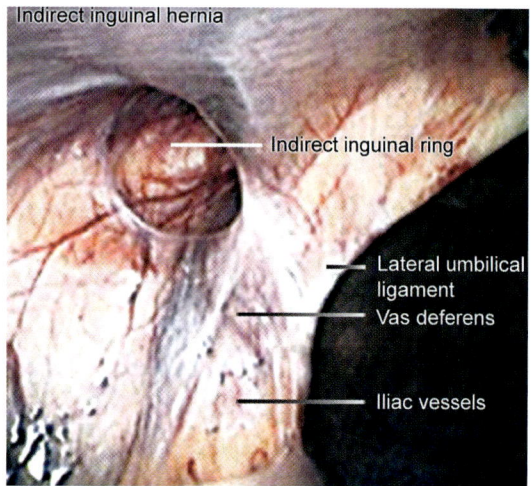

Important anatomical landmarks of inguinal hernia repair

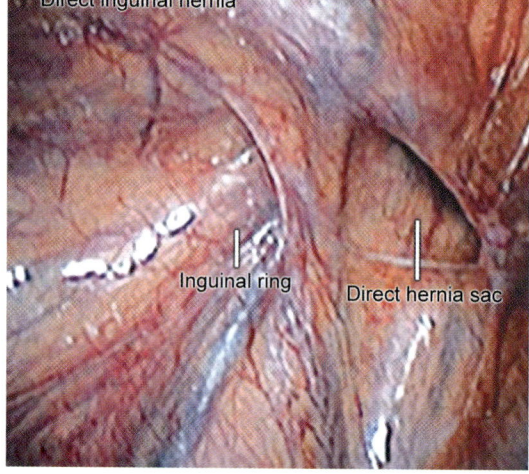

Laparoscopic view of inguinal hernia

Step 5: Mesh placement: A mesh 10 × 6 cm can cover the defect of direct hernia, deep ring and femoral ring in one side. Roll the mesh into a compact cylinder and pass through umbilical trocar. Temporary ties around the cylinder can facilitate handling. Keep the cylinder inferiorly unroll the mesh toward anterior abdominal wall. Tucking the corner of the mesh underneath the peritoneal flap (place the mesh over the cord structure, no need to make it slit). Good cover all the hernial defects, specially myopectineal orifice of Fruchaud. The mesh may be placed simply or can be stapled along the superior border of the mesh and at the medial part of contralateral pubic tubercle and laterally along the superior border of anterosuperior iliac spine (ASIS). Staple the inferior border to ligament of Cooper. And close to pubic tubercle or instead of stapler simple running intracorporeal suture with 3-0 vicryl (the aim is to isolate the mesh from the viscera).

Step 6: Excise the extra-mesh and close the peritoneal flap over the mesh with sutures or staples without any tension.

Step 7: Hemostasis to be ensured. Remove all the trocars. Desufflate pneumoperitoneum. Close the rectus sheath with 2-0 vicryl. Skin is closed with 3-0 nylon. Bilateral hernias may be repaired using one long transverse peritoneal incision from one ASIS to another. Two pieces of mesh 10 × 6 cm each are preferable as it is easier to manipulate, bladder function is preserved.

Complications for both TEP and TAPP

1. Vascular injury: Inferior epigastric, and gonadal vessels are prone to be injured.
2. Urinary tract infection (UTI), urinary retention, hematuria, etc. due to catheterization, preperitoneal dissection, general anesthesia (GA), intravenous (IV) fluids, etc.
3. Nerve injury: Femoral branch of genitofemoral nerve, lateral femoral nerve, lateral cutaneous nerve of thigh may be injured during the procedure.
4. Bladder injury: More common with the patient of previous prostate surgery. Otherwise bladder injury is one of the common complications of laparoscopic hernia repair.
5. Injury to vas deferens, testicular vessels.
6. Mesh migration and failure of hernia repair, i.e. recurrence. Erosion of abdominal viscera, etc.
7. Pelvic or pubic ostitis as a result of staple placement directly into the bone. And last not the least is wound infection.

	Difference between TEP and TAPP	
Criteria	*TEP*	*TAPP*
• Entry into peritoneum	No	Yes
• Anatomy	Not familiar usually	Familiar
• Detection of bilateral sacs	Needs clear dissection	Easier to identify
• For irreducible or sliding hernia	Difficult procedure	Preferred procedure
• Bowel injury vascular injury	Rare	Common
• Port site hernia	Very rare	Common
• Conversions	More common	Less common
• Mesh fixation	Only medial fixation is enough	Proper all side fixation is required
• Recurrence	Same 1–5%	Same 1–5%
• Return to work	Early and similar	Early and similar
• Learning curve	Very steep	Relatively less steep

10.2.3 VENTRAL HERNIA REPAIR (INCISIONAL, EPIGASTRIC, PARAUMBILICAL, ETC.)

Indications

1. Early repair of a small ventral hernia as it is a simple procedure.(<3 cm defect, anatomical repair is acceptable)
2. Symptomatic ventral hernia which brings the patient to you.

Pitfalls

1. Many time surrounding tissues are too weak to hold the sutures
2. Excessive tension on the suture line
3. Failure to achieve complete repair
4. May be multiple defects
5. Postoperative hematoma and infection.

Preoperative Preparation

1. Ultrasonography (USG) abdominal wall to see the size of the defect or multiple defects
2. Nasogastric (NG) tubes, antibiotics, etc.

Procedure

1. General anesthesia
2. Supine position
3. Cleaning and draping.
4. *Incision:* Usually, a midline vertical incision is made when the defect is 4 cm and more or multiple defects and mesh repair is desirable. Many surgeons make transverse elliptical incision even in a large defect. Three centimeters or less than 3 cm defect, transverse incision is enough and anatomical repair is acceptable.

Incision

Make an elliptical incision along the axis of the hernia ring and go down to the sac.

Step 1: Dissection of sac: Dissect all around the sac and the skin away from the sac and expose entire circumference of the sac. And make it free from the sheath all sides completely. Remove the pad of fat from the base of the hernial sac.

Nature does not hurry, yet everything is accomplished.

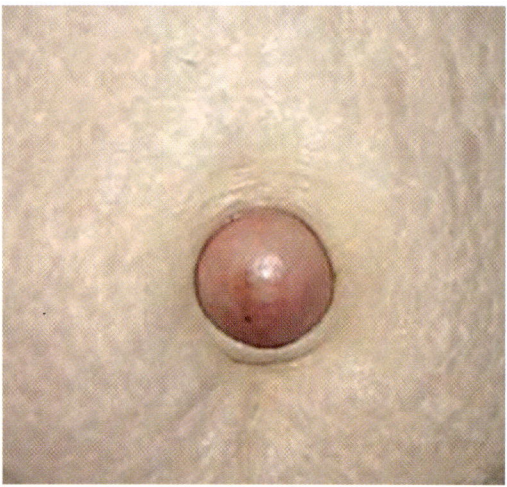

Hernial sac is visible after opening through elliptical incision

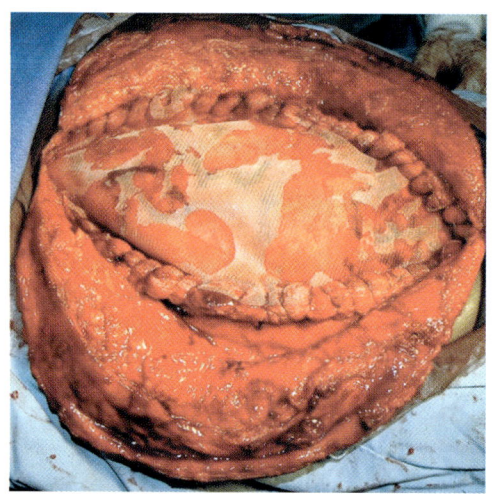

Sandwich repair of ventral hernia

Step 2: Exposure of the surrounding sheath: Minimum 2 cm width of sheath from the margin of the defect to be exposed by retracting the skin flap all around the defect.

Step 3: Resecting the hernial sac: Now, the hernial sac to be separated from the underlying coils of intestine after incising the sac along the apex of it. Sac to be preserved in case of onlay mesh repair no incision made. And intestine or omentum, the content of the sac is reduced to abdominal cavity. (In case of small sac, usually content is reduced back to abdominal cavity along the sac). Now, total sac and all around 2/3 cm width of peritoneum will be free from all kind of adhesions.

Step 4: Mesh repair: Sandwich repair (two pieces of mesh): The size should be 2 cm larger than the defect. One sheet of mesh is placed inside the abdominal cavity and hold it with mosquito after spreading the omentum below the defect to protect underlying intestine from the mesh. And other one on the defect and 2 cm beyond over the sheath. Take 2-0 prolene pass through the top sheet then go through full thickness of the abdominal wall and then go to the deep sheet and returns as a mattress stitch and again through the full thickness of abdominal and finally through the top sheet and tie the knot.

(Sandwich repair is feasible only when the omentum is present adequately and it is usually for larger or recurrent ventral hernia and in an obese patient. If omentum is not adequate underlying, non-erosive vicryl mesh may be placed inside and outside the prolene mesh.)

Onlay mesh repair: When sandwich repair is not suitable as mentioned above onlay mesh repair is preferable.

- Here, hernial sac is preserved
- Excess sac may be excised and repair with 2-0 vicryl
- Place the prolene mesh over the defect and 2 cm beyond over the sheath then fix the mesh with 1-0/2-0 prolene, to the dense fibrous tissue at the margin of the defect continuous or intermittently. Same stitches are taken with the sheath all around with 2-0 prolene.

Mesh fixation over the defect

It is not important in life that who is ahead or behind us. What truly matters in life is—who is besides us.

Step 5: Hemostasis to be achieved completely and insert a closed suction drain through a puncture wound and close subcutaneous tissue with vicryl 2-0 to obliterate dead space. Close skin with 2-0/3-0 nylon.

Preoperative Care

- Prophylactic broad-spectrum antibiotics, like II/III generation cephalosporin, aminoglycoside for 3 doses.
- Promote early ambulation
- Remove the drain after 5 days or drainage is less than 30 mL.

Complications and Management

1. *Wound infections:* With prophylactic antibiotics, it is rare. If infection develops in subcutaneous tissue, give suitable antibiotics as per culture sensitivity report. No need to remove the mesh as you know monofilament like prolene mesh usually resists infections, if the skin incision is properly opened for drainage.
    - Keep the moist guaze pack daily till the granulation tissue appears over the mesh.
    - The secondary suturing may be required or if the gap is small allow it to heal by secondary intention.
2. *Hematoma:* Small hematoma absorbs so observe. Large hematoma or progressing—evacuation and secondary closure.

Laparoscopic ventral hernia repair is the trend nowadays. The ports placement of laparoscopic ventral hernia repair has given in figure below.

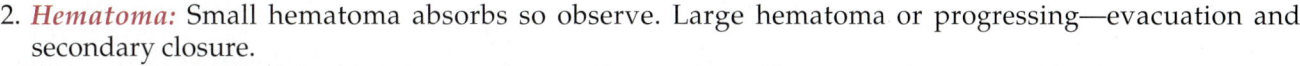

Overline tissue is closed with continuous suture

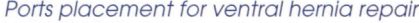
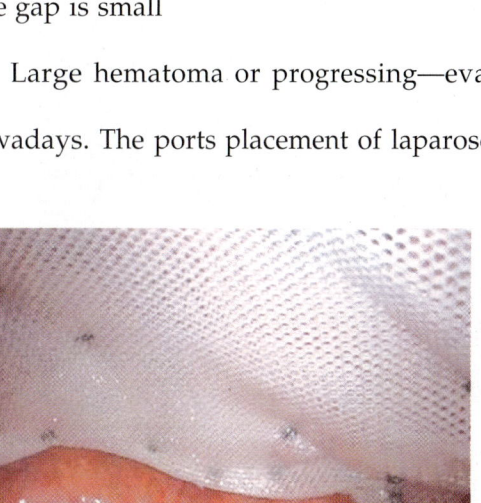

Ports placement for ventral hernia repair   *Laparoscopic mesh placement for ventral hernia*

10.3 SPECIALLY FOR UNDERGRADUATE STUDENTS

10.3.1 OPERATIONS FOR HYDROCELE

Indications

- Moderate to large size hydrocele
- Symptomatic and psychosocial reason.

Try to become a man of value, rather than a man of success because valuable man is always superior than a successful man.

Pitfalls

- Hemorrhage: During and after surgery
- Hematoma formation.

Procedure

1. Supine position
2. Local/spinal anesthesia
3. Cleaning and draping (If local anesthesia is given, take 1% lignocaine HCl and infiltrate into the spermatic cord and along the longitudinal line of incision.)
4. Incision: A vertical incision is made 2–3 cm parallel to the median raphe of the scrotum.

Step 1: The incision is deepened to cut the dartos muscle, the scrotal fascia, external spermatic, cremasteric and internal spermatic fascia—layer by layer and reach to the sac.

Step 2: By finger dissection, a space is created between the dartos and the sac of tunica vaginalis.

Step 3: Make a nick over the avascular part of the sac, caring the testis, epididymis and cord structures and all fluid to be drained out.

Step 4: The sac is then cut longitudinally and testis is delivered from the sac of tunica vaginalis. The cut margin of the sac is now everted around the testis and sutured behind the testis and lower part of spermatic cord.

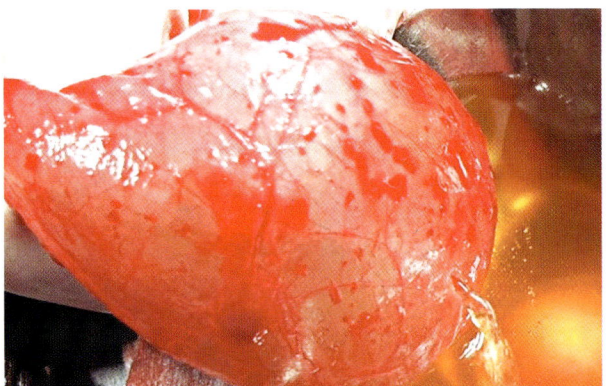

Hydrocele fluid is being drained out

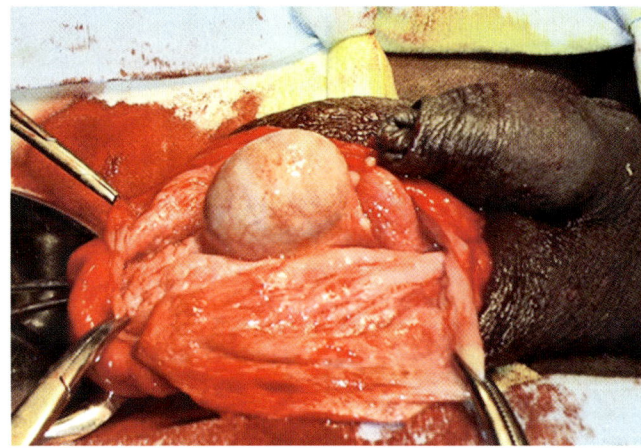

Testis is delivered out from tunica vaginalis

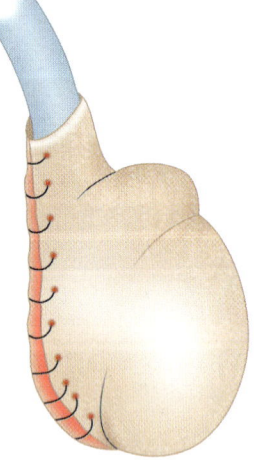

Sac everted and sutured behind the testis and lower part of spermatic cord

Only happiness does not follow the rule of mathematics. When you divide it to others it never reduced rather it multiplies always.

Step 5: Hemostasis to be achieved meticulously and the everted sac is placed in the subdartos pouch. The cut edges of the dartos muscle are sutured with 2-0 absorbable suture like chromic cat gut or vicryl. Put a corrugated rubber drain. The skin is closed with interrupted polymide or silk suture. A coconut bandage must be applied. (In case of bilateral hydrocele, the incision is made either on the median raphe or a separate incision is made parallel to the median raphe opposite to the first incision.)

10.3.2 LORD'S PROCEDURE

Indication

Small size hydrocele.

Procedures

1. Supine position
2. Local/spinal anesthesia
3. Cleaning and draping (If local anesthesia is given, take 1% lignocaine HCl and infiltrate into the spermatic cord and along the longitudinal line of incision.)
4. *Incision:* A vertical incision is made 2–3 cm parallel to the median raphe of the scrotum.

Step 1: The incision is deepened to cut the dartos muscle, the scrotal fascia, external spermatic, cremasteric and internal spermatic fascia—layer by layer and reach to the sac.

Step 2: By finger dissection, a space is created between the dartos and the sac of tunica vaginalis.

Step 3: Make a nick over the avascular part of the sac, caring the testis, epididymis and cord structures and all fluids to be drained out.

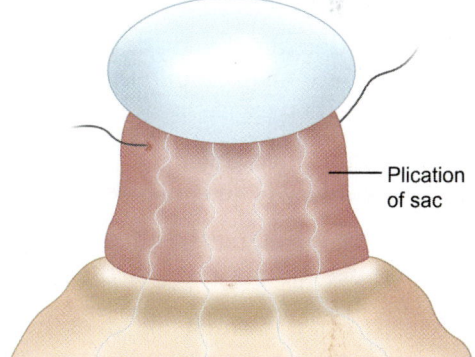
Plication of sac

Step 4: The sac is to cut longitudinally and the cut margins of tunica vaginalis are then plicated with tunica albuginea interrupted suture in such a way that there will be no empty space to accumulate fluid. When these sutures are tied, the edges of the sac will lie as a cuff behind the testis.

Plication of sac to obliterate dead space

Step 5: The dartos and the scrotal skin are drawn back all over the testis. Hemostasis to be achieved completely. Place a corrugated rubber drain and the skin is closed with 3-0 polymide or silk suture as usual.

10.3.3 CIRCUMCISION

Indications

- Congenital and acquired phimosis
- For religious purposes: Muslims/Jews
- Paraphimosis: When cannot be reduced.

Procedure

1. Supine position
2. Local anesthesia or field block for adult and general anesthesia for children
3. Cleaning and draping.

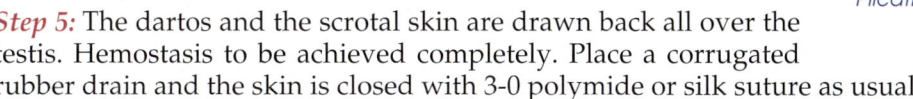

To establish order around oneself helps to bring order within oneself.

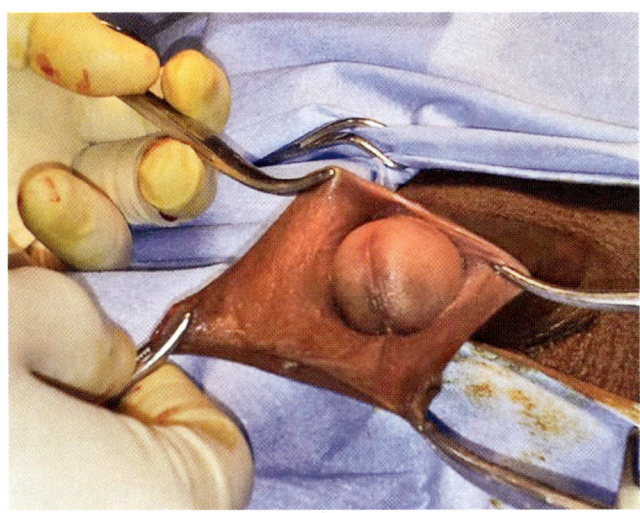

Procedure of circumcision

Step 1: Hold the prepuce at 12, 3, 6 and 9 O'clock positions with mosquito forceps. Adhesiolysis between the glans and prepuce to be done.

Step 2: A dorsal cut is made in the prepuce with scissors extending 5 mm beyond the corona glandis. The prepuce is to cut all around the penis. At the ventral aspect, frenulum to be tied with 3-0 vicryl to tie the small artery and then excise the whole prepuce.

Step 3: Evert the skin edges and control all bleeding points with 3-0 vicryl or cat gut suture. (Never use the bipolar cautery to control bleeding points. Monopolar may be used.)

Step 4: After complete hemostasis, use 3-0/4-0 absorbable suture is used to oppose inner and outer cut edges of the prepuce. Initially appose the layers at 12, 3, 6, 9 O'clock positions and then in between of all clocks.

Step 5: Keep paraffin gauge over the wound and apply light pressure bandage.

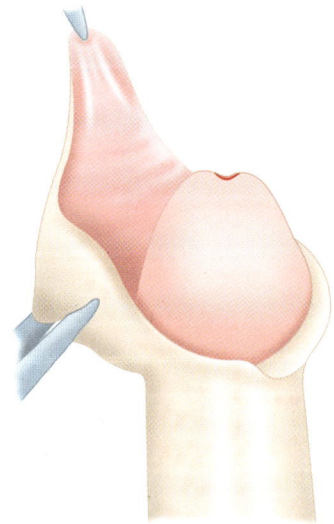

Prepuce is cut all around

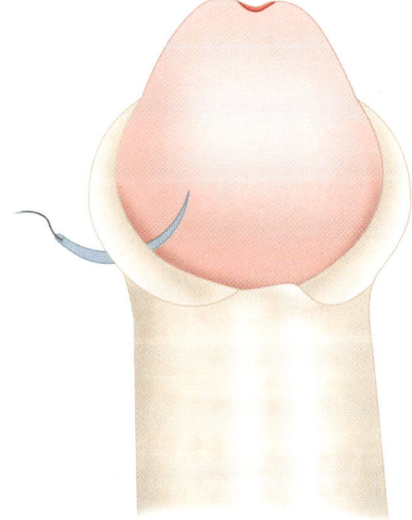

Suturing of the cut edges of prepuce

To do with care all that one does is the basis of all progress.

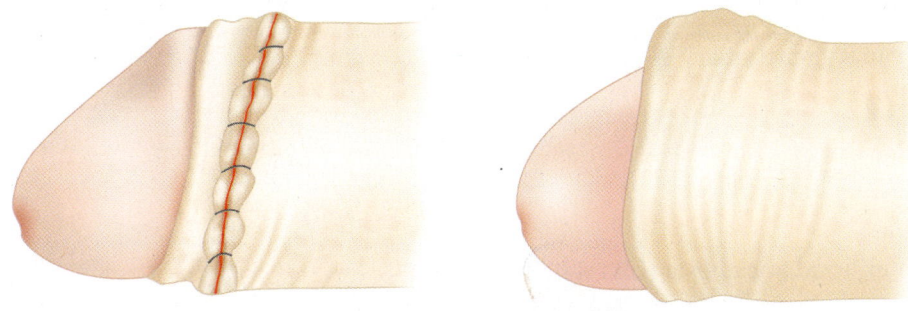

Completion of circumcision

10.3.4 HEMORRHOIDS (PILES)

Surgical Anatomy (Open Surgery (Milligan-Morgan))

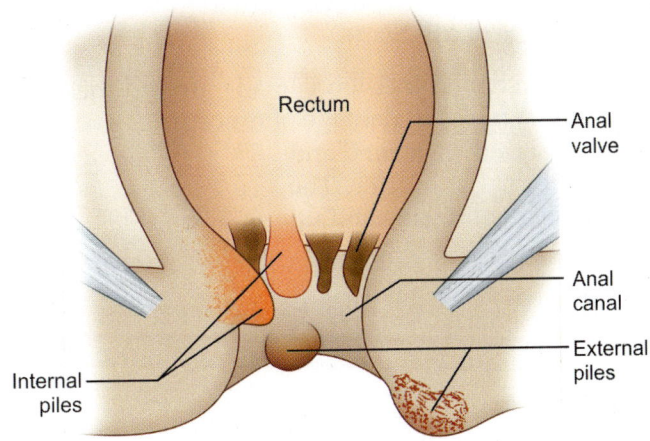

Anatomy of internal and external piles

Hemorrhoids are nothing but dilated internal venous plexus along with anal cushion enlargement. The primary piles are usually located at 3, 7, 11 O'clock positions. The secondary hemorrhoids are other than primary.
1. Internal hemorrhoids: Located above the dentate line covered by both transitional and columnar epithelium.
2. External hemorrhoids are located below the dentate line and covered by squamous epithelium.
3. Interoexternal hemorrhoids are the combination of both internal and external hemorrhoids.

Internal hemorrhoids are classified into four degrees:
1. First degree: Eearly dilation of venous plexus without any displacement.
2. Second degree: During defecation, it prolapses, but it reduces again automatically.
3. Third degree: Prolapses during defecation and requires manual reduction.
4. Fourth degree: Remains prolapsed all the time.
   Externally, the third and fourth looking the same but in third degree, manual reduction is possible but in fourth, the prolapse is permanent.

Indications

1. Third and fourth degree hemorrhoids
2. Failure of sclerotherapy/banding for first and second degree hemorrhoids

---

It is in the silence of your heart that the divine will speak to you and will guide you and will lead you to your goal.

Pitfalls

1. Hemorrhage: Primary reactionary even secondary
2. Retention of urine
3. Anal stenosis.

Procedure

1. Position: Lithotomy
2. Anesthesia: Spinal/local anesthesia (LA) with sedation.

Step 1: Position of all piles to be inspected first and to exclude any other abnormalities. Mild anal stretching to dilate the passage.

Step 2: Hold the skin at the side of piles with Allis or artery forceps just outside of mucocutaneous junction. Pull the skin so that the mucosa, covering the piles, will be protruding out and now hold the piles with another artery forceps and pull gently downward. It appears like a triangle (exposure triangle of Milligan).

Step 3: Incision and dissection: A "V" shaped incision is made around the pile and the lower edge of "V" would be toward the mucosa aiming to minimal damage of mucosa.

Now the hemorrhoidal mass is dissected all around and from the transverse fibers of the internal sphincter. The dissection to be continued beyond the dentate line and up to the apex of the piles.

Step 4: Ligation and excision: The pedicle of the piles is doubly ligated at the apex with silk/vicryl and excises it distal to the ligature.

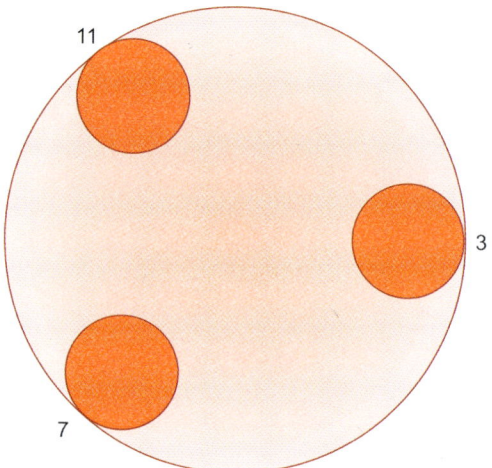

Typical location of primary piles

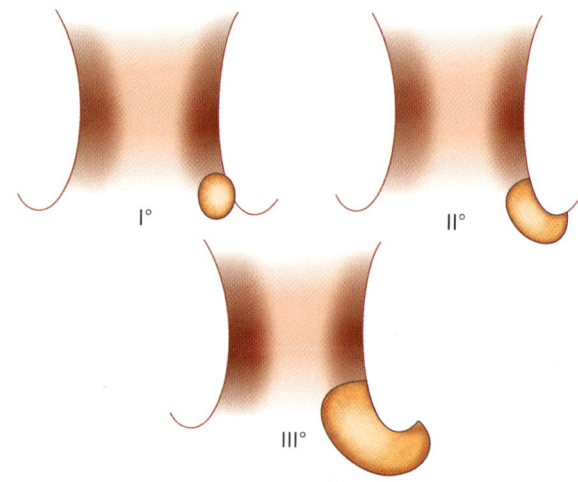

Different degrees of hemorrhoids

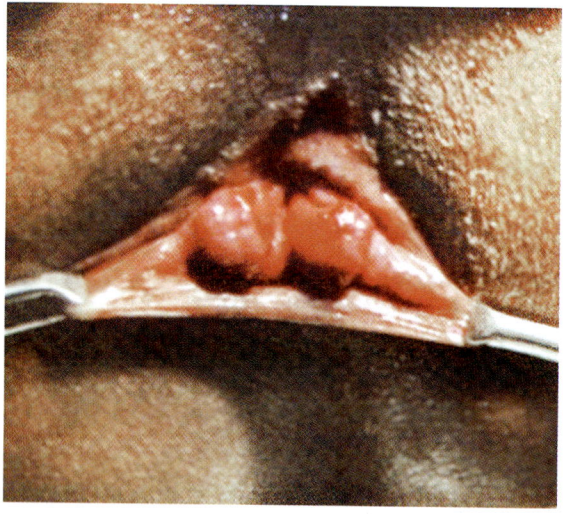

Excision of primary hemorrhoids

Never hold yourself solely responsible for any misfortune in life because no single raindrop is ever alone responsible for any flood.

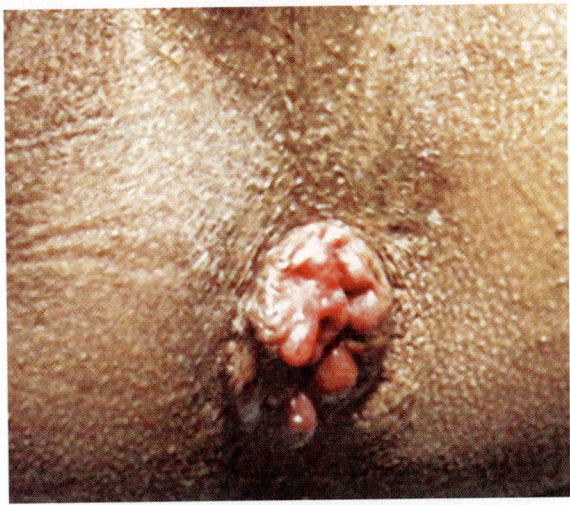

Excision of secondary hemorrhoids

The procedure to be repeated for the other major piles. Excise all the piles in such a way that mucosa and skin bridge in between must be preserved.

(Remember the dictum: Make a clover, the trouble is over.)

Step 5: Secondary hemorrhoids excision: Additional or secondary piles can be removed by dividing/undermining the skin bridges and excise the underlying dilated vein after ligating properly and stitch the trimmed flap back into position, i.e. in between mucosa and skin will be intact. Skin tag at anal verge may be excised too.

Step 6: Hemostasis: In each step, hemostasis to be achieved. An adequate pad of roller gauge, mixed with xylocaine gel and betadine lotion is to be placed at anal canal and be secured with T bandage.

Postoperative Care

1. Ask the patient to have Sitz bath after 24 hours and remove the pack. Then, advice for twice daily Sitz bath.
2. Analgesic, purgatives for 5–7 days.
3. Finger dilatation to prevent stenosis.

Complications and their Management

1. Pain: Adequate analgesis to be prescribed.
2. Reactionary hemorrhage: Padding if not controlled retransfixation is necessary.
3. Secondary hemorrhage: Antibiotics for 5 days. Blood transfusion, if required.
4. Retention of urine: The most common complication. To manage this remove pack→ privacy → hot and cold compression over hypogastrium → Catheterization for 2 more days.
5. Anal stenosis
   Prevention: Manual regular stretching with xylocaine gel application may prevent the stenosis. If developed→ stretching under anesthesia or anal dilatation by serial dilators.
6. Other complications are anal fissure formation, recurrence, etc.

It is only when we are not disturbed that we can always do the right thing at the right time in the right way.

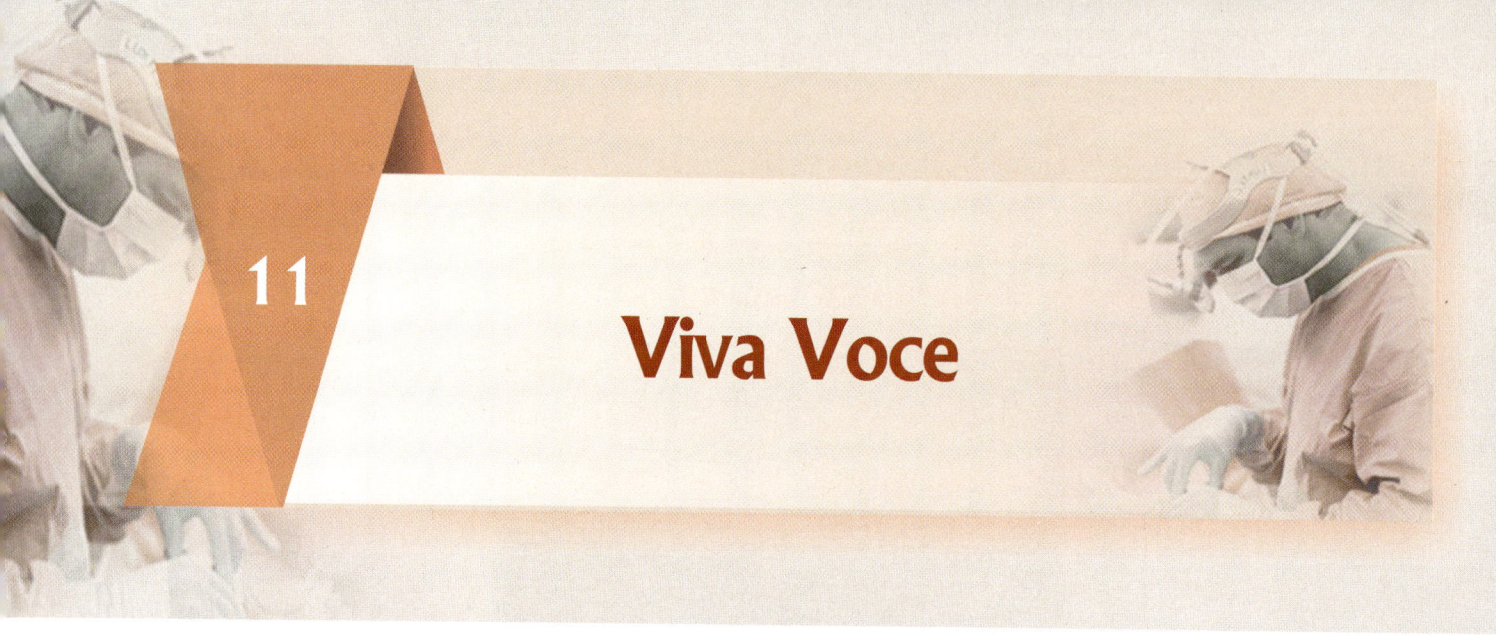

11

Viva Voce

COMMON X-RAYS

"We Diagnose What We Look for and Look for What We Know"

1. This is a posteroanterior (PA) view of chest X-ray and the X-ray of upper part of the abdomen showing free gas under right dome of diaphragm which is considered abnormal and under the left dome there is a fundal gas shadow of the stomach which is considered normal.

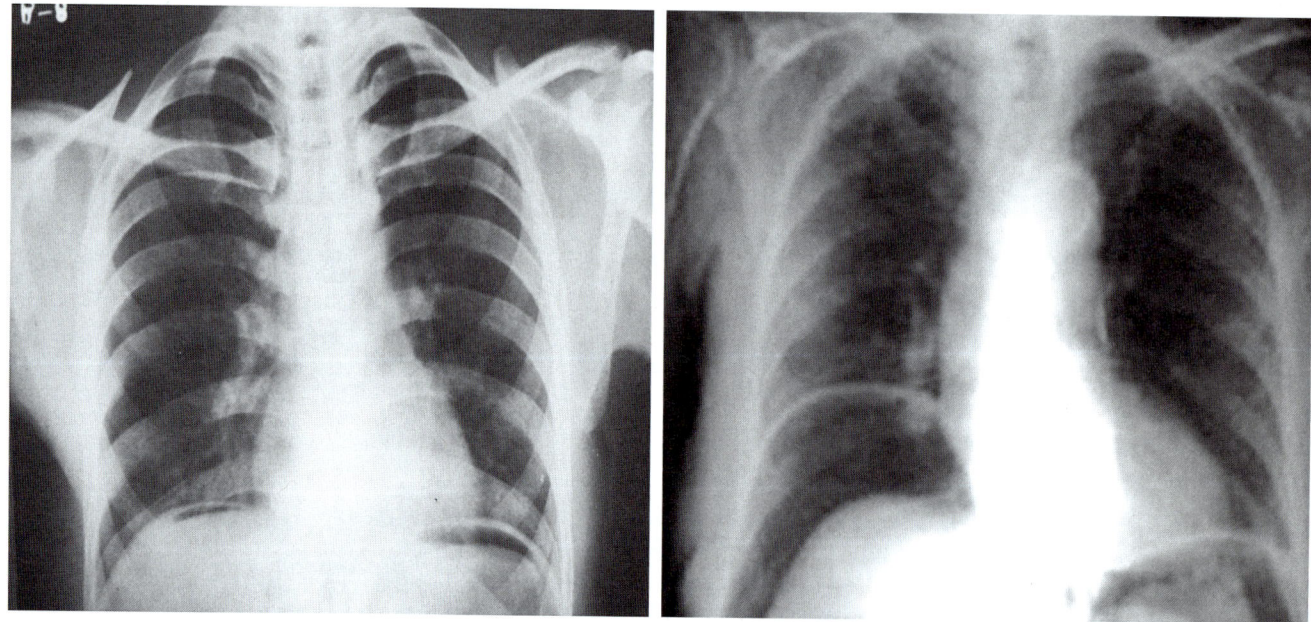

1. X-rays of free gas under right dome of diaphragm

Causes of Gas Under Diaphragm

a. Any abdominal hollo viscus perforation due to various reasons, like ulcers, trauma, malignancy, etc.

b. Postoperative period, like after laparotomy or laparoscopy. The gas under right dome of diaphragm considered normal for 3–7 days.

No one in this world is rich enough to buy his past. So, enjoy each moment before it gets beyond reach.

c. Raptured subdiaphragmatic abscess
d. Chilaiditi's syndrome in which colonic gas shadow comes in between diaphram and liver
e. After histosalpingography and following tubul insufflations for tubul patency.

Remember: Only 60–70% cases free gas under diaphragm is noticed following a hollow viscus perforation.

2. Chest X-ray, PA view, showing multiple fracture in the right side resulting in a flail chest along with the fracture of lateral end of right clavicle. There is a homogenous opacity in the right side of the chest with a horizontal fluid level and hypertranslucent right lung field and absence of bronchovascular markings are suggesting right-sided hemopneumothorax. There is a surgical emphysema noticed.

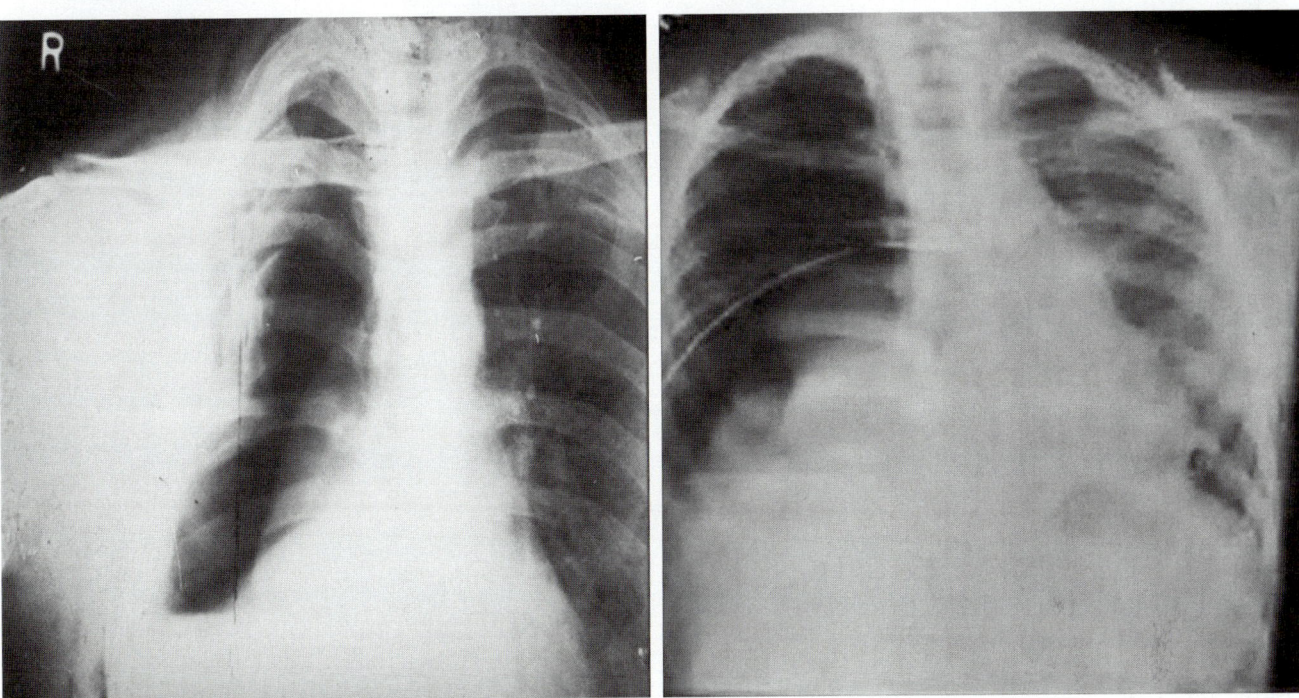

2. X-rays of chest injury

3. The X-ray chest, PA view, showing there are multiple rounded opacities in both lung fields called cannonball metastasis (*see* Fig. 3).

Cannonballs

Neoplasms with rich vascular supply draining directly into the systemic venous system often present in this fashion.

Miliary Pattern

This presentation is seen in patients with the following:
- Thyroid carcinoma
- Renal cell carcinoma
- Sarcoma of the bone.

Be in today, believe in today, behave in today, be alive in today, because yesterday died for today and tomorrow takes birth from today.

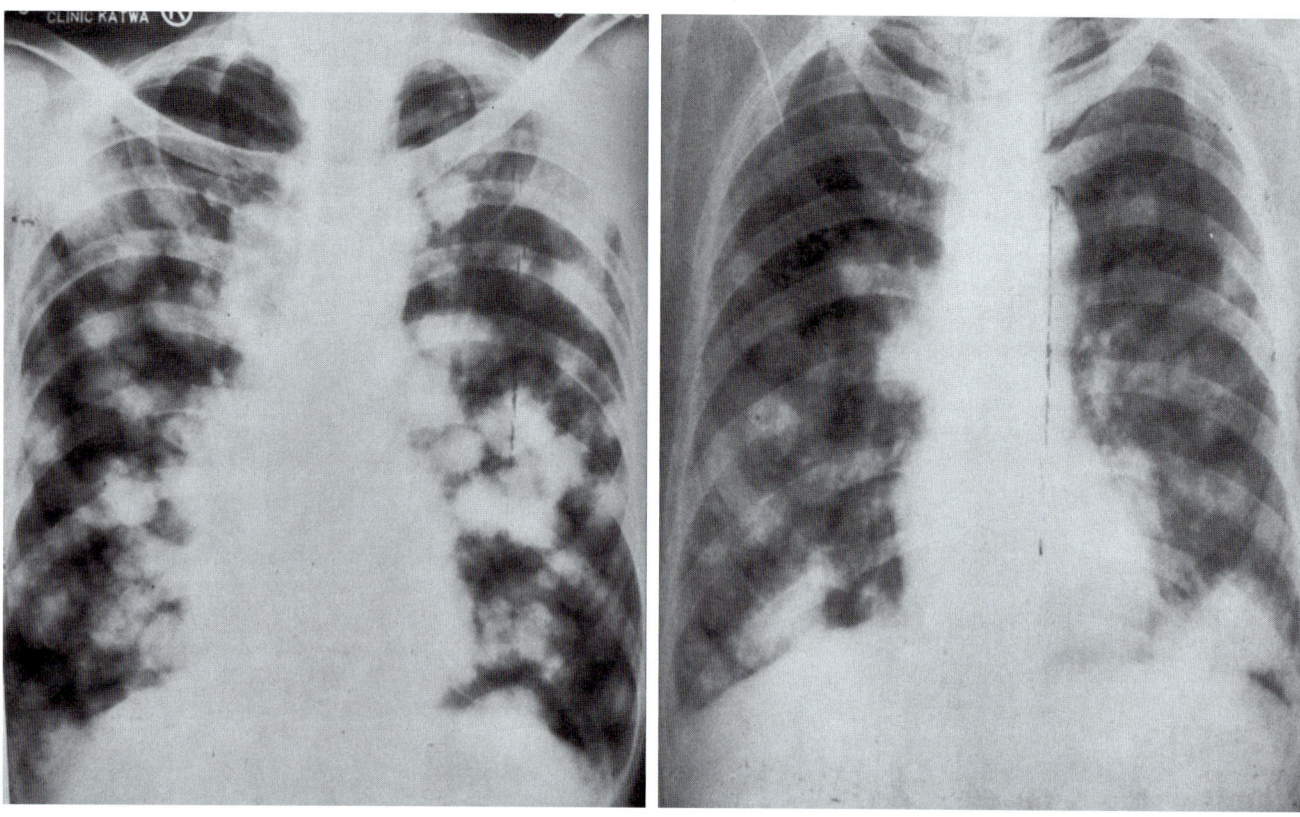

3. X-rays of cannonball appearance

Common benign causes of cannonball metastasis:
• Trophoblastic disease, like hydatid cyst, filariasis
• Fungal infection, like histoplasmosis, aspergillosis
• Sarcoidosis
• Wegener's granulomatosis

4. The straight X-ray abdomen in erect posture showing multiple air fluid levels. The dilated bowel loops are located at the central part of the abdomen. The inner wall of the bowel loops showing the step ladder fashion and having the concertina effect (valvulae conniventes) suggestive of small bowel obstruction (*see* Fig. 4).

5. The straight X-ray abdomen in erect posture showing multiple air fluid levels. The dilated loops are located more periphery in the abdomen. There are haustrations in the walls and incomplete mucosal folds are placed at different levels (not continuous like in small bowel) (*see* Fig. 5).

6. Subdiaphragmatic abscess: The straight X-ray chest (PA view) with upper part of the abdomen showing the fluid collection in the right subdiaphragmatic region suggestive of right subdiaphragmatic abscess and there is a pneumonic patch in the right middle zone of the lung (*see* Fig. 6).

Remember: There are four intraperitoneal and three extraperitoneal subphrenic spaces.

Intraperitoneal subphrenic spaces are:
a. Left anterior and superior intraperitoneal space
b. Left posterior and inferior intraperitoneal space
c. Right anterior and superior intraperitoneal space

A little true love does more than the most beautiful speeches.

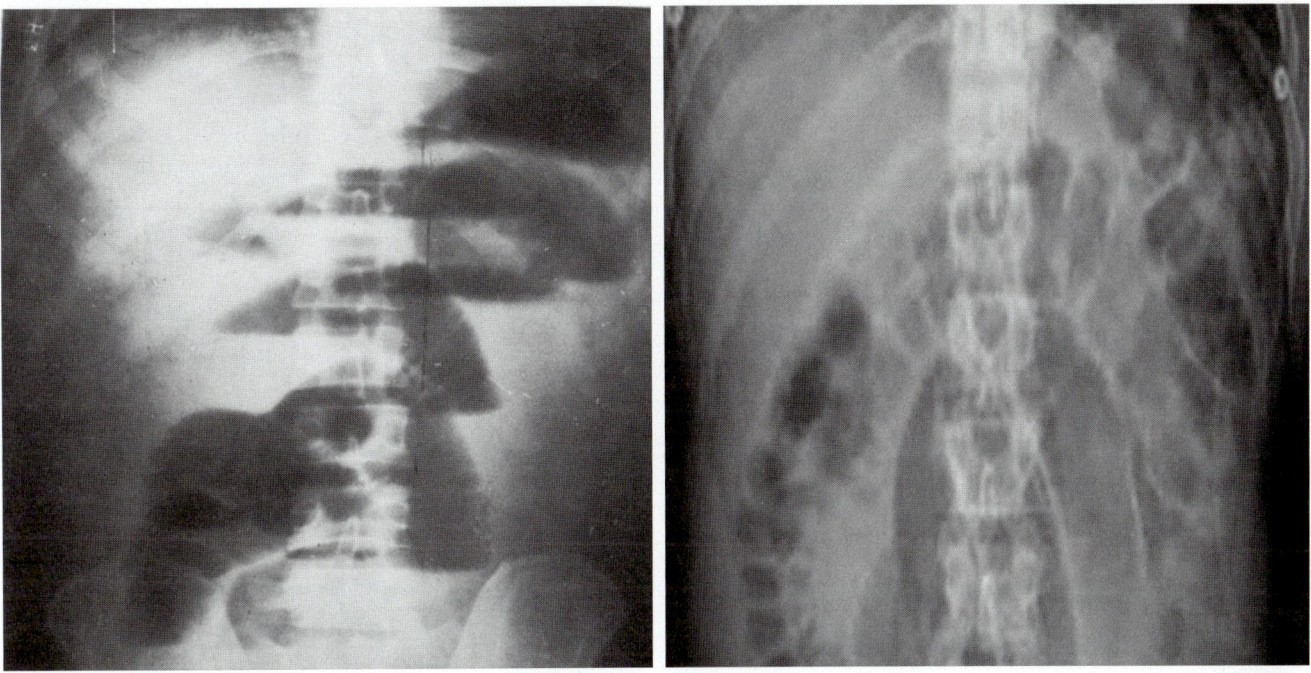

4. X-rays of small bowel obstruction

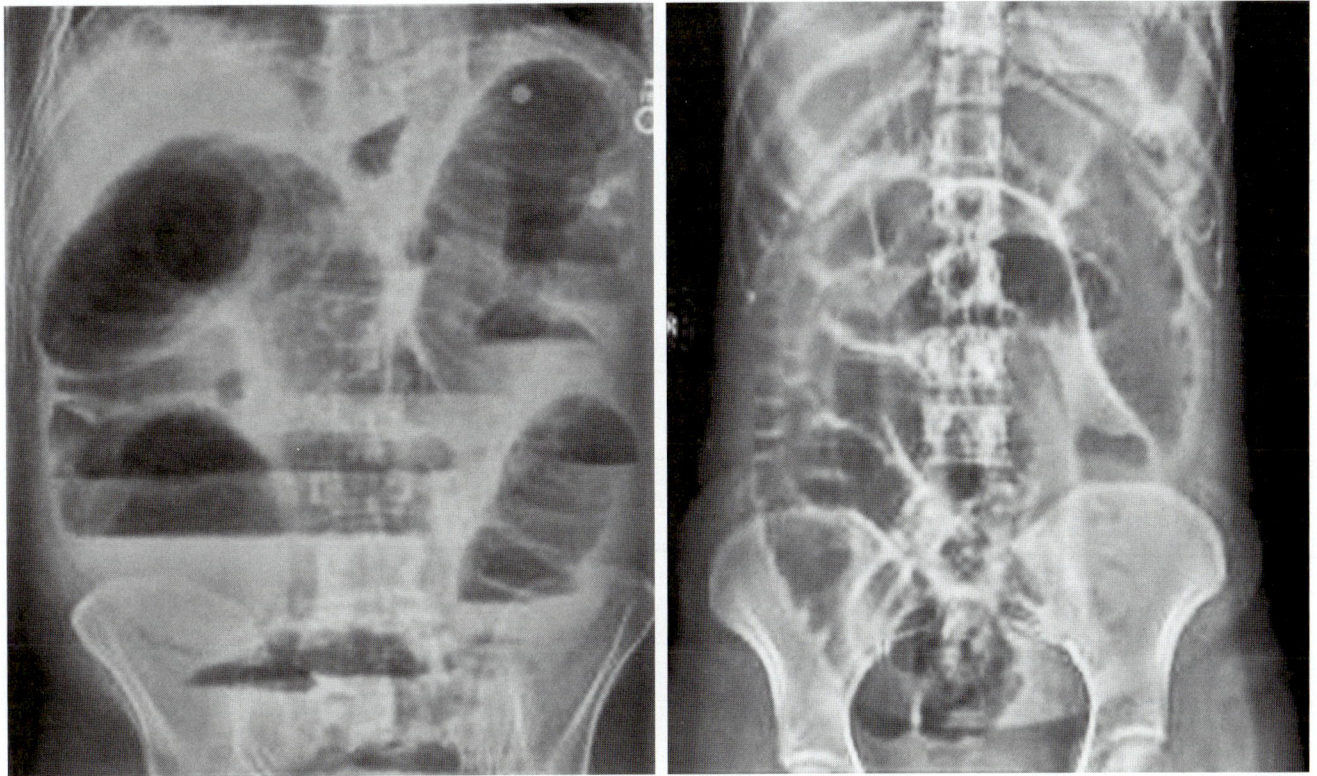

5. X-rays of large bowel obstruction

Zeal without knowledge is fire without light.

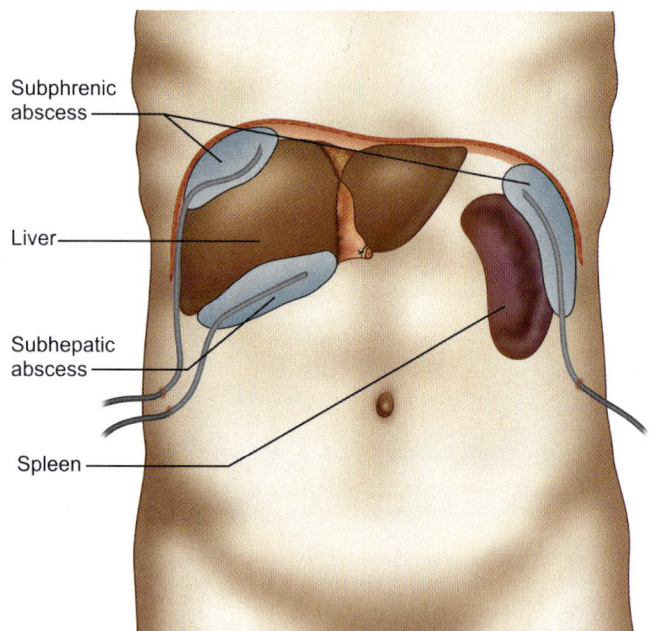

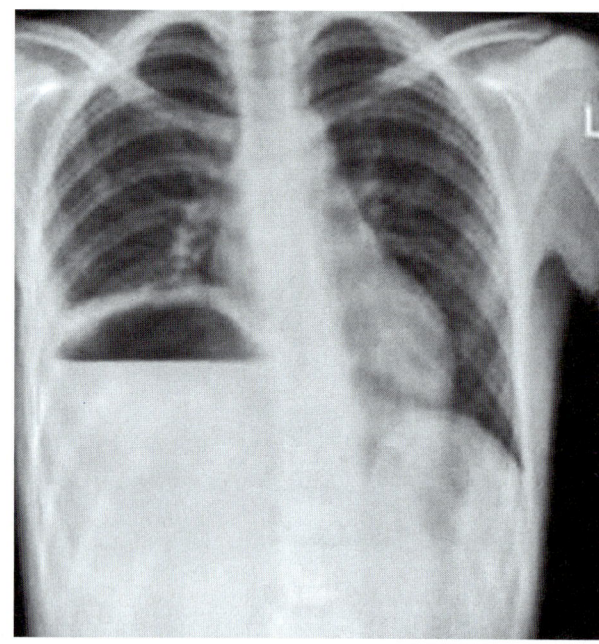

Subphrenic abscess

Liver

Subhepatic abscess

Spleen

6. X-ray of subphrenic (subdiaphragmatic) abscess

d. Right posterior and inferior intraperitoneal space. (The space is called right subhepatic-hepatorenal pouch of Morrison. This is the most dependent part of the body in supine position.)

The extraperitoneal spaces are:
a. The right subphrenic spaces
b. The left subphrenic spaces
c. Middle subphrenic spaces. (This area is corresponding to bare area of the liver.)

Causes of Subdiaphragmatic (Subphrenic) Abscess

a. Perforated duodenal or gastric ulcer
b. Rupture of liver abscess
c. Perforation of gallbladder, intestinal perforation, appendicular perforation, etc.
d. Duodenal stump blow out
e. After major abdominal operations, like surgery of the pancears, spleen, liver, stomach, colon, etc.

7. The straight X-ray of abdomen, erect position showing a usually dilated large bowel loop extending from the pelvis toward the upper abdomen. The loops are clearly seen with outer borders and intervening wall formed by the inner walls of the large bowels, converging toward the pelvis suggestive of large bowel obstruction due to sigmoid volvulus (*see* Fig. 7).

Remember: Sigmoid is a common site for development of volvulus because there may be: Long, redundant sigmoid colon; the presence of more bands; long sigmoid mesocolon which has the narrow attachment; frequently fecal loaded sigmoid colon.
   Read details about the volvulus.

Coffee never knew it would taste so nice and sweet, before it met milk and sugar. We are good as individuals but become better when meet the right person.

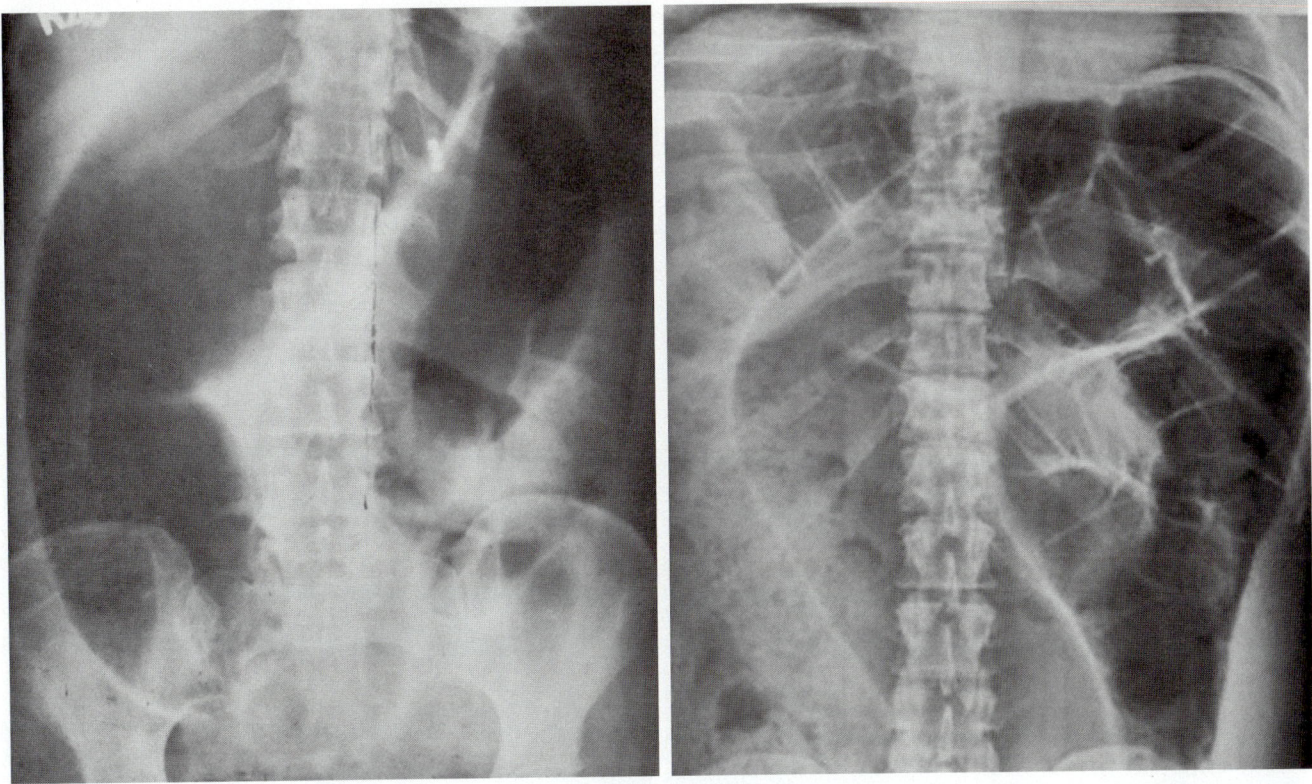

7. X-rays of sigmoid volvulus

8. Straight X-ray abdomen shows multiple closely packed small radiopaque shadows in the right hypochondrium below 12th rib suggestive of multiple gallstones.

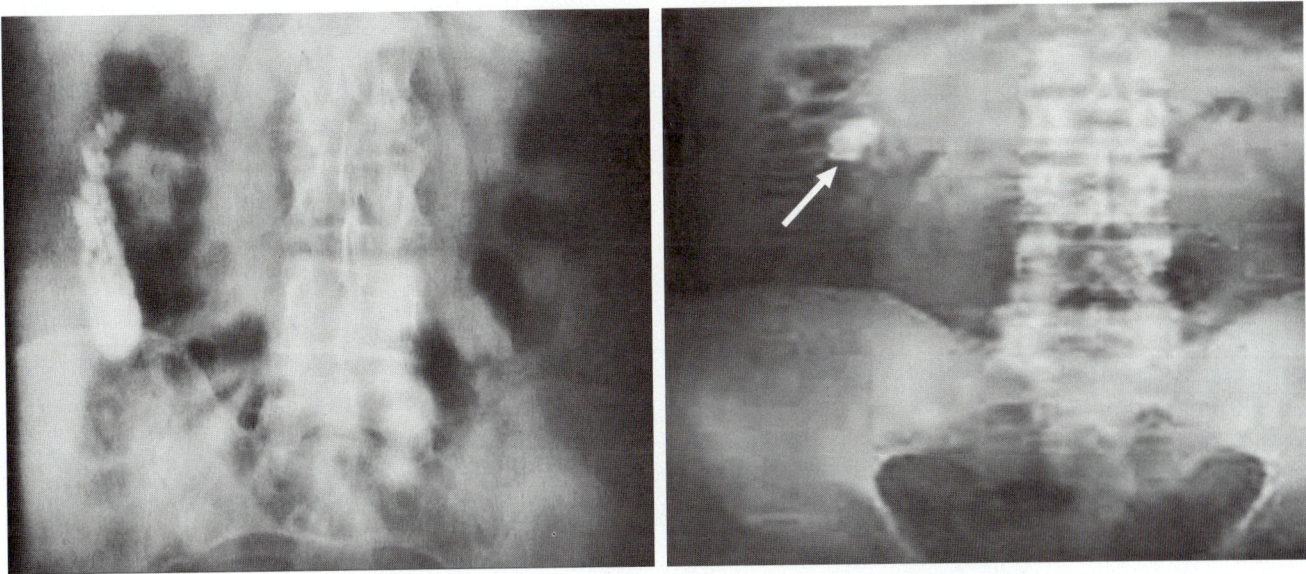

8. X-rays of gallstones (Remember: only 10% gallstones are radiopaque)

Two things to remember in life: 1. take care of your thoughts when you are alone, and 2. take care of your words when you are with people.

9. Straight X-ray KUB (kidney, ureter, bladder) showing radiopaque shadow at the right lumbar region. Right one showing a Denas of staghorn type radiopaque shadow suggestive of staghorn calculus and left one is suggestive of other renal calculus.

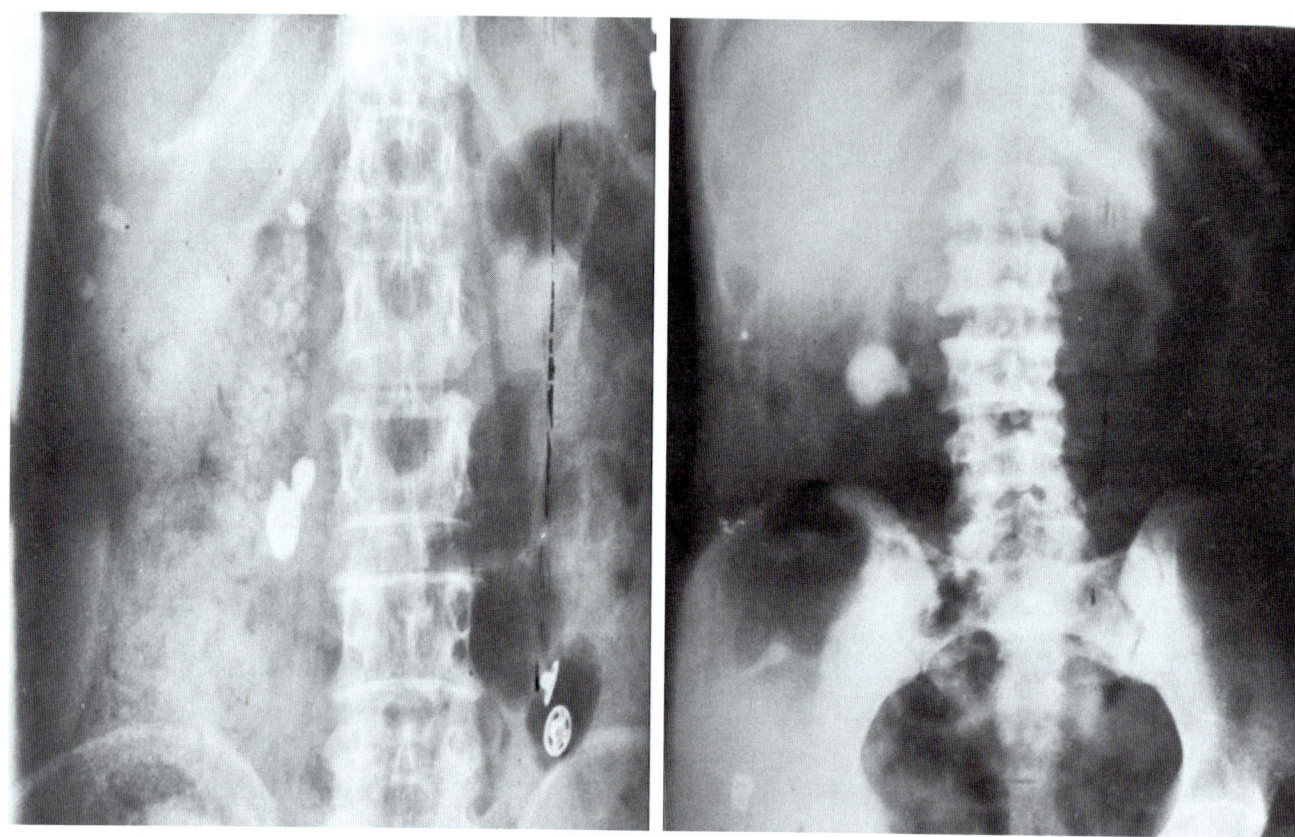

9. X-rays of radiopaque kidney stones (Remember: 90% kidney stones are radiopaque)

Note: Easy way to differentiate kidney stone and gallstone is to do a lateral view X-ray. The gallstone lies anterior to the vertebral body and the kidney stone lies posterior to the vertebral body or superimposed/ overlaps the vertebral body. This is confirmed by ultrasound abdomen.

10. Differential diagnosis of radiopaque shadow at right upper quadrant of abdomen (*see* Fig. 10):
   a. Renal stones
   b. Gallstones
   c. Foreign body
   d. Fecolith, phlebolith
   e. Calcified lymphnodes
   f. Calcified renal tuberculosis
   g. Calcified suprarenal gland
   h. Calcified pancreatic head/pancreatic calculus
   i. Calcified costal cartilage
   j. Fracture transverse process of vertebra.

Control your thought process when you are alone. Control your speech process when you are together.

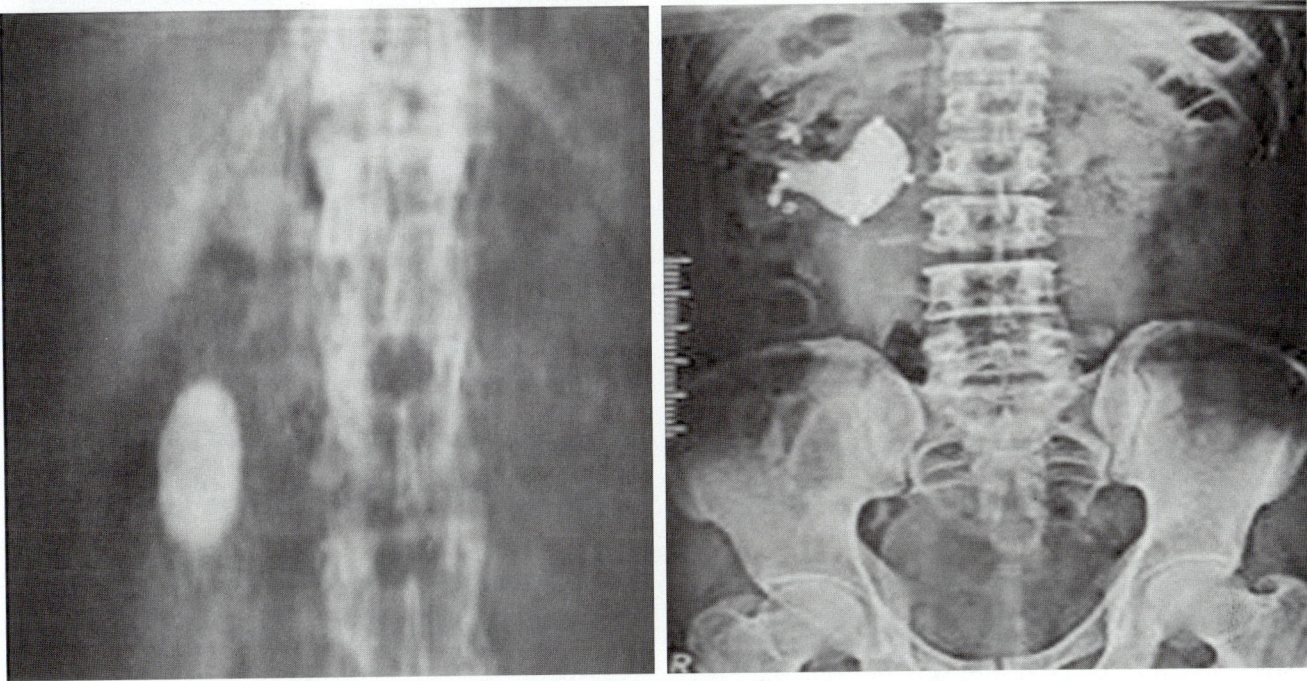

10. X-rays of radiopaque shadow at right upper quadrant of abdomen

11. X-ray KUB showing: **I.** a small radiopaque shadow in the left lower quadrant of abdomen in the left paravertebral region suggestive of ureteric stone; **II.** a large round-shaped radiopaque shadow in hypogastric region suggestive of urinary bladder stone.

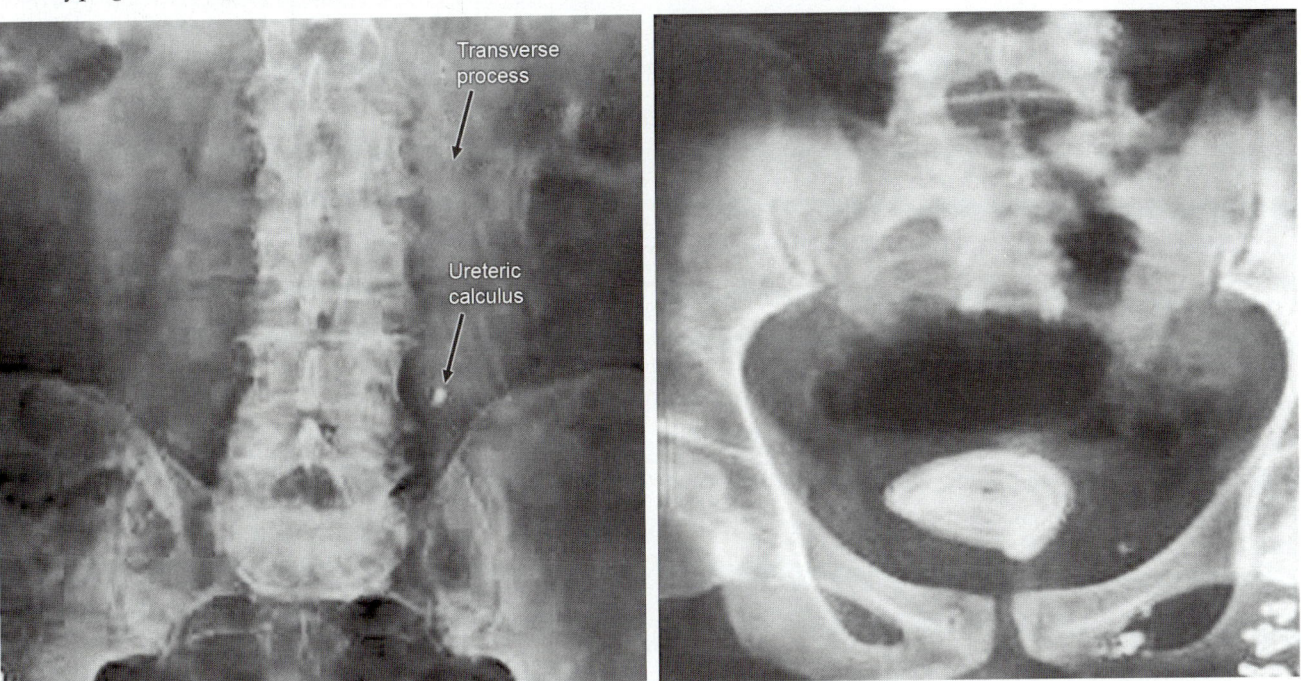

11.I X-ray of ureteric calculus   *11. II X-ray of bladder calculus*

A fool can become a genius when he understands he is a fool but a genius can become a fool when he understands he is a genius.

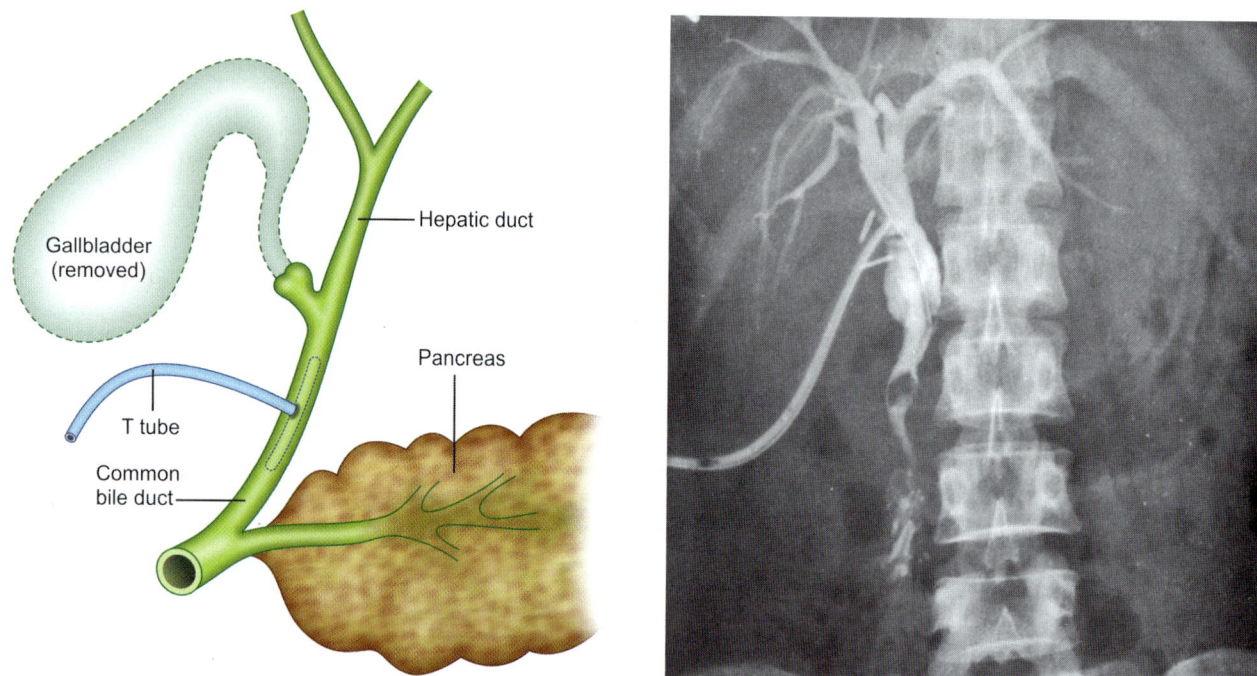

12. X-ray of T-tube cholangiography

12. The film of T-tube cholangiography showing there is a big filling defect within the bile duct which suggests above radiolucent stone. The intrahepatic biliary radicals, both common hepatic ducts and common bile duct, appear to be dilated. The dye has not passed below the defect appears to be an obstruction due to an impacted stone in the bile duct.

Note: T-tube cholangiography is a commonly asked question please read details about it.

13.I. The plates of endoscopic retrograde cholangiopancreaticography (ERCP) showing the endoscopy are in situ. The pancreatic duct appears normal. The right and left ducts, the common hepatic duct and the common bile duct appear to be dilated. There is a radiolucent filling defect at the lower end of the bile duct suggests above bile duct calculus.

II. The plate of ERCP showing the dilated common bile duct and hepatic duct. There is a radiolucent filling defect in the upper part of the bile duct suggests above bile duct stone. The gallbladder shows multiple radiolucent opacities inside the lumen suggests multiple gallstones (*see* Fig. 13).

14. The plate of ERCP showing the normal gallbladder bile duct, no filling defect but there is a dilatation of the main pancreatic duct is suggestive of chronic pancreatitis (*see* Fig. 14).

15. The barium swallow X-ray of esophagus showing irregular narrowing of the esophagus at the lower end and the proximal part is dilated suggest above carcinoma lower end of esophagus (*see* Fig. 15).

16. Barium swallow X-ray showing smooth tapering at the lower end of the esophagus without any irregularity, and there is a gross dilatation of the esophagus proximal to the site of narrowing suggestive of achalasia cardia (*see* Fig. 16).

17. The barium meal X-ray of stomach and duodenum showing there is a large ulcerative area at the lesser curvature. The ulcer crater projecting outward from the outline of the lesser curvature. The surrounding mucosal fold converging toward the base of the ulcer suggestive of chronic gastric ulcer (*see* Fig. 17).

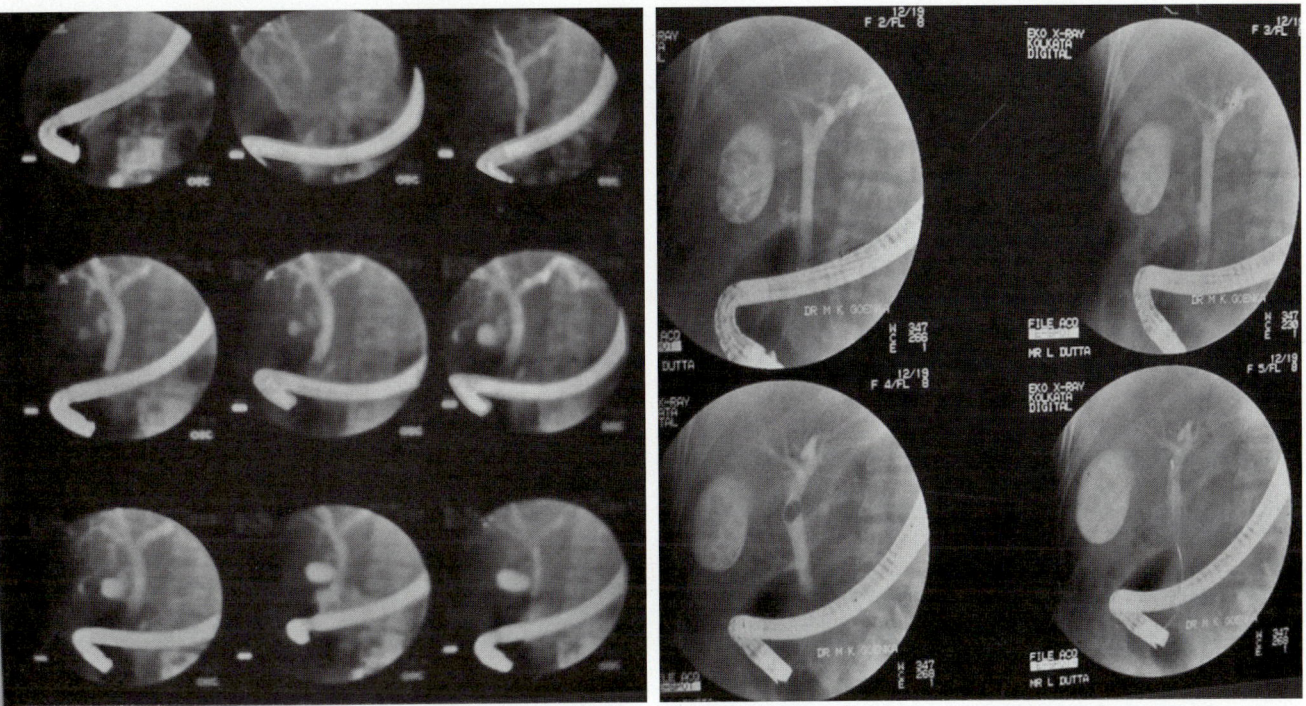

13. Plates of endoscopic retrograde cholangiopancreaticography (ERCP)

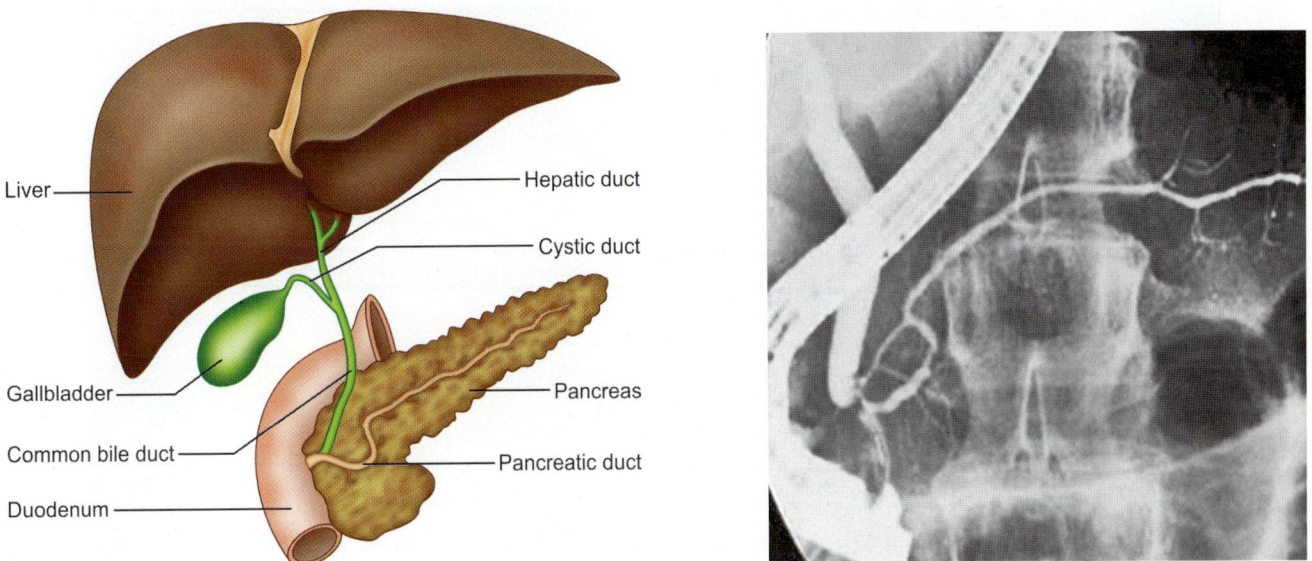

14. ERCP features of chronic pancreatitis

18. In malignant ulcer, usually there is a gap between the mucosal folds and the ulcer and it is located mostly at the greater curvature of the stomach (*see* Fig. 18).

Strength in the nature, wisdom in the mind, love in the heart complete the trinity of glorious manhood.

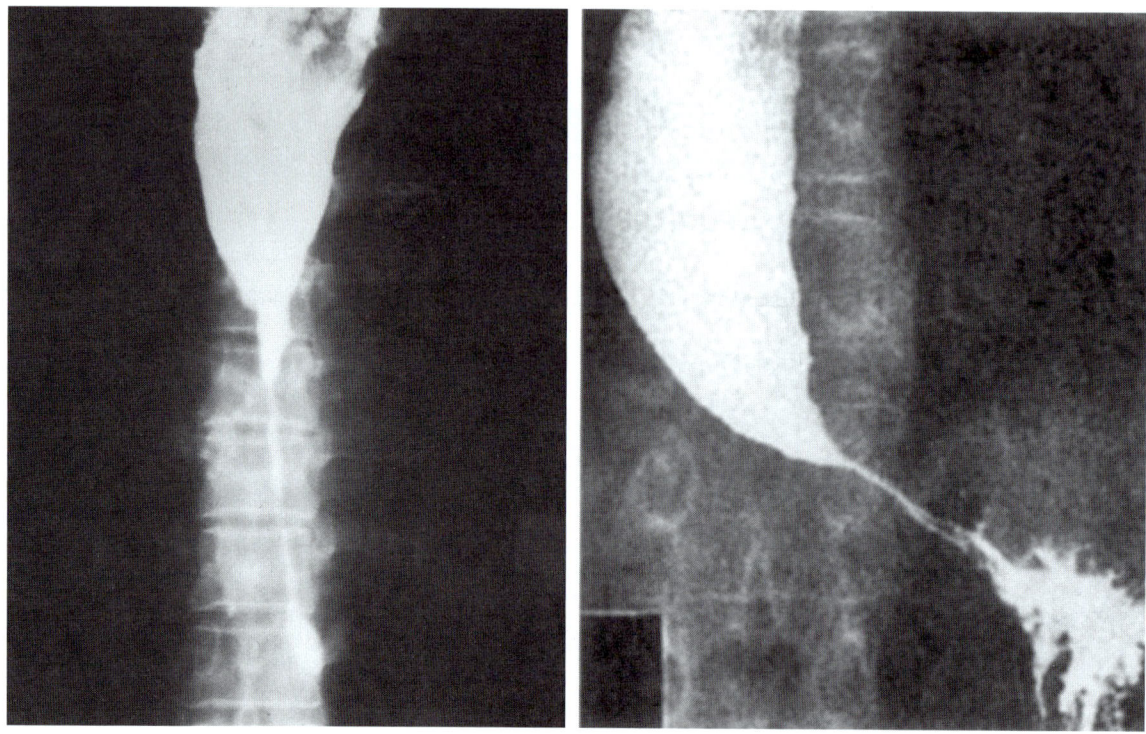

15. The barium swallow of carcinoma esophagus

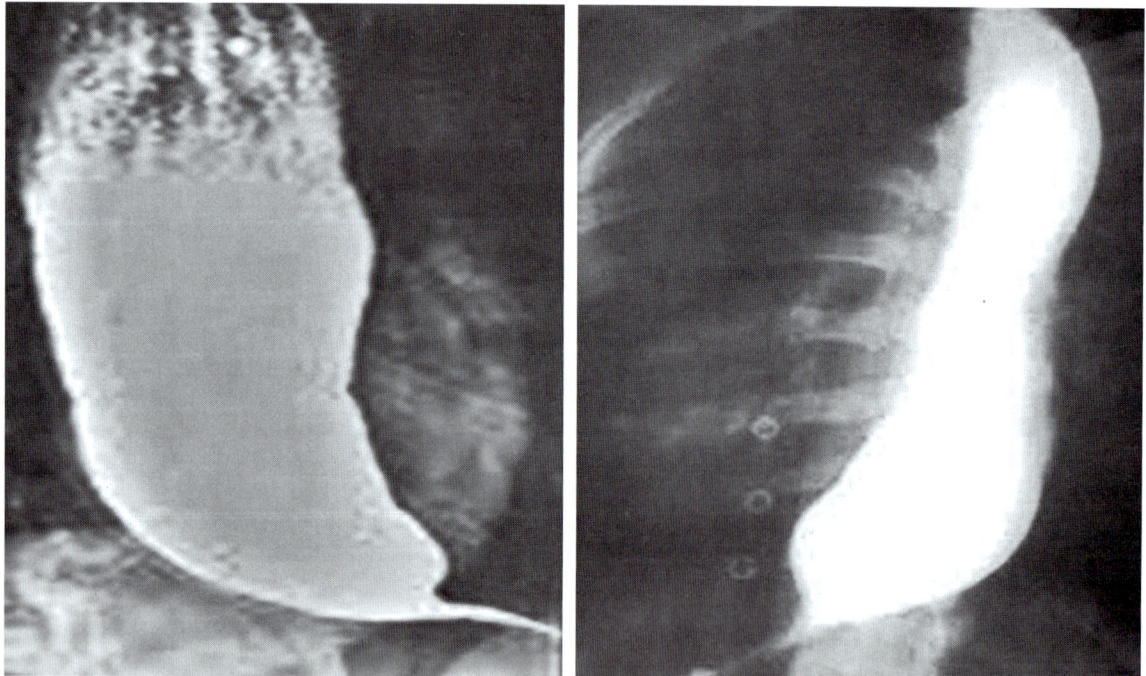

16. Barium swallow X-rays showing achalasia cardia

Whatever work you do, do it as perfectly as you can. That is the best service to the divine in man.

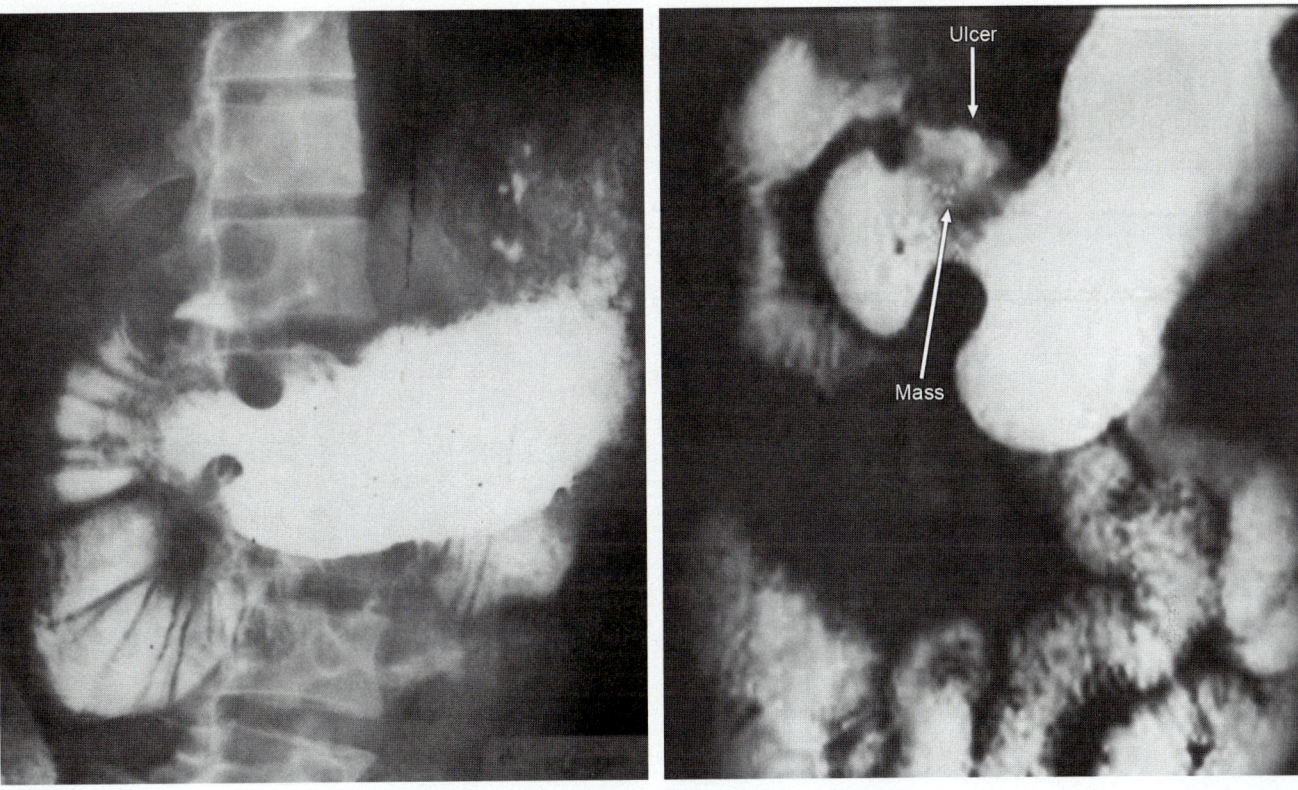

17. Barium swallow X-rays of chronic gastric ulcer at the lesser curvature

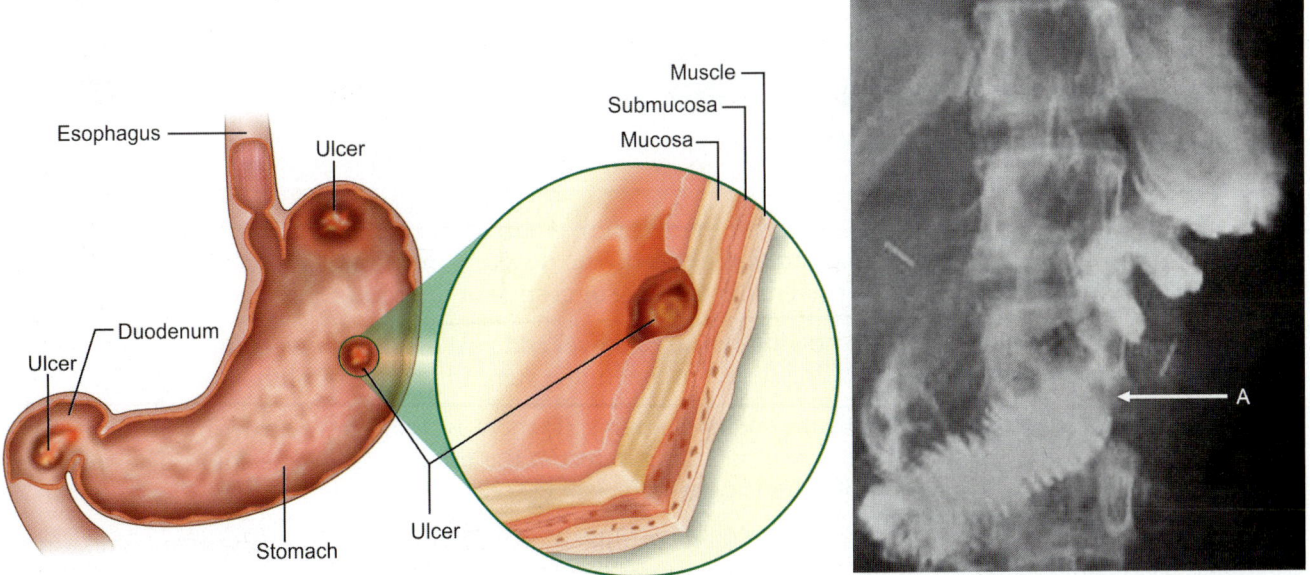

18. Barium meal X-ray of stomach showing the irregular ulcer at the greater curvature. It may be a malignant ulcer

The one thing quite indispensable is to persevere in the resolve to reach the goal.

Remember: Benign gastric ulcers are round or oval with regular margin. Usually, the mucosal folds converge toward the base of the ulcer and there is no gap in between the folds and ulcer and it is located at the lesser curvature and projects beyond the lumen of the ulcer.

19. The barium meal X-ray of the stomach showing gross dilatation of the stomach and the duodenal bulb and duodenum are not visible suggestive of gastric outlet obstruction.

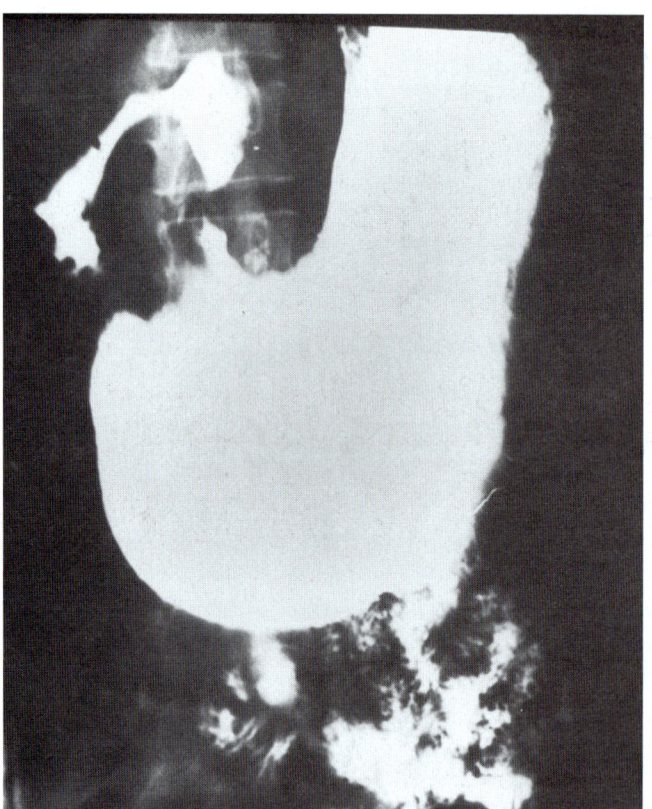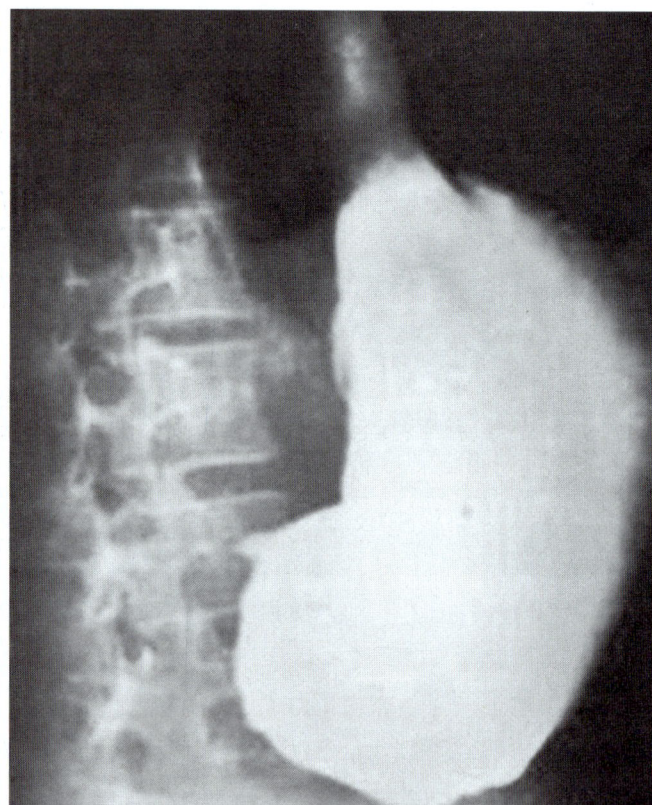

19. Barium meal X-rays of gastric outlet obstruction

20. Barium meal follow through X-rays showing there is a gross narrowing of the terminal ileum and proximal to the narrowing, there is a gross dilatation noticed. The ileocecal junction is drawn higher up and the cecum is deformed and loss of normal distensibility suggestive of ileocecal tuberculosis (*see* Fig. 20).

21. The barium meal follow through showing the large bowel and part of small bowel with ileocecal region. The appendix showing multiple filling defect in the lumen suggests above fecoliths (*see* Fig. 21).

22. The X-rays of double contrast varium enema showing (I) there is a sudden narrowing at the level of hepatic texture and (II) there is an irregular filling defect at the mid of transverse colon. The stenosing lesion of both X-rays suggestive of colonic carcinoma (*see* Fig. 22).

23. The intravenous urography (IVU) showing there are dilatation and clubbing of the calyces in right kidney. There is abrupt narrowing at the pelviureteric junction and the right ureter is not visualized. The IVU picture suggestive of right-sided hydronephrosis due to left pelviureteric junction obstruction. The left kidney appears normal (*see* Fig. 23).

You are great if you can find your faults. You are greater if you can correct them. But, you are greatest if you accept and love someone with their faults.

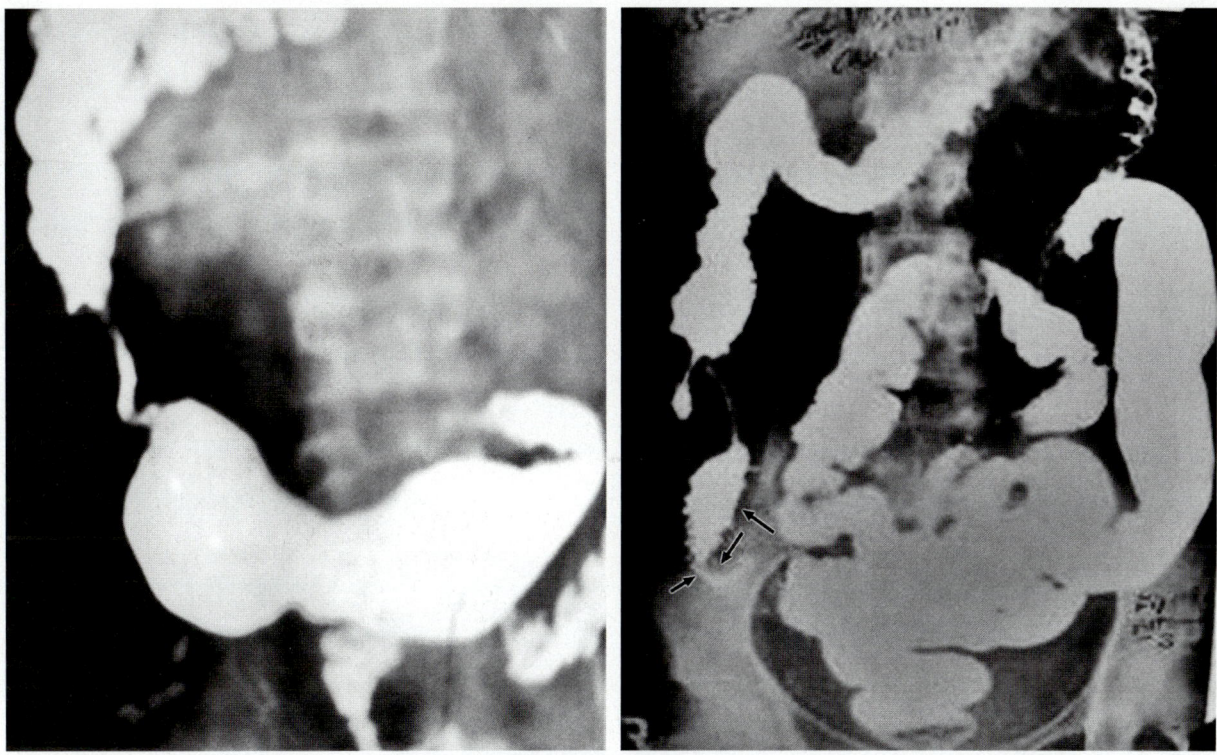

20. X-rays of barium meal follows through suggestive of ileocecal tuberculosis

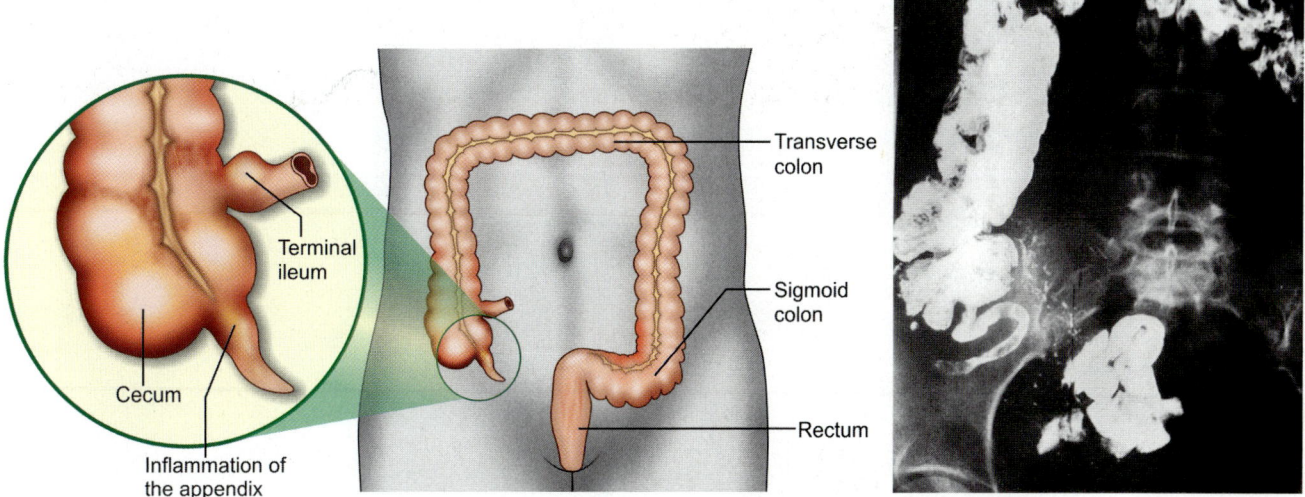

Transverse colon

Terminal ileum

Sigmoid colon

Cecum

Rectum

Inflammation of the appendix

21. Barium meal follow through showing multiple filling defects in the appendix

24. Multiple X-rays of pneumoperitoneum: "The radiological signs of pneumoperitoneum are among the most important signs in radiology, indeed in medicine. Sometimes, the amount of free gas is small and you may have to work to demonstrate it. Miss it and the patient may die" (*see* Fig. 24).

There is no greater courage than that of recognizing one's own mistakes.

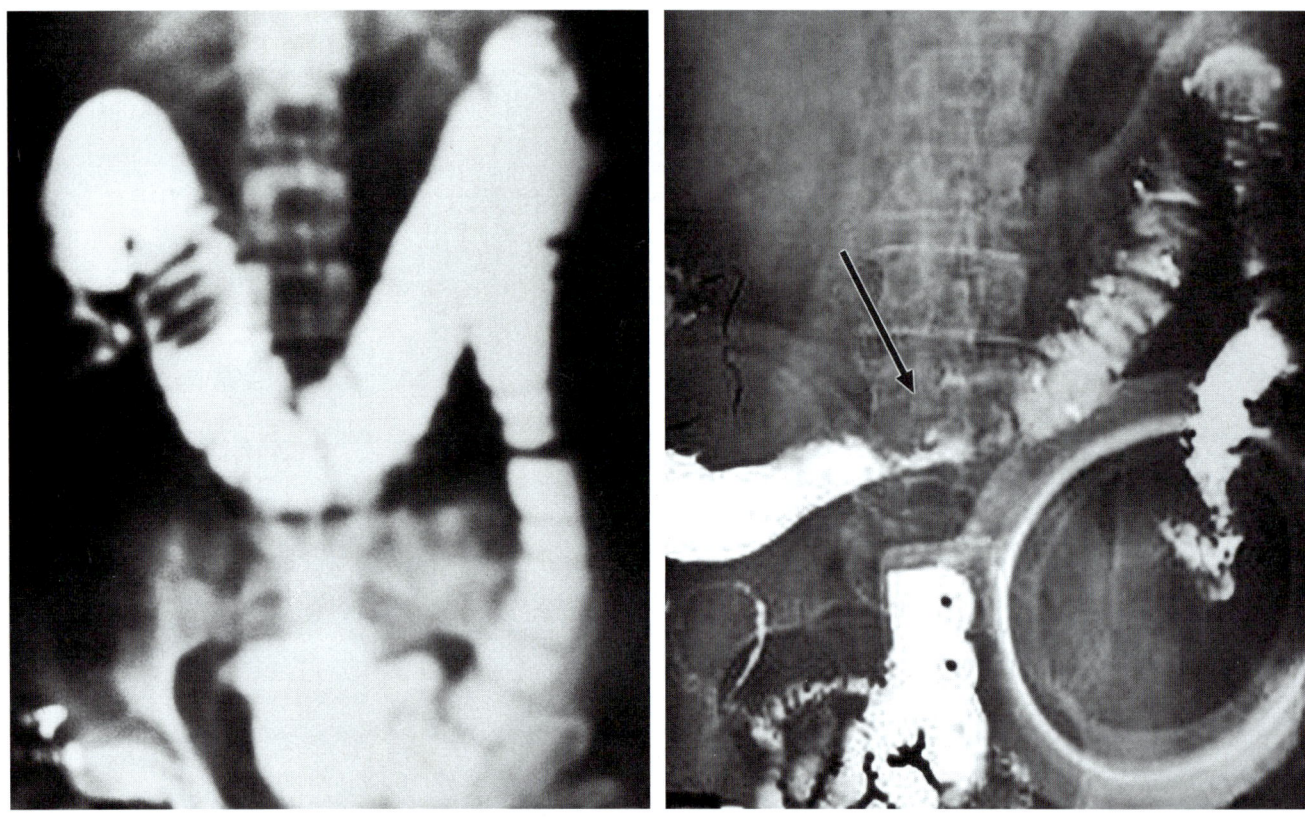

22. Barium enema X-rays of colonic cancer

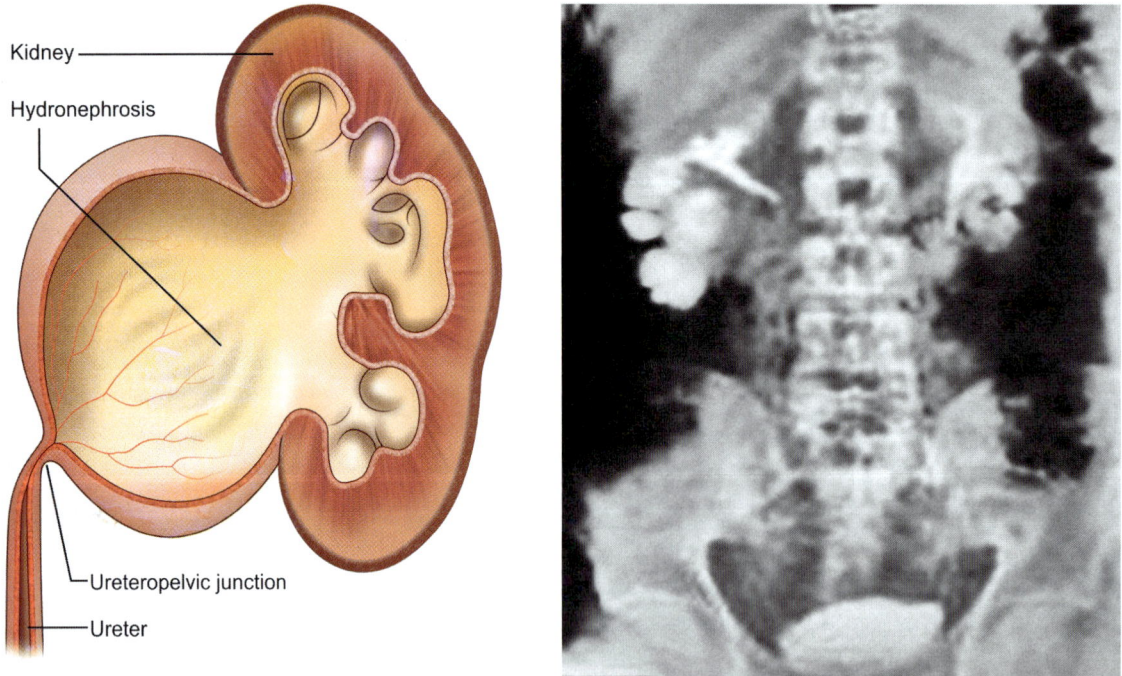

Kidney

Hydronephrosis

Ureteropelvic junction

Ureter

23. IVU of hydronephrosis

Forward, ever forward, without fear and without hesitation.

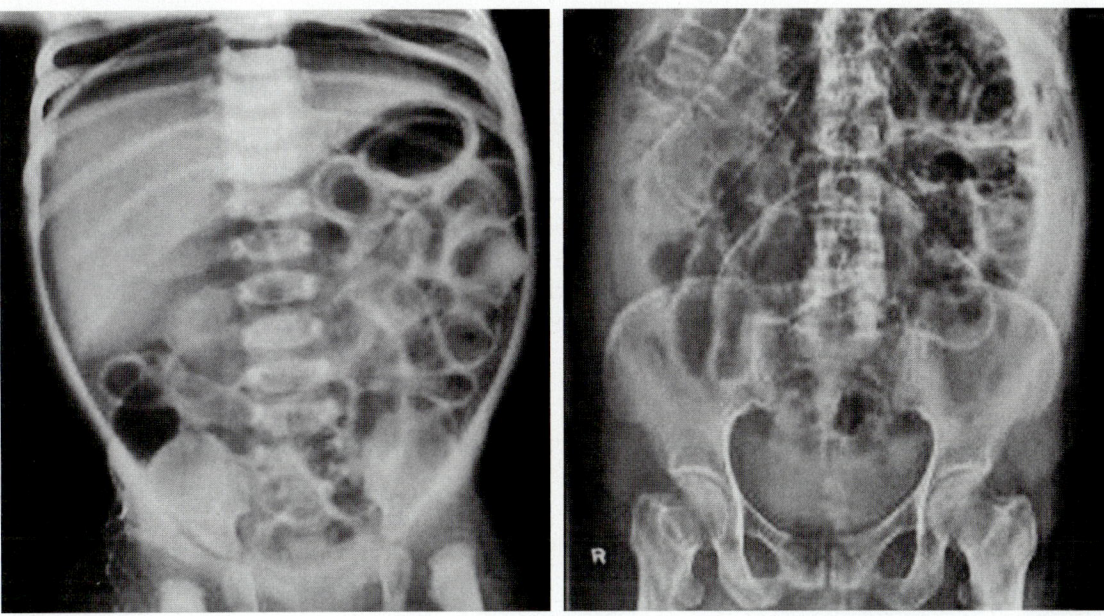

24. X-rays of pneumoperitoneum

The straight X-ray abdomen showing multiple air pockets inside the peritoneal cavity suggestive of pneumoperitoneum.

Anterior Subhepatic Space Free Air

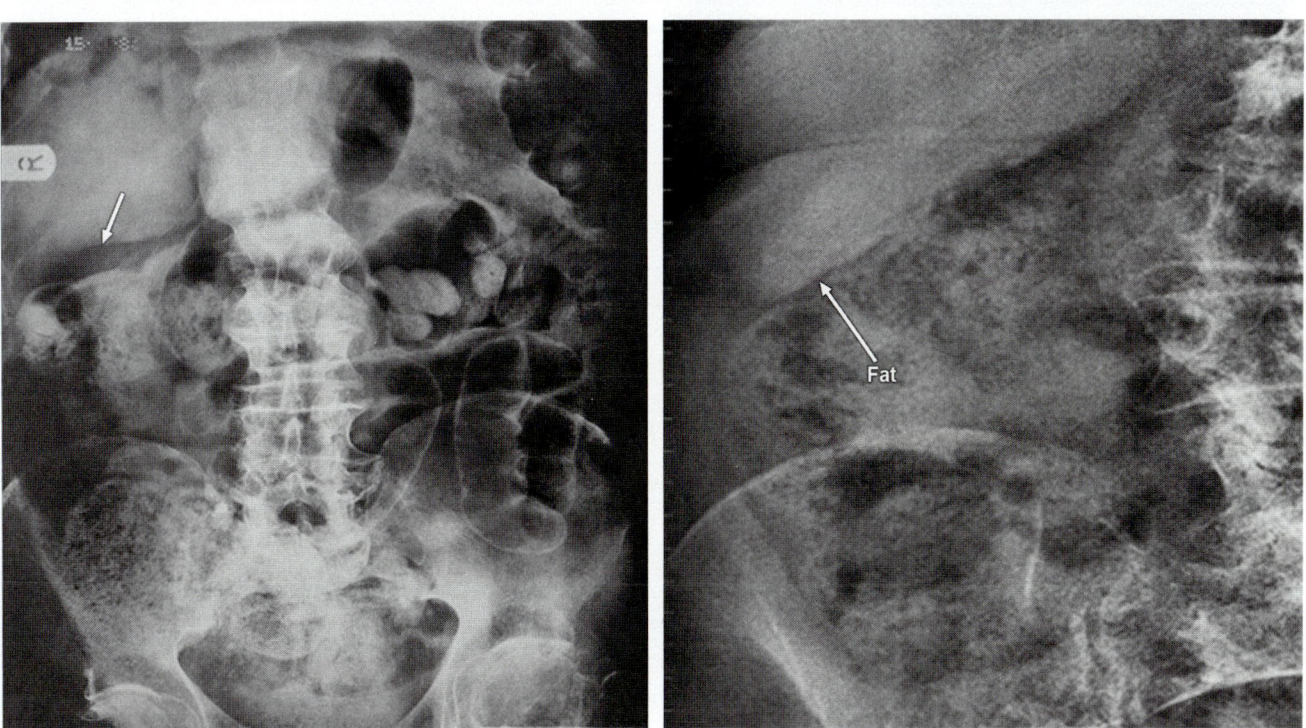

Free air of subhepatic space

Do not look behind, look always in front, at what you want to do—and you are sure of progressing.

Anterior subhepatic space free air tends to be vaguely linear in shape as shown by arrow. A visible medial border of the liver is often seen outlined by fat. The left image shows the subhepatic density is the air density rather than fat density. This image of normal fat surrounding the liver shows a consistent density continuous with the properitoneal fat stripe.

Air Anterior to Ventral Surface of Liver

Air sitting against the ventral surface of the liver can be any shape but here it is "geographical" in shape. The liver is a homogenous organ and should be homogenous in density on plain film. If the liver is seen as an uneven density, pneumoperitoneum should be considered. Note also Rigler's sign.

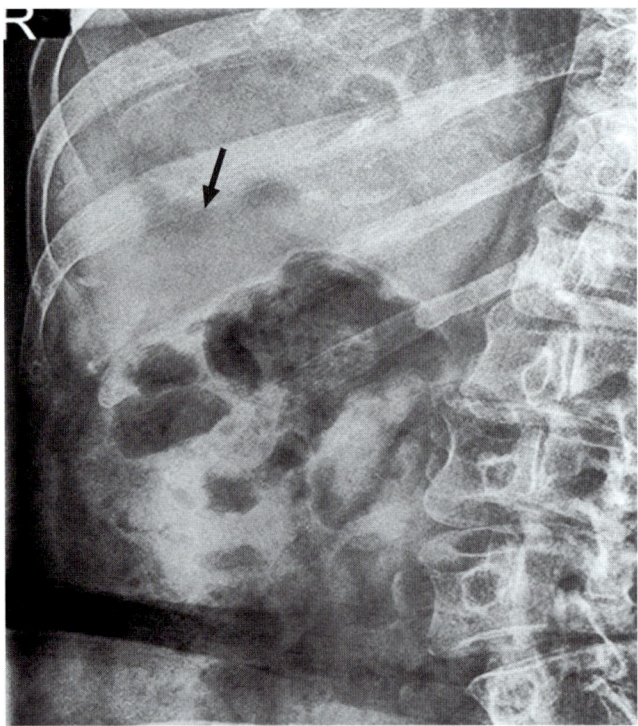

Air at anterior to ventral surface of liver

Decubitus Abdomen Sign

This patient is in the left lateral decubitus position. There is an evidence of free air between the abdominal wall and the liver (white arrow). There is also evidence of free fluid in the peritoneum (black arrow).

Rigler's Sign on Supine X-Ray

Rigler's sign is named after Leo G Rigler. The sign refers to the appearance of the bowel wall on plain film when it is outlined by intraluminal and extraluminal air as shown by arrow. The extraluminal air is free peritoneal gas.

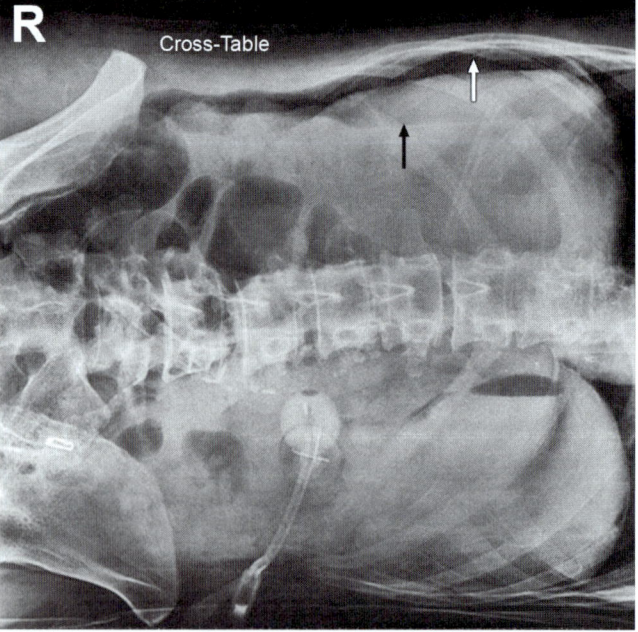

Decubitus abdomen sign

Have faith in your destiny and your road will be lit.

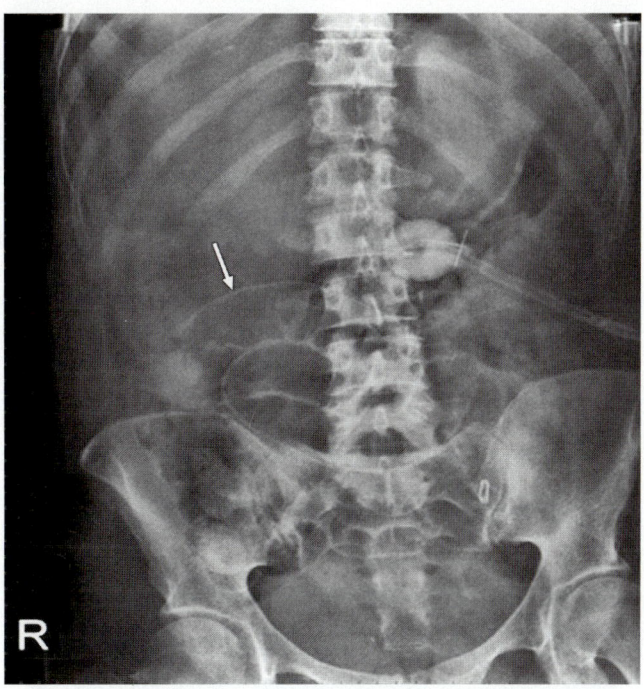

Rigler's sign

Falciform Ligament Sign

The falciform ligament connects the anterior abdominal wall to the liver. The ligament continues to extend inferiorly beyond the liver where it becomes the round ligament as shown by the arrow. Given that the falciform ligament is situated against the anterior abdominal wall, it is not surprising that it becomes outlined with air in a supine patient with free abdominal gas. This is an axial computed tomography (CT) scan image of a patient with pneumoperitoneum. The free gas is seen outlining the anterior abdominal wall and several loops of bowel. The arrowed structure is the falciform ligament surrounded by free intraperitoneal gas.

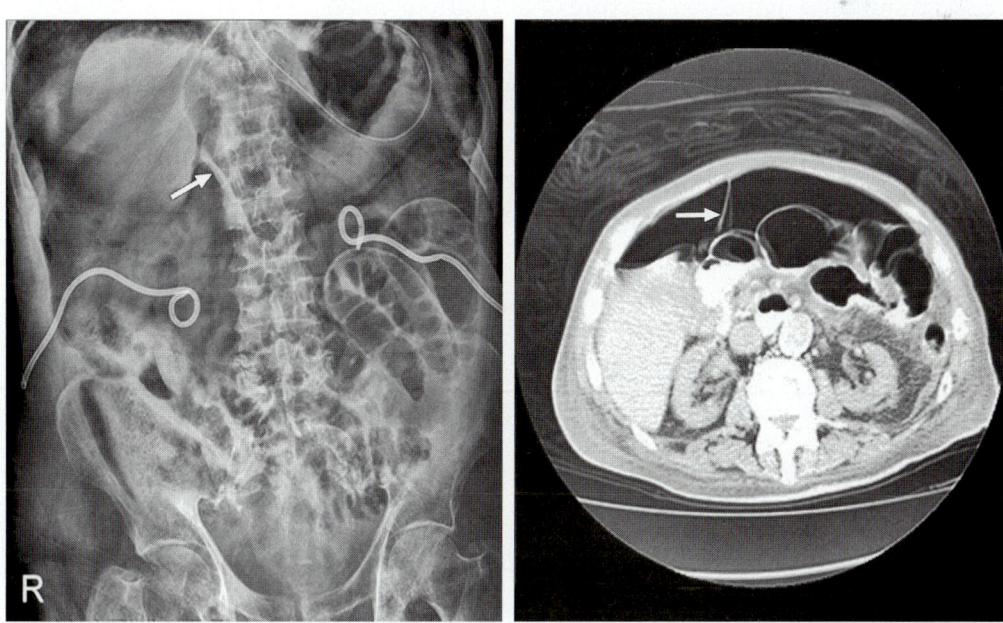

Falciform ligament sign

Those who are weak wait for miracles and those who are strong create miracles.

The "Football" Sign

The football sign likens the massively air-filled peritoneum to an American football. To extend the simile a little further, the falciform ligament has been likened to the seam in the football, and the rarely seen medial and lateral umbilical ligaments are likened to the football laces.

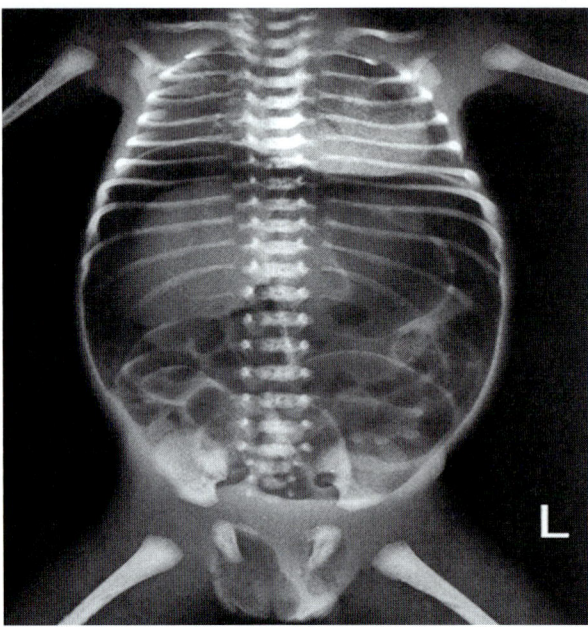

Football sign

25. The X-rays of skull both AP and lateral views, showing a comminuted fracture in the left parietal bone. The AP view showing the fracture fragments is depressed inward. So, the X-ray skull suggestive of comminuted depressed fracture of left parietal bone.

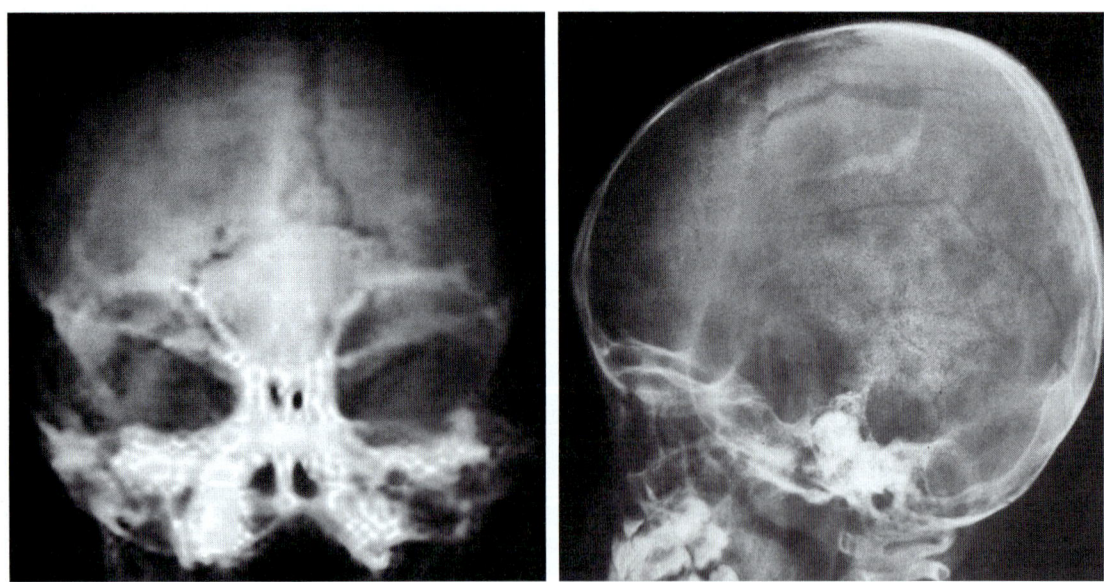

25. X-rays skull showing a comminuted fracture in the left parietal bone

It takes around two years to learn to speak. But, it takes our lifetime to learn what not to speak. Strange but true.

26. *Contrast-enhanced computed tomography (CECT) abdomen:* Few commonly asking CT films are described below. So that students can get idea how to describe CT scan in the examination.

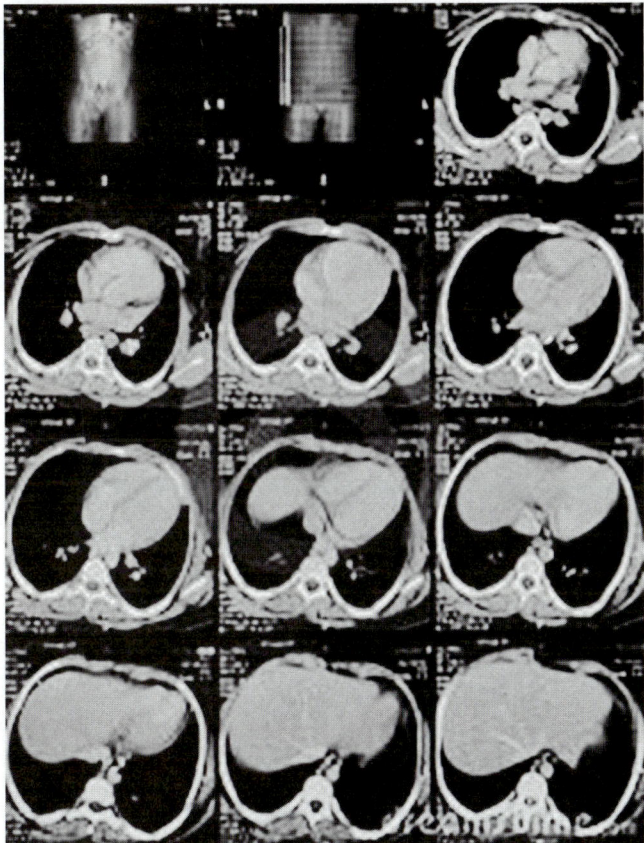

26. I. CECT abdomen how it looks like

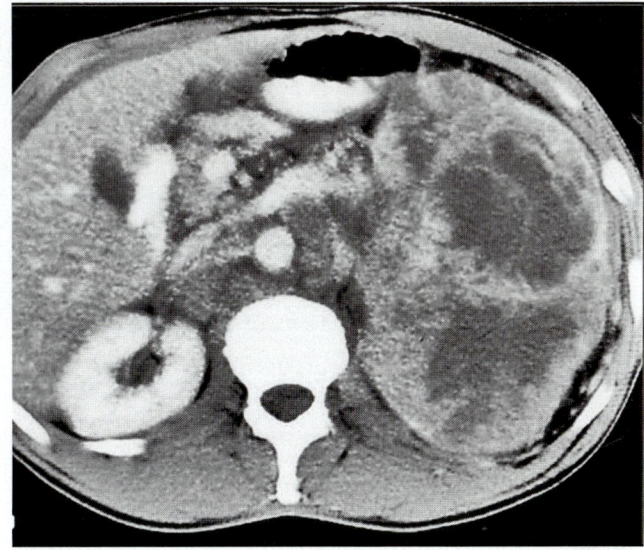

26. II. CECT abdomen shows RCC left kidney

Abdomen CT scan of the left-sided renal cell carcinoma: Axial CT scan of the abdomen showing the large well-defined heterogeneously enhancing mass seen arising from the left kidney showing areas of necrosis within. It is reaching up to the hilum with involvement of left renal vein. Associated retroperitoneal lymphadneopathy seen as well.

27. *Abdomen CT scan of gallbladder carcinoma:* Axial CT scan of the abdomen showing irregular heterogeneously enhancing mass seen arising from fundus and body of gallbladder with infiltration of adjacent segment 4b of the liver. Fat plane with other adjacent structures appear maintained. Few enlarged periportal lymphnodes seen as well.

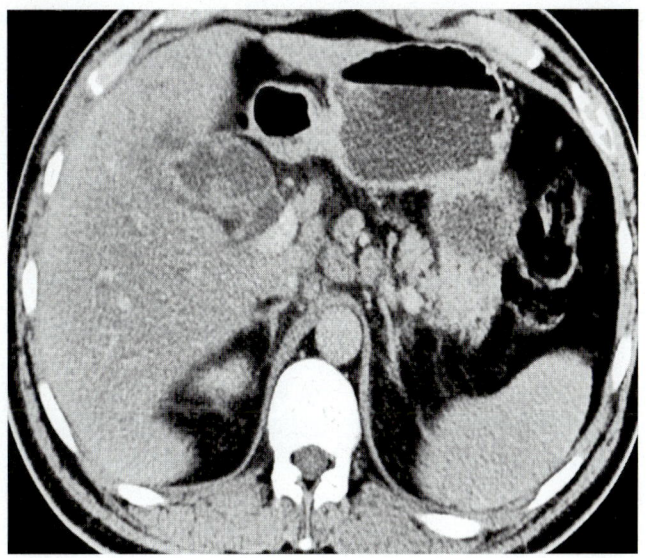

27. CECT abdomen shows carcinoma gallbladder

River cuts a rock not because of its power, but because of its consistency so never loose hope, keep walking toward the goal.

28. *Abdomen CT scan of pancreatic head carcinoma:* Axial and coronal CT scan of the abdomen showing irregular heterogeneously enhancing mass seen arising from head of the pancreas resulting in the dilatation of the main pancreatic duct with infiltration of adjacent second part of the duodenum. Fat plane with superior mesenteric artery and veins, other adjacent structures appear maintained.

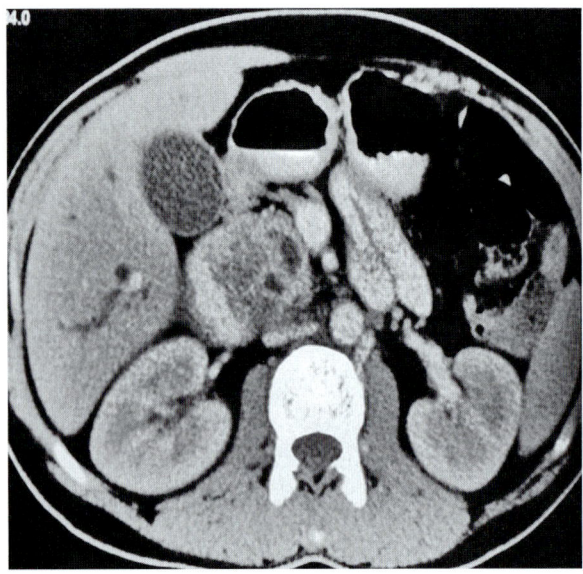 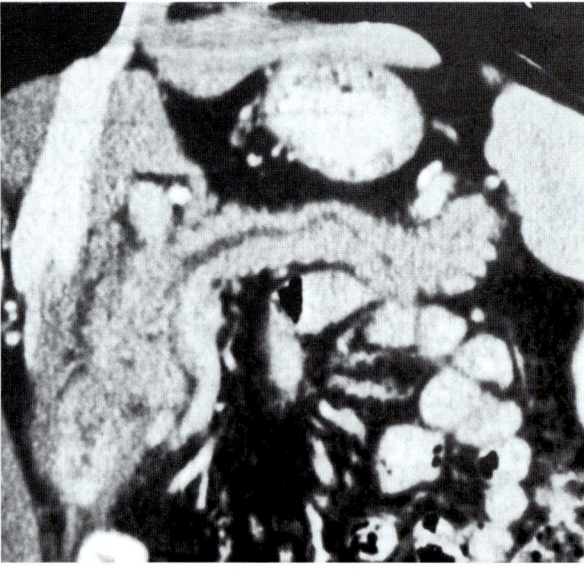

28. I. CECT shows gallbladder   *28. II. CECT shows carcinoma head of pancreas*

29. *Multiphase CT scan of hepatic cell carcinoma:* Axial CT scan of the abdomen showing well-defined heterogeneously enhancing mass seen in the segment 7 of the liver. It shows enhancement in the arterial phase, show wash out in venous phase and reveals capsule formation in the delayed phase. Thrombosis in the right branch of the portal vein adjacent to the mass also seen in the venous phase

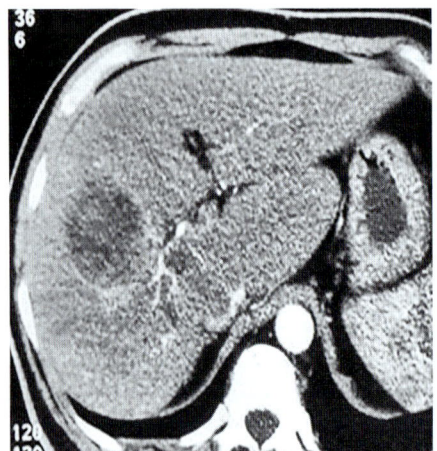 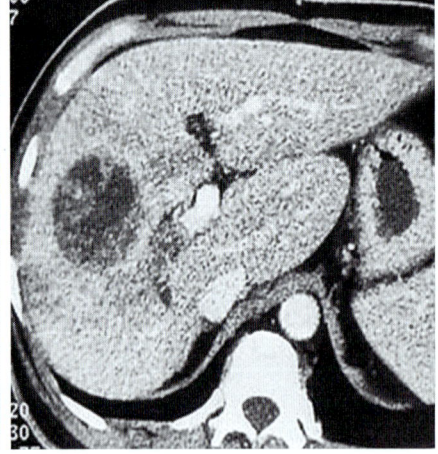 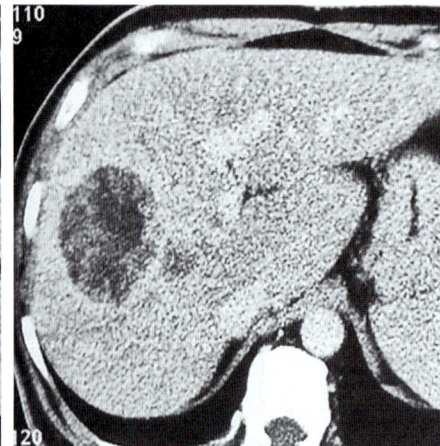

29. CECT shows hepatocellular carcinoma

The hopes of today are the realization of tomorrow.

COMMONLY USED INSTRUMENTS

You know in examination you have to just identify the instrument and you have to tell the uses of the instrument. Then the examiner will lead you to the concerned operation steps. Usually, how you are identifying the instrument is not asked by the examiner.

1. RAMPLEY'S SWAB HOLDING FORCEPS

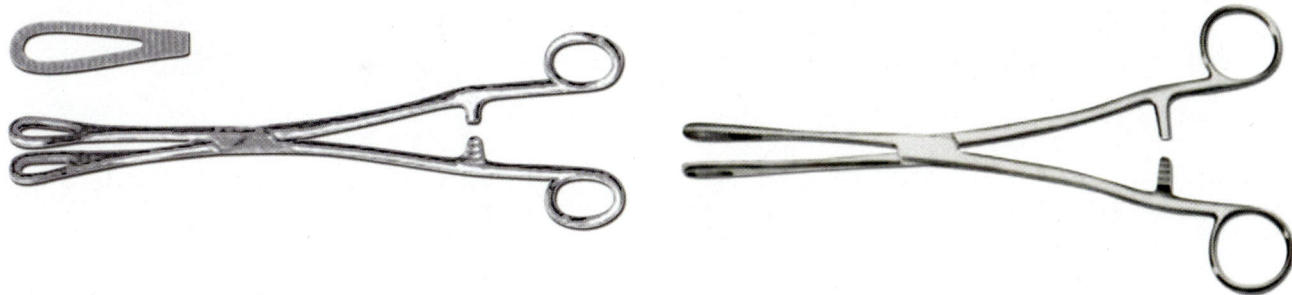

2. HEMOSTATIC ARTERY FORCEPS

a. Mosquito forcep (Halsted forcep)—curve and straight

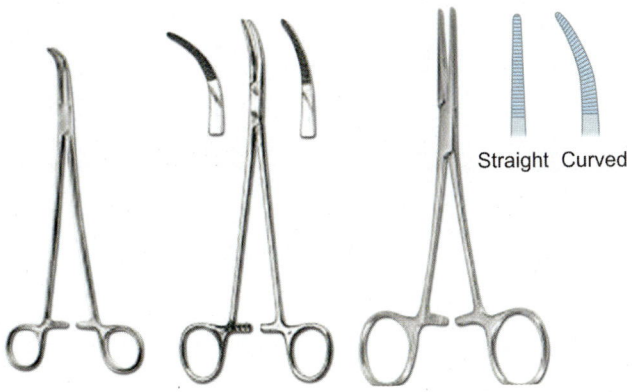

b. Spencer Wells artery forceps

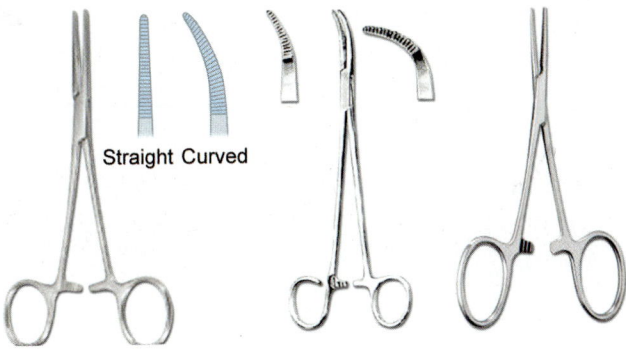

Character is not about honesty and integrity alone. It's more about doing the right thing when tempted to do the wrong.

c. Kocher's hemostatic artery forceps

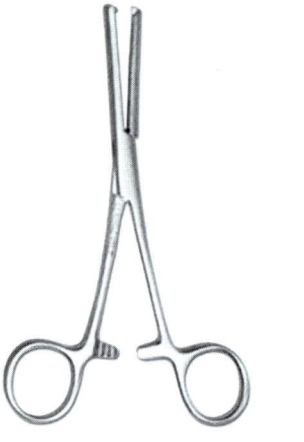
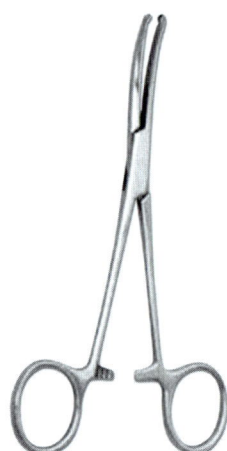

3. LISTER'S SINUS FORCEPS

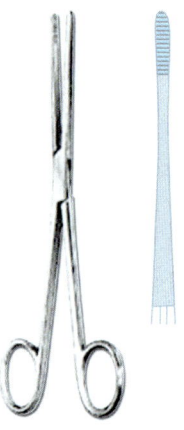
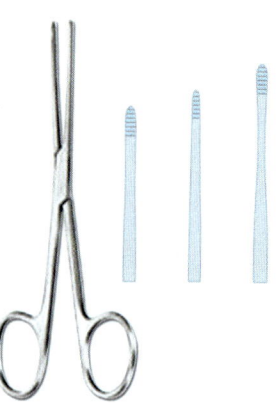

4. ALLIS TISSUE FORCEPS

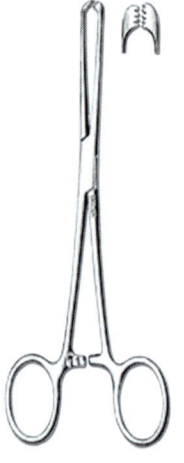
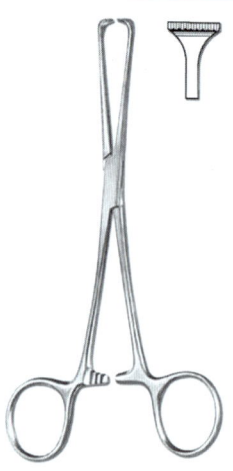

Never grumble. All sorts of forces enter you when you grumble and they pull you down. Keep smiling.

5. BABCOCK'S TISSUE FORCEPS

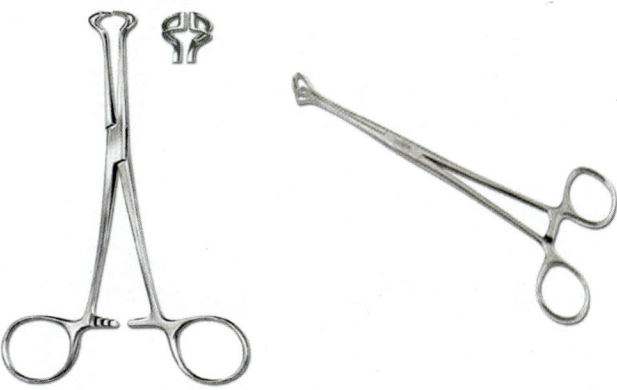

6. LANE'S TISSUE FORCEPS

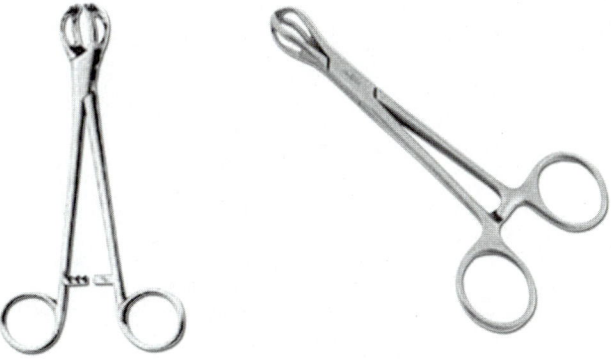

7. RETRACTORS

a. Langenbach's
b. Morris
c. Deaver's
d. Harringtons
e. Doyen's
f. Joll's thyroid retractors
g. Kelly's
h. Czerny retractors
i. Self-retaining abdominal retractors
j. Volkman's retractors—Cat's paw

None can reach heaven who has not passed through hell.

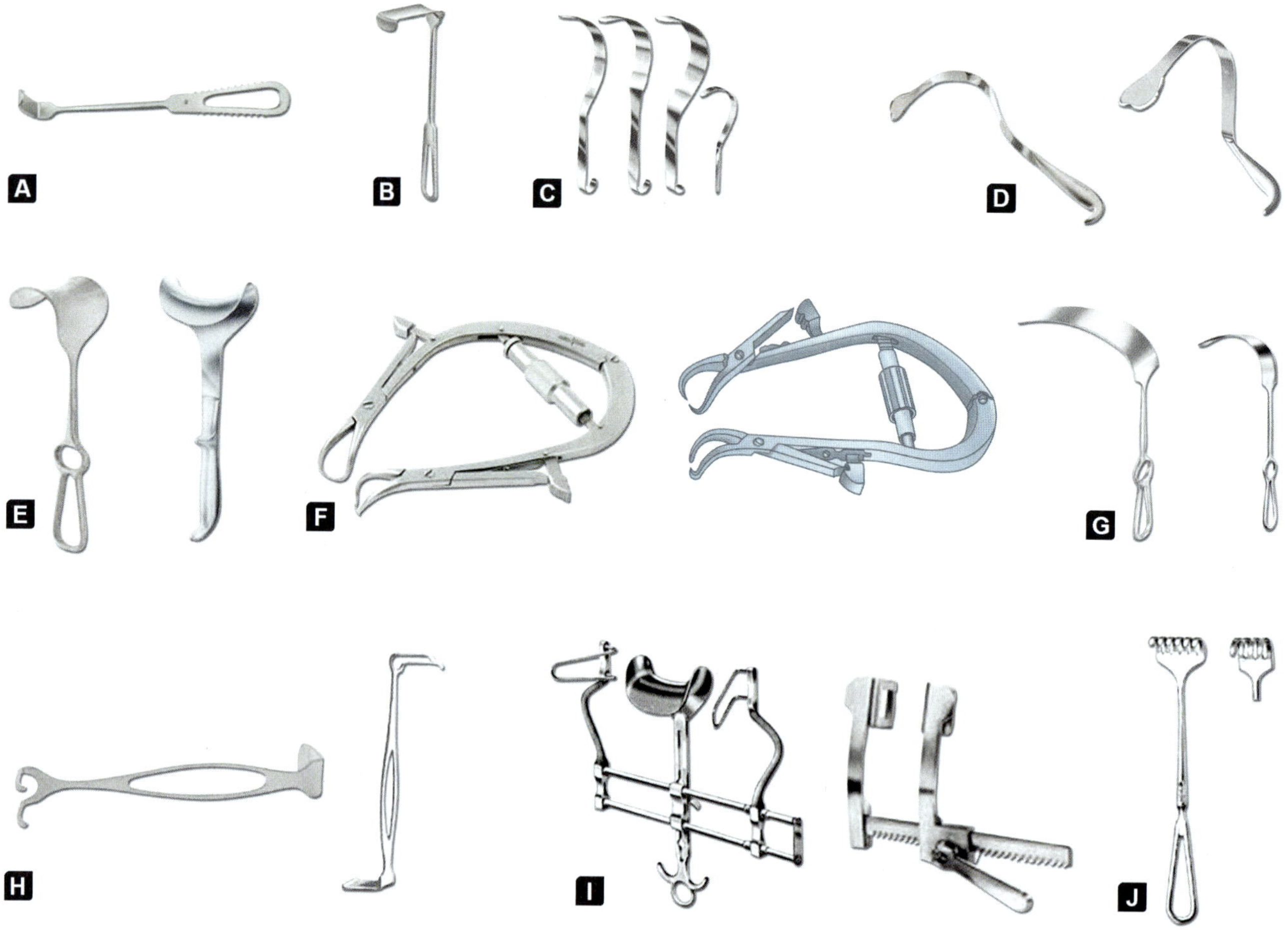

A

B

C

D

E

F

G

H

I

J

8. RIGHT-ANGLED FORCEPS (LAHEY'S FORCEPS)

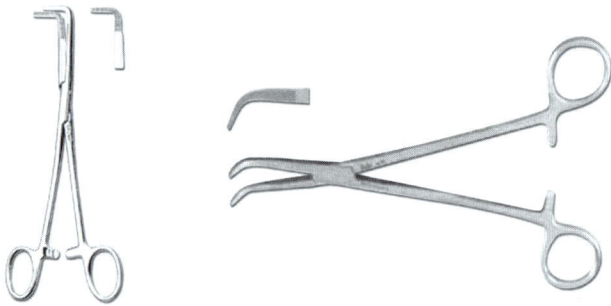

9. MIXTER RIGHT ANGLE FORCEPS (WESTPHAL FORCEPS)

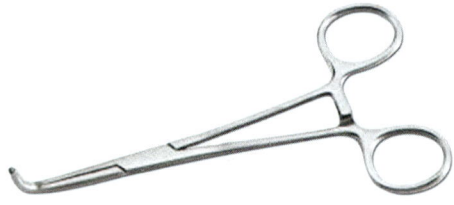

Take truth for your force, take truth for your refuge.

10. DESJARDIN'S CHOLEDOCHOLITHOTOMY FORCEPS

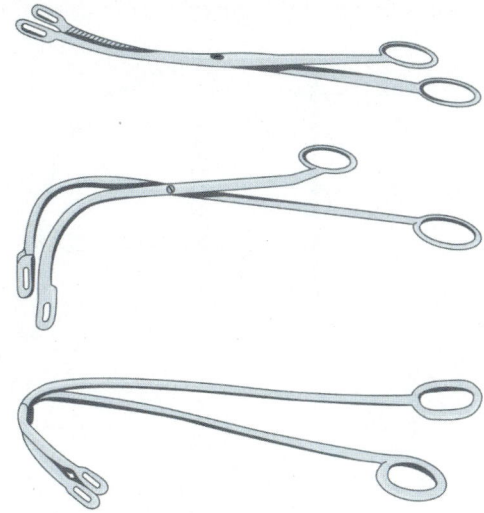

11. GASTRIC OCCLUSION CLAMPS

Kocher's gastric occlusion clamps—the stout blades having vertical serrations

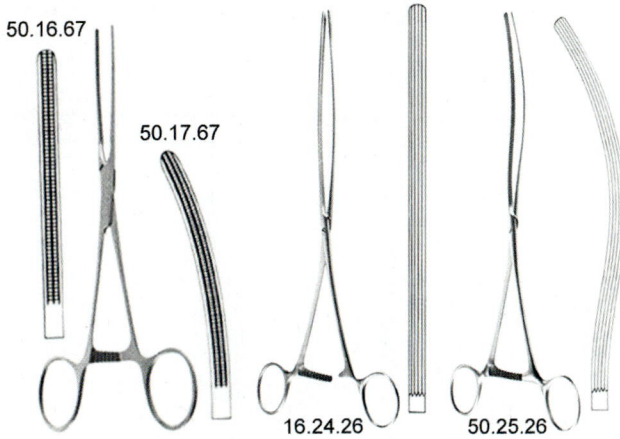

Moynihan's straight and curve gastric occlusion clamps—the blades having transverse serrations with linear fenestration along the center of each blade.

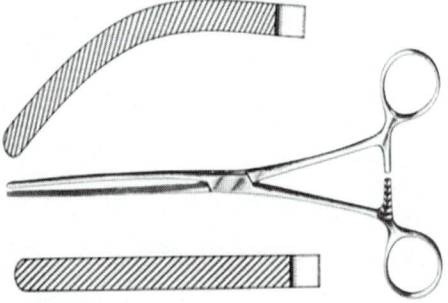

12A. DOYEN'S INTESTINAL OCCLUSION CLAMPS

Doyen's occlusion clamps—these are lighter than the gastric occlusion clamps having the vertical serrations.

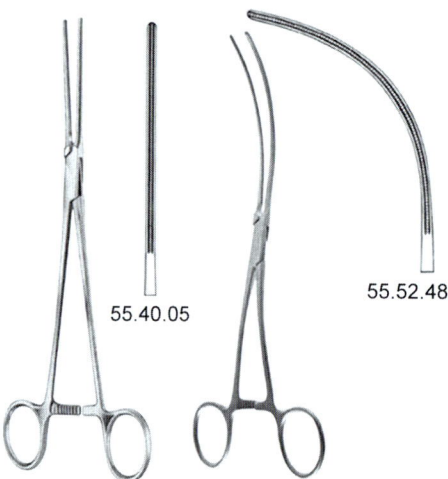

55.40.05   55.52.48

12B. PAYR'S INTESTINAL CRUSHING CLAMPS

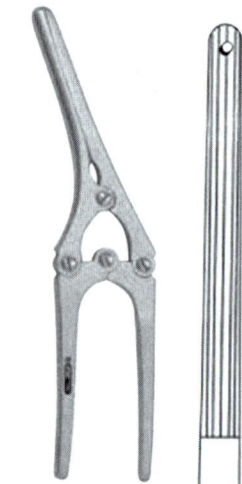

13. PYELOLITHOTOMY FORCEPS

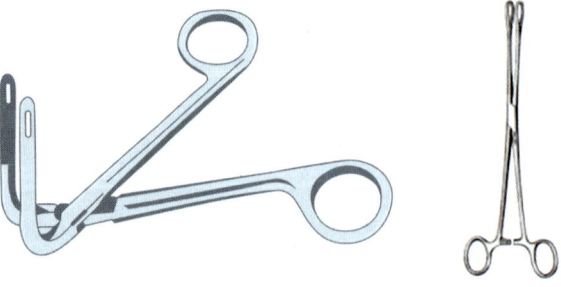

The impossible is the hint of what shall be, Mortality to immortality.

14. RENDAL'S NEPHROLITHOTOMY FORCEPS

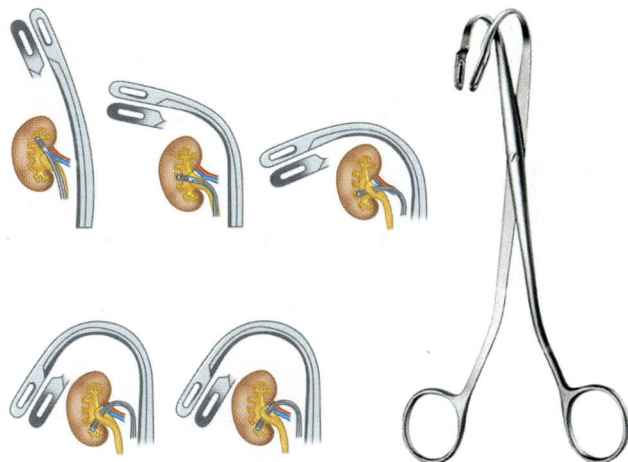

15. CYSTOLITHOTOMY FORCEPS

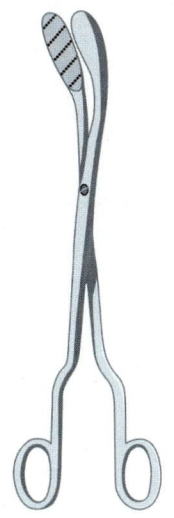

16. CATHETERS AND TUBES

a. Kehr's T-tube

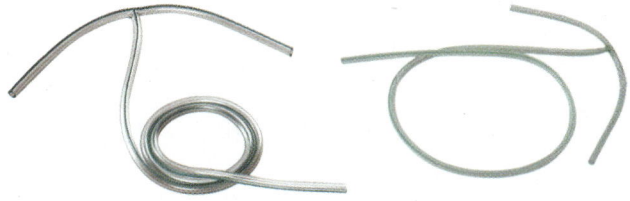

We find in others what is in us. If we always find mud around us, it proves that there is mud somewhere in us.

b. Foley's catheter

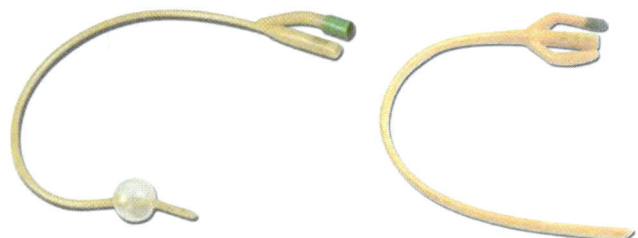

c. Malaecot's catheter

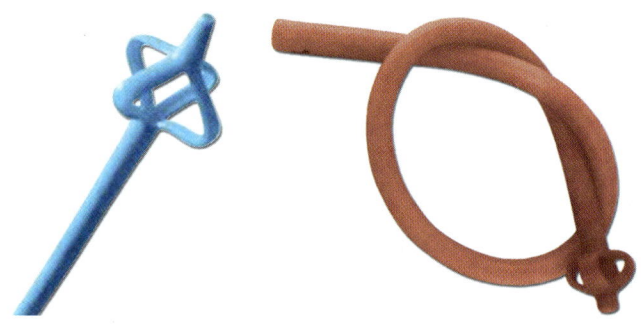

17. AIRWAY TUBES

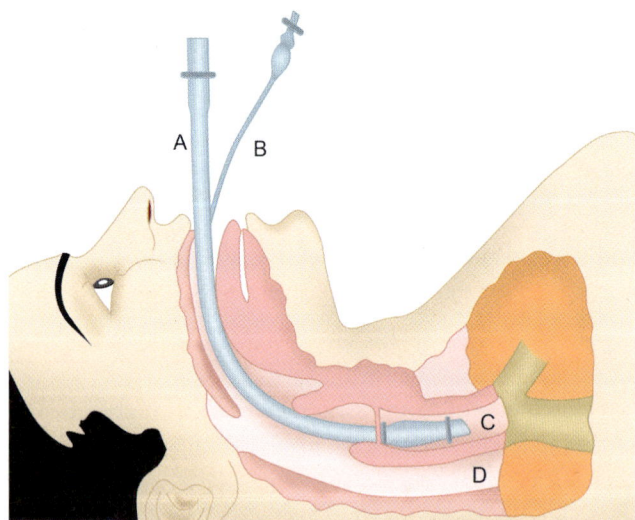

Cuffed endotracheal tube (red rubber)

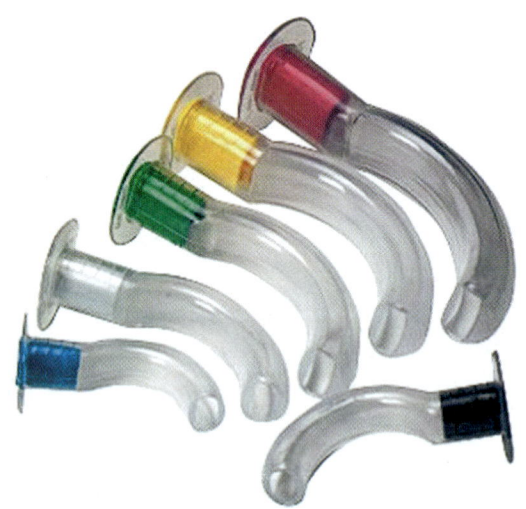

Guedel's oropharyngeal airway

All here must learn to obey a higher law; our body's cells must hold the Immortal's flame.

18. TRACHEOSTOMY TUBE

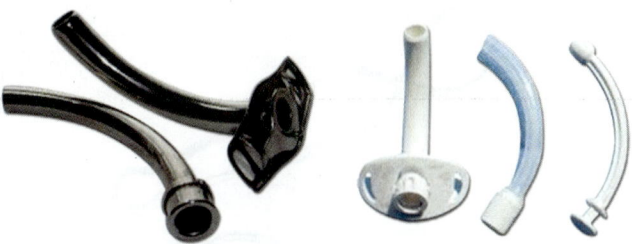

Percutaneous tracheostomy set

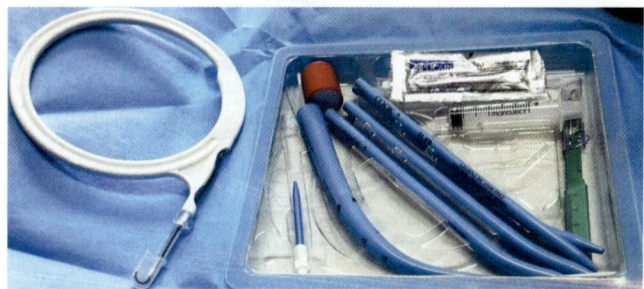

Percutaneous tracheostomy set, fiberoptic bronchoscope, laryngoscope and tracheostomy tube

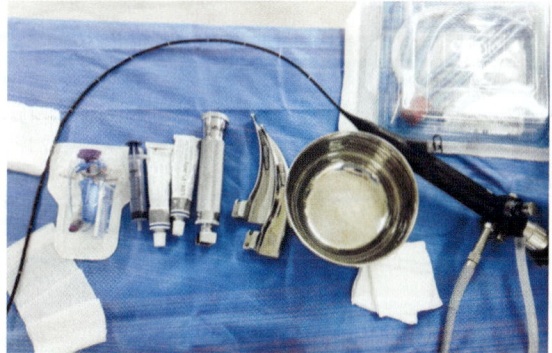

19. PLAIN AND TOOTHED DISSECTING FORCEPS

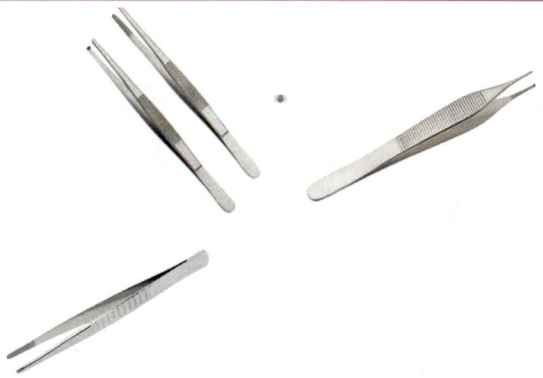

If you want peace upon earth first establish peace in your heart.

20. TOWEL CLIP

1. Doyen's cross towel clip
2. Backhaus towel clip

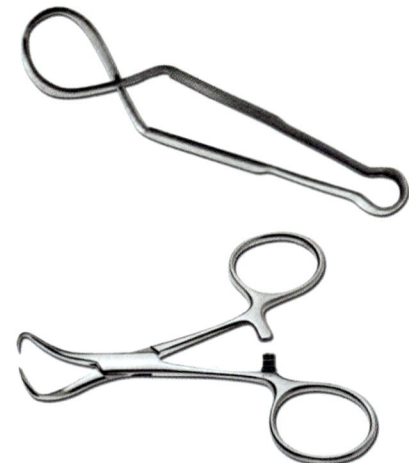

21. DISSECTING SCISSORS

• Mayo's tissue cutting scissors
• Straight scissors

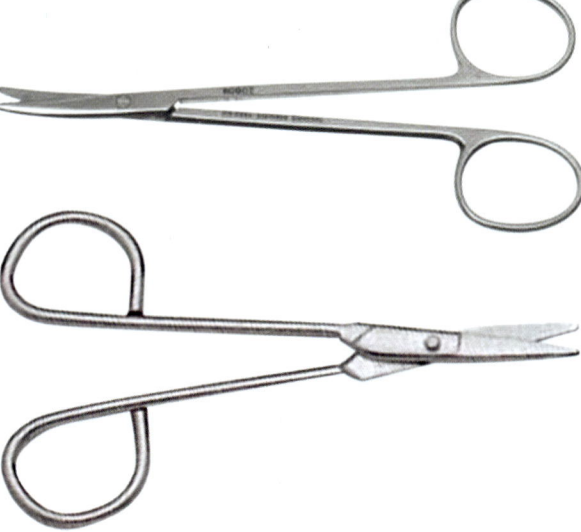

22. NEEDLE HOLDER

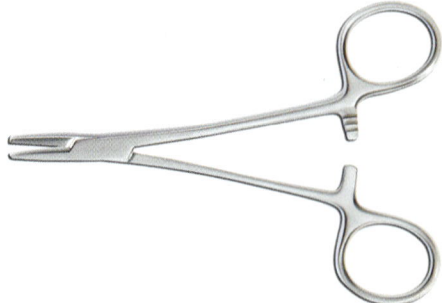

From step to step, from truth to truth, we shall climb ceaselessly until we reach the perfect realization of tomorrow.

23. BARD PARKER HANDLE

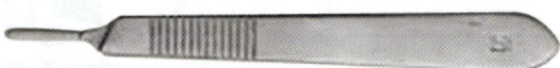

24. LAPAROSCOPY AND ITS EQUIPMENT

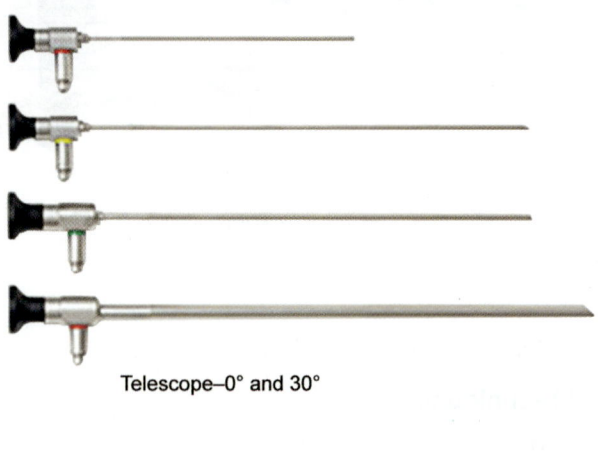

Telescope–0° and 30°

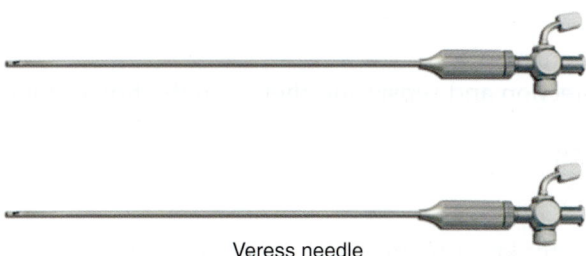

Veress needle

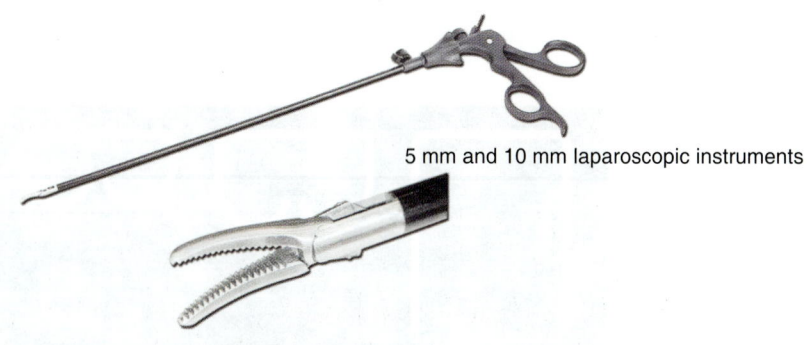

5 mm and 10 mm laparoscopic instruments

Merryland dissecting forceps

Change yourself and then only the circumstances will change.

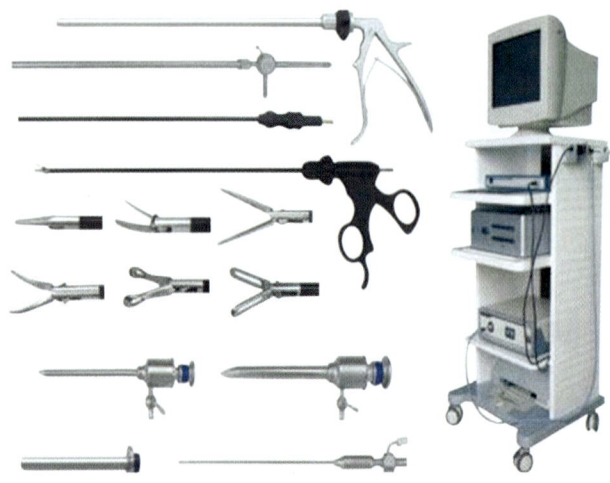

Laparoscopic surgery set

NOTES ON STAPLER, GASTROINTESTINAL (GI) STAPLER AND SUTURE

Primary Goals of the Surgical Techniques

- Restoration of the continuity of the gut and function of the affected part
- Reduction of tissue trauma
- Effective hemostasis to be achieved
- Reduction of morbidity, infection and sepsis and thereby reduction of mortality.

HISTORY OF STAPLING DEVICES

Hutl's Stapling Principles

- A "B-shaped" staple eliminates knotting problems when using surgical steel suture
- "B-shaped" staple configuration helps in hemostasis.
- Use of fine-diameter wire reduces the quantity of foreign objects inserted in the tissues
- Use of fine-diameter wire and a double-staggered staple line provides hemostasis and leakproof.

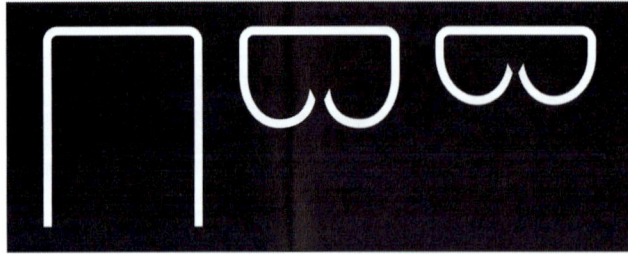

Configuration of surgical stapler

You have no right to judge a man unless you are capable of doing what he does better than himself.

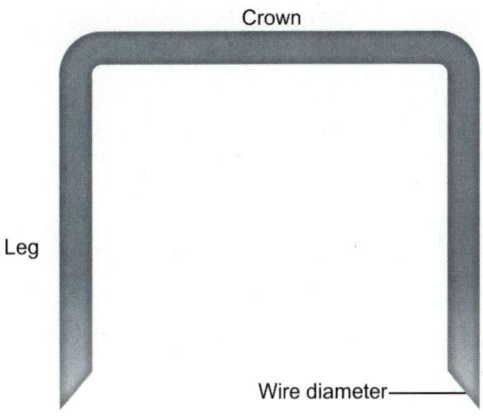

Anatomy of a staple

History of Surgical Stapling

- In 1908, Dr Humer Hütl, Hungarian surgeon, first person who used the surgical stapling device and till date we are following the same principles.
- In 1924, Dr Petz Aladar, another Hungarian surgeon, discovered gastrointestinal stapling device. Each staple was individually loaded. One firing per surgery and reusable are accepted widely globally.
- In 1934, Dr H Friedrich, German Surgeon, modifies "Von Petz" instrument, and creates the concept of reuse of stapler in surgery, designs a reusable cartridge, allowing multiple uses of one instrument in one surgical procedure.

Along with Russian and USA Contributions, the Ethicon Contributes a Lot

- In 1978, Ethicon introduced the first disposable stapling device
- The disposable instruments became standard because of following advantages:
  - Time savings
  - Cost control
  - Reliability
  - Less potential for infection, etc.

ADVANTAGES OF SURGICAL STAPLING

- The use of surgical staplers—especially disposables—can be faster than traditional techniques for suturing and anastomosis, thus reducing total operating time and anesthetic time
- Faster recovery
- Less tissue manipulation, which reduces tissue trauma
- Surgical staplers allow for reach into areas of difficult access, allowing procedures that otherwise could not be performed like ultra-low and low anterior resection.
- Accessibility in relatively non-accessible areas
- Stapled tissue and anastomosis heal as reliably and rapidly as sutured anastomoses
- Reliability
- Uniform quality and quality control-instrument by instrument
  - Sterilization, assembling, packaging, etc.
- Nosocomial infection control and cost control.

Do not think of what you have been, think only of what you want to be and you are sure to progress.

ANASTOMOSIS

SIDE-TO-SIDE GASTROJEJUNOSTOMY

- Skeletonization of the gastric greater curvature
- Elevation of a jejunal loop
- Gastrostomy, jejunostomy
- Introduction of a TLC55 or TLC75 linear cutter
- Firing of the device
- Placement of three traction and guide sutures
- Closure of the common opening using a TL60 linear stapler and the procedure to be completed.

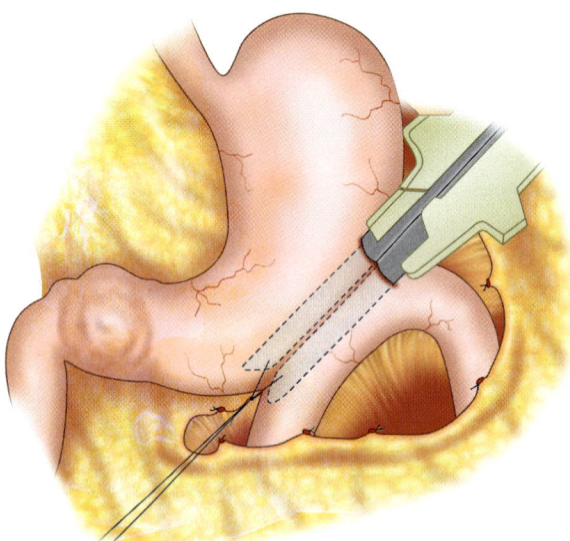

Side-to-side gastrojejunostomy by linear cutter stapler

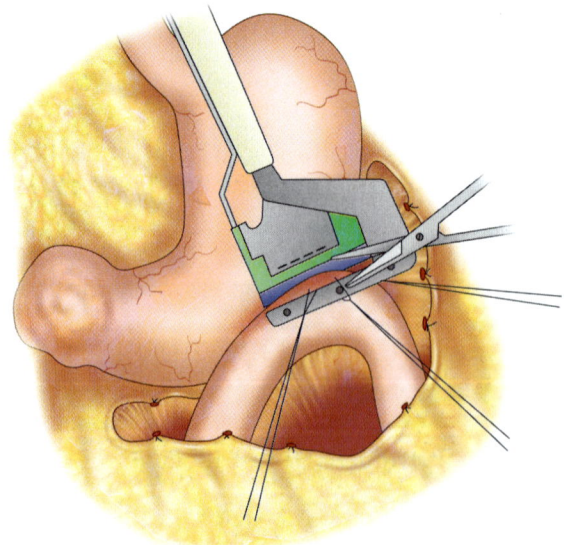

Closure of the common opening using a TL60 linear stapler

The smile within my heart makes all my strength.

END-TO-END FUNCTIONAL

- Closure of a temporary colostomy
- The closed colostomy is detached from the abdominal wall
- A window is opened in the mesocolon
- Both segments are occluded using an intestinal clamp
- Two antimesenteric colostomies
- Introduction of the jaws of a TLC55 or TLC75 linear cutter
- Placement of a seromuscular traction and guide suture closure and firing of the device
- Introduction of the jaws of a TLC55 or TLC75 linear cutter
- Placement of a seromuscular traction and guide suture
- closure and firing of the stapler
- Closure of the common opening using a TL60 linear stapler
- Colon section using the device as a cutting guide.

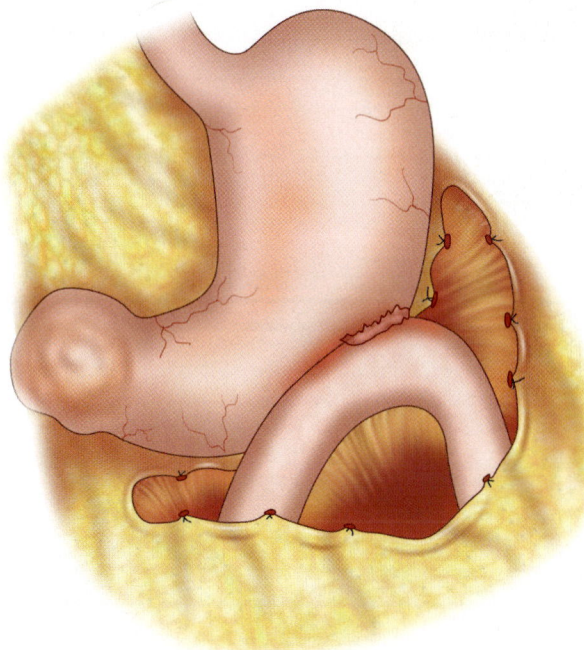

Side-to-side gastrojejunostomy completed

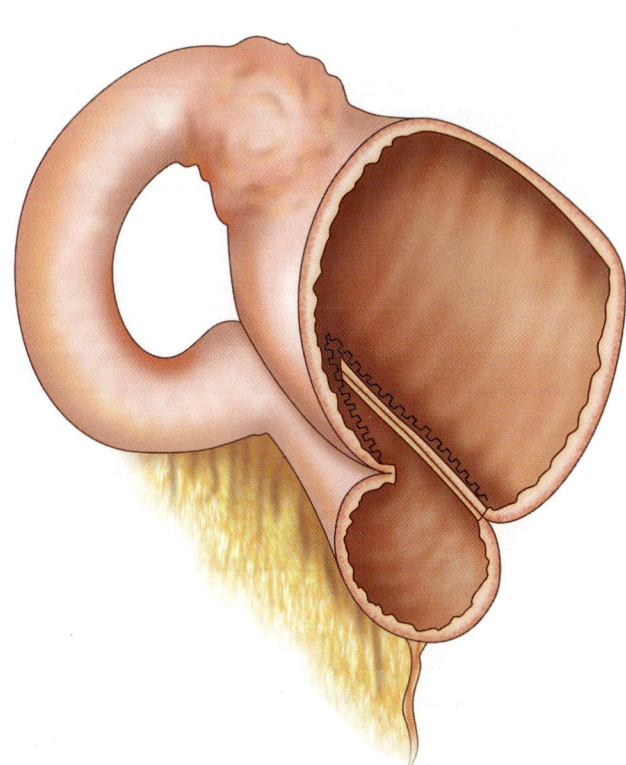

Interior view gastrojejunostomy

A businessman who lost everything in a fire, place a sign board: "Everything burnt but luckily faith and confidence undamaged. Business starts tomorrow.

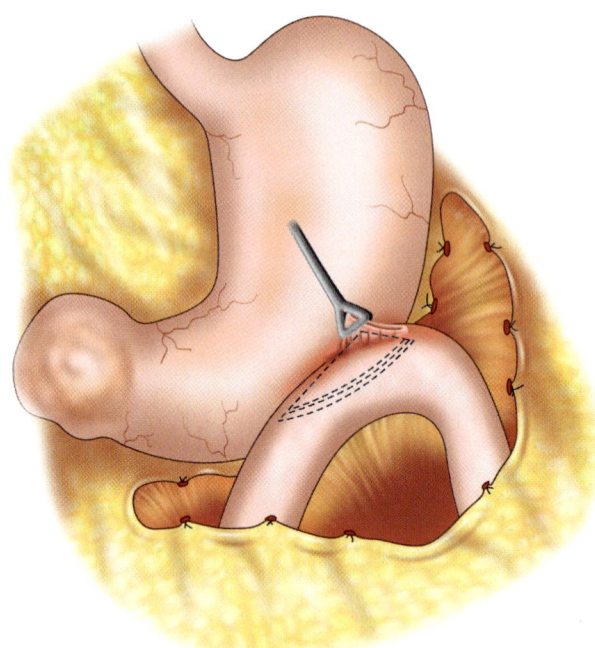

Gastrojejunostomy stoma

END-TO-SIDE ILEOCOLIC ANASTOMOSIS

- Terminal ileectomy
- Right hemicolectomy
- A purse-string suture is placed in the terminal ileum
- The anvil of a CDH25 or CDH29 circular stapler is introduced in the ileal end
- Closure of the purse-string suture on the integral trocar
- Elimination of excess tissue
- Introduction of the device through the proximal colonic end
- Perforation of the antimesenteric border with the integral trocar
- A purse-string suture is placed
- The instrument is assembled
- Closure and firing of the instrument
- The integrity of the anastomosis to be checked
- Placement of three traction and guide sutures
- Closure of the common opening using a TL60 linear stapler or hand sewn.

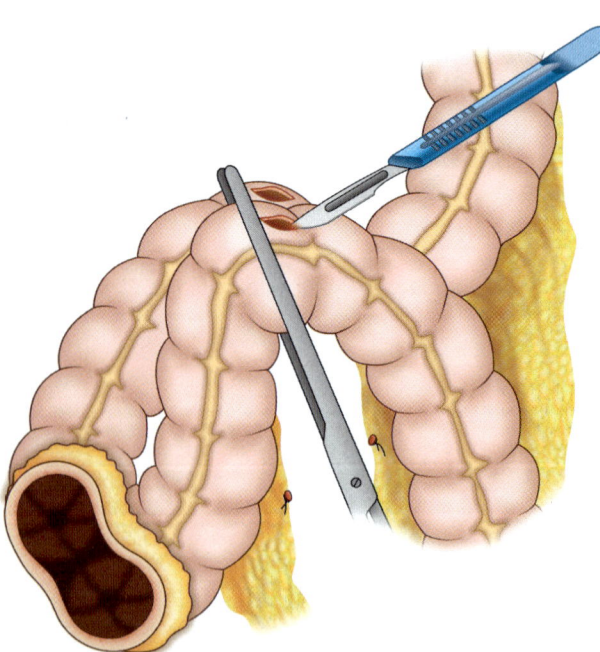

The openings for introduction of linear cutter stapler

Let us keep flaming in our heart, the fire of progress.

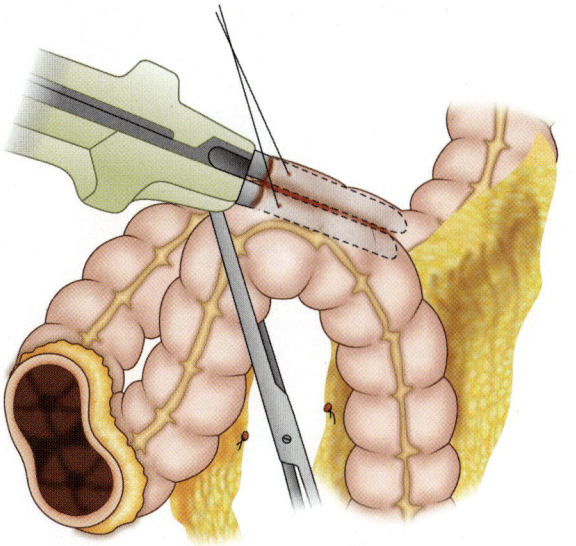

Closure and firing on the stapler

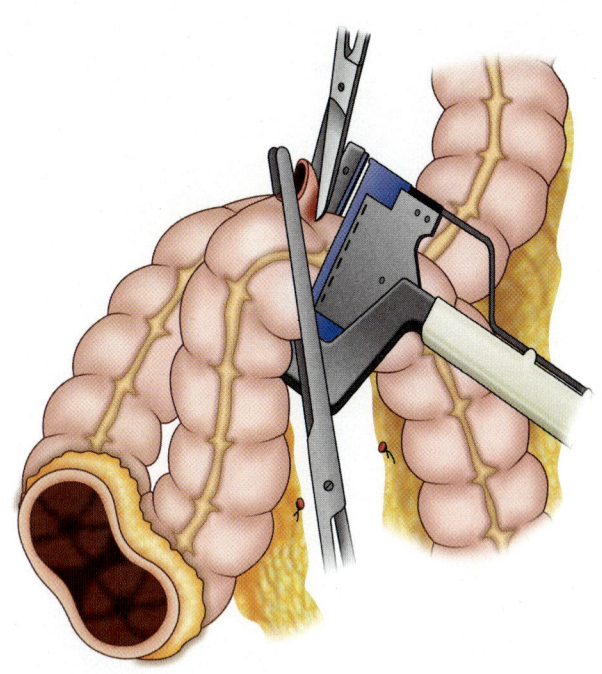

Close the common opening in the gut using a TA60 linear stapler

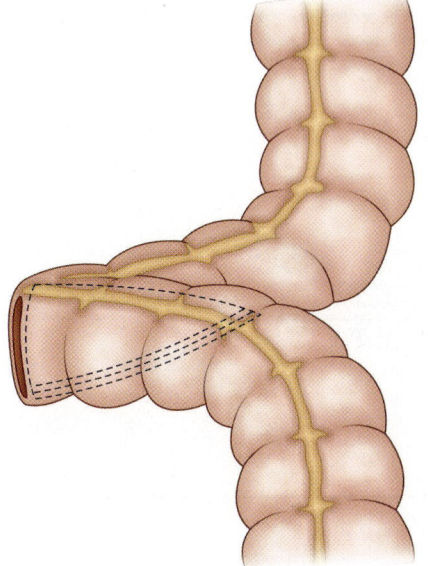

The image shows a projection of the stoma of the functional end-to-end

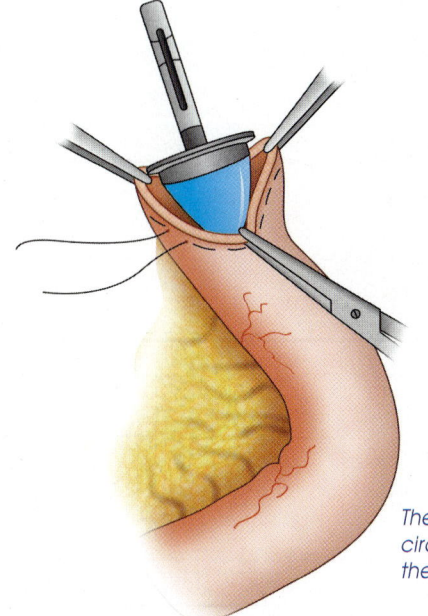

The anvil of a CDH25 or CDH29 circular stapler is introduced in the ileal end

One mighty deed can change the course of things; a lonely thought becomes omnipotent.

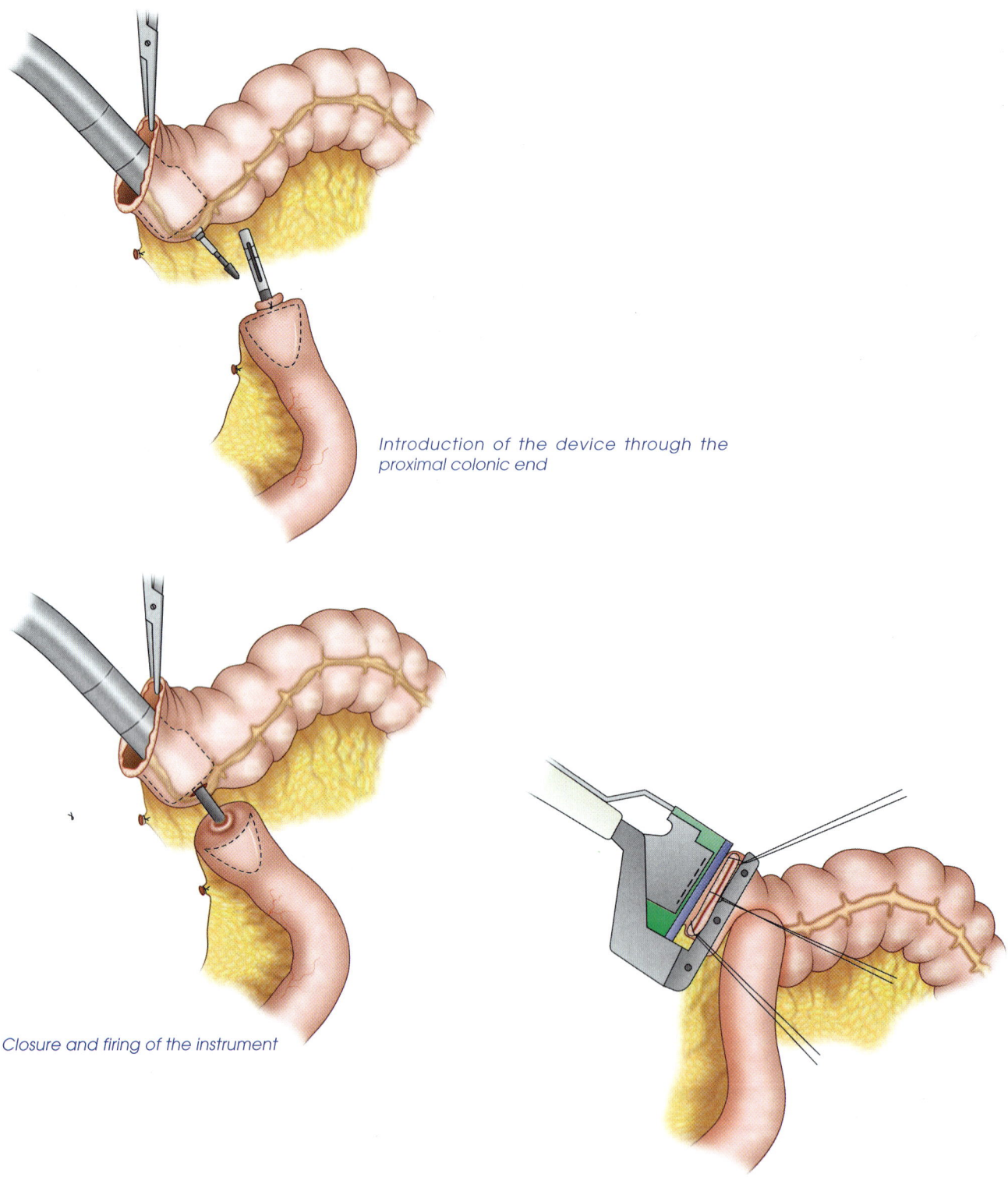

Introduction of the device through the proximal colonic end

Closure and firing of the instrument

Closure of the common opening using TL60 linear stapler

Old man T-shirt quote: "I am not 60, I am 16 with 44 years of experience. Think different. Problems are common to all, but attitude makes the difference".

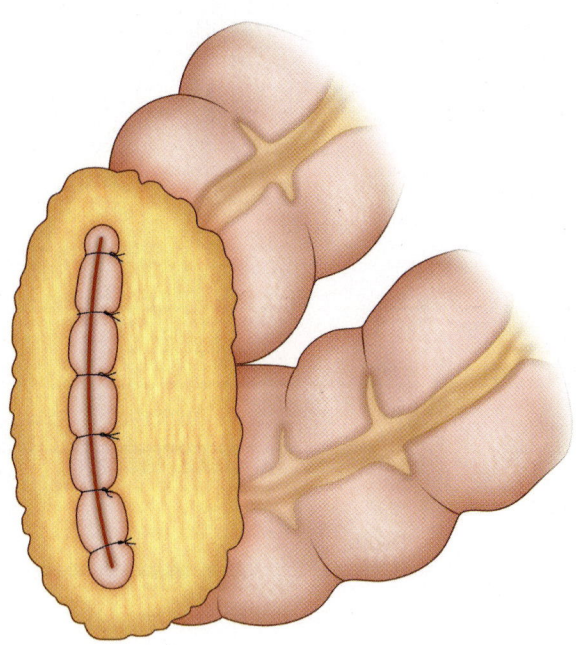

Closure of temporary colostomy

TYPES OF SURGICAL STAPLERS

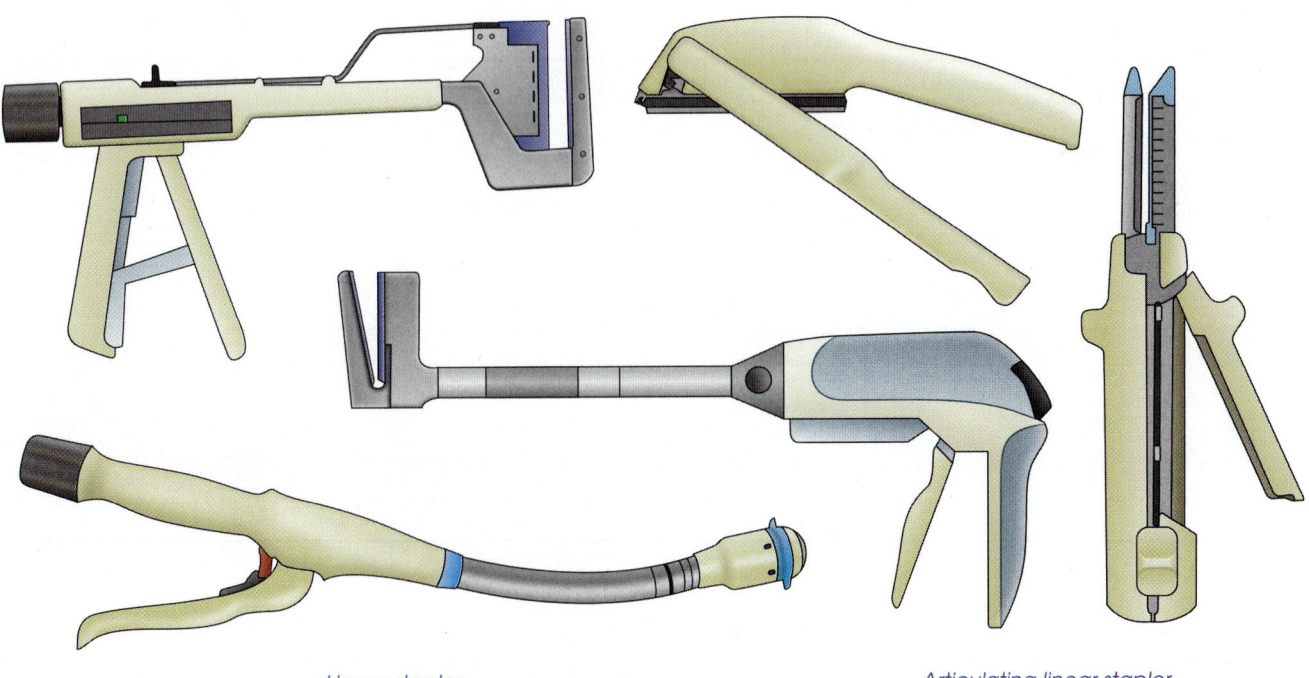

Linear stapler   *Articulating linear stapler*

When you start your day, keep three words in mind: TRY, TRUE and TRUST. Try for better future, true with your work and trust in yourself then success will be your way.

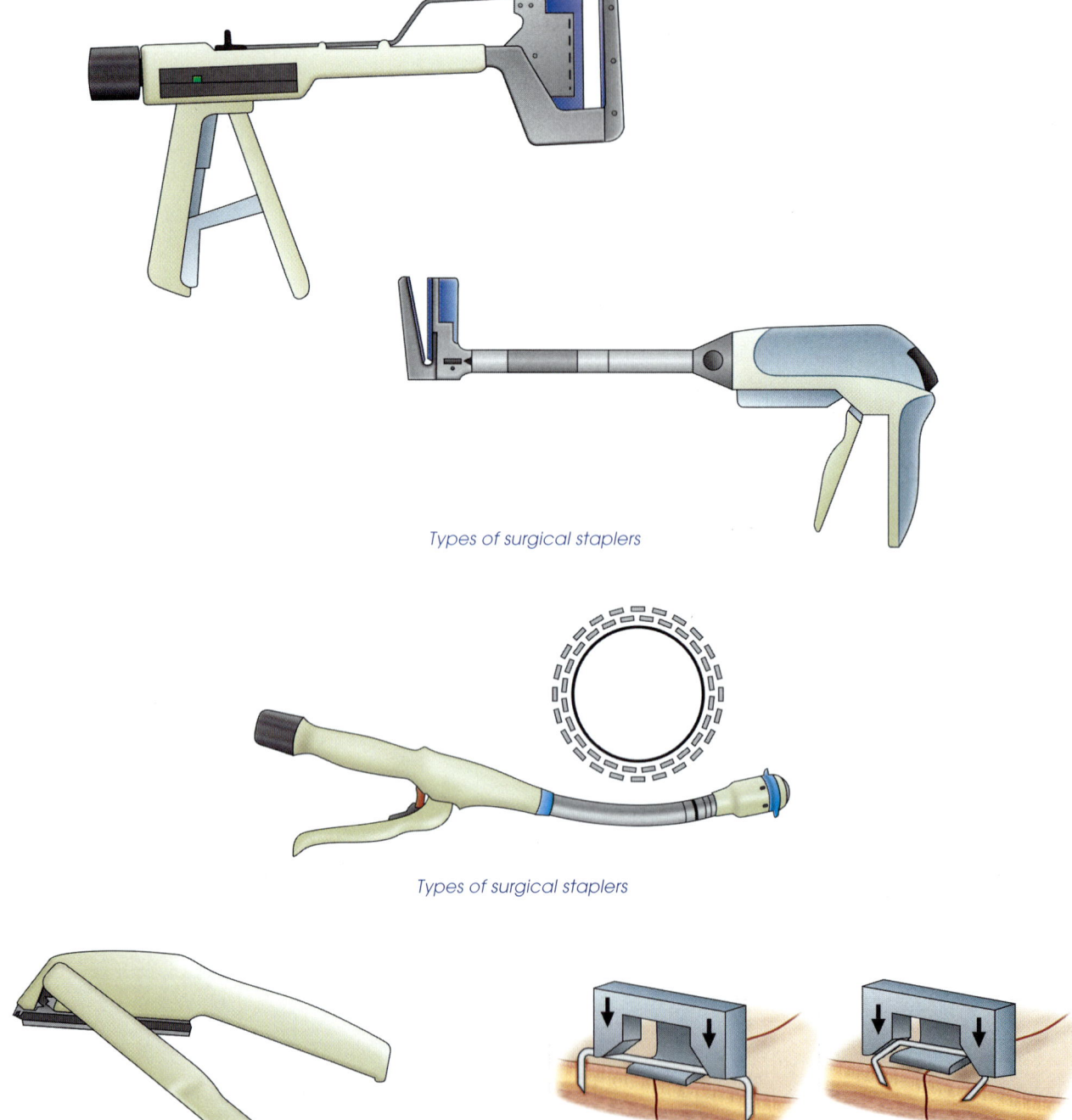

Types of surgical staplers

Types of surgical staplers

Skin stapler: staple formation

Success is never permanent. Failure is never final. So always do not stop effort until your victory makes a history.

GASTRIC SURGERY

Antrectomy with a Billroth Type I Gastroduodenal Reconstruction (usually not recommended nowadays for its inherent drawbacks)

- Skeletonization of the lesser and greater curvatures
- Proximal transection using a TLC75 linear cutter of stomach. If needed, the device can be reloaded for further firing to complete the duodenal transection using a TLC55 linear cutter
- The distal line of transection can be made first
- A gastrotomy is made in the distal staple line, toward the greater curvature
- Placement of guide sutures
- Stabilization of the line to be sutured with a Babcock forceps
- Posterior wall anastomosis using a TL60 linear stapler
- The device is reloaded
- Closure of the anterosuperior edge of the anastomosis using the same TL60 linear stapler
- The device can be reloaded
- Closure of the anteroinferior edge of the anastomosis using the same TL60 linear stapler and completed procedure
- Gastroduodenal anastomosis can be performed by using a CDH25 or CDH29 circular stapler by placement of the anvil in the duodenum
- And closure of the purse-string suture around the integral trocar
- Gastrostomy with a TLC55 linear cutter
- Perforation of the posterior gastric wall, joining of the instruments
- The device is closed and fired
- Verification of anastomotic site
- Placement of traction and guide sutures
- Closure of the gastrostomy with a TL60 linear stapler
- Completed procedure
- Alternative technique using a circular stapler
- Duodenal transection
- Placement of the anvil in the duodenum
- Alternative technique using a circular stapler
- Duodenal transection
- Placement of the anvil in the duodenum
- Closure of the purse-string suture around the integral trocar and elimination of excess tissue
- A gastrostomy is made
- Introduction of the body of the CDH25 or CDH29 circular stapler through the gastrostomy
- Perforation of the posterior wall of the stomach
- Joining of the device components
- Firing of the device and check the integrity of the anastomosis
- Gastric transection using one or two firings of a TLC75 linear cutter
- The antrectomy has been made
- A jejunal loop is selected and antimesenteric jejunostomy made
- Gastrostomy in the posterior gastric surface
- Gastrojejunal anastomosis with the firing of a TLC75 linear cutter
- Placement of traction and guide sutures
- Closure of the common opening using a TL60 linear stapler

With goodwill and faith, nothing is impossible

ALTERNATIVE TECHNIQUE USING A CDH25, A CDH29 OR CDH33 CIRCULAR STAPLER

- A jejunal loop is passed retrocolic and jejunostomy and placement of the anvil
- Closure of a purse-string suture around the integral trocar and elimination of excess tissue
- A gastrostomy is made
- Introduction of the body of the stapler through the gastrostomy
- Perforation of the posterior wall of the stomach
- Joining of the device components and fire
- Check the integrity of the anastomosis
- Placement of traction and guide sutures
- Closure of the common opening using a TL60 linear stapler.

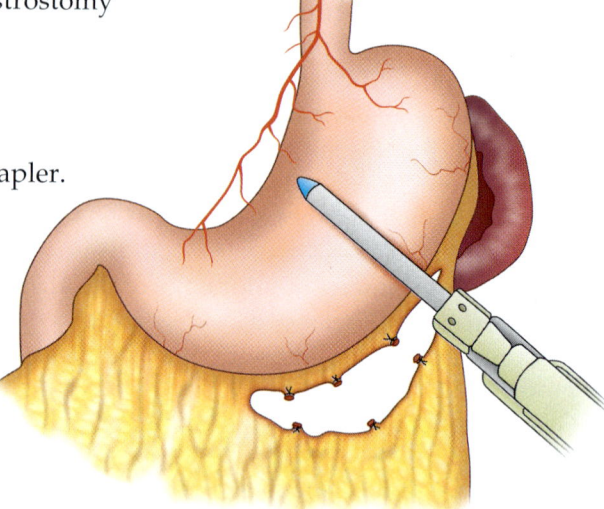

Proximal transection of stomach using TLC75 linear cutter

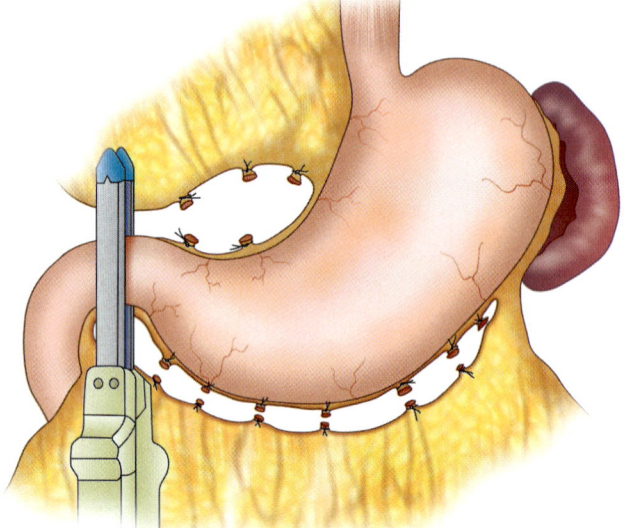

Duodenal transection using a TLC55 linear cutter

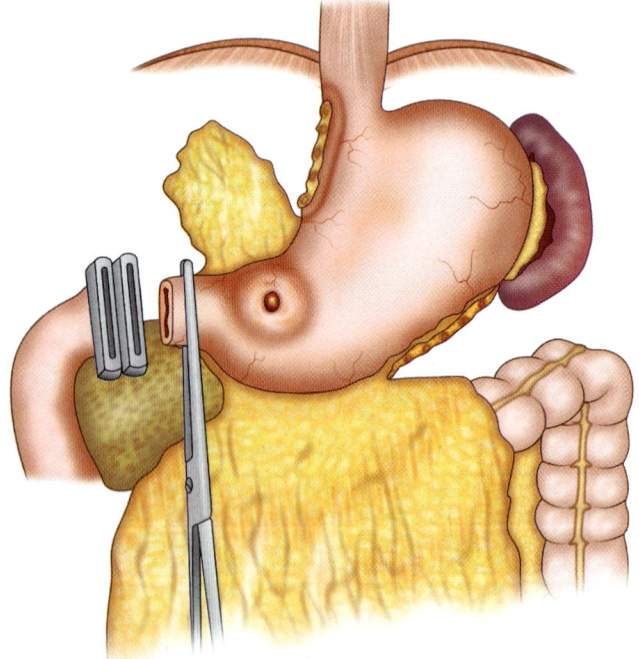

Preparation for a triangulation anastomosis

Remembering is easy for those who have brains, but forgetting is hard for those who have heart.

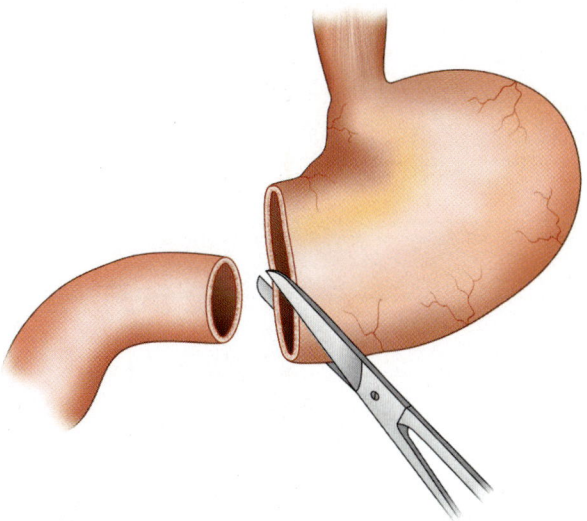

A gastrotomy is made in the distal staple line, toward the greater curvature

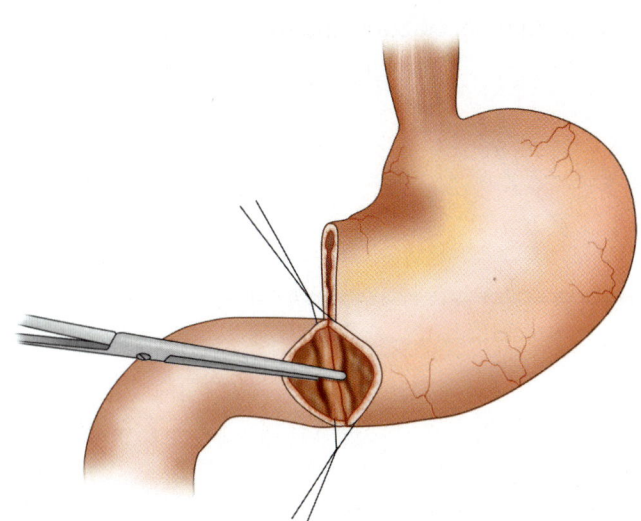

Stabilization of the line to be sutured with a forceps

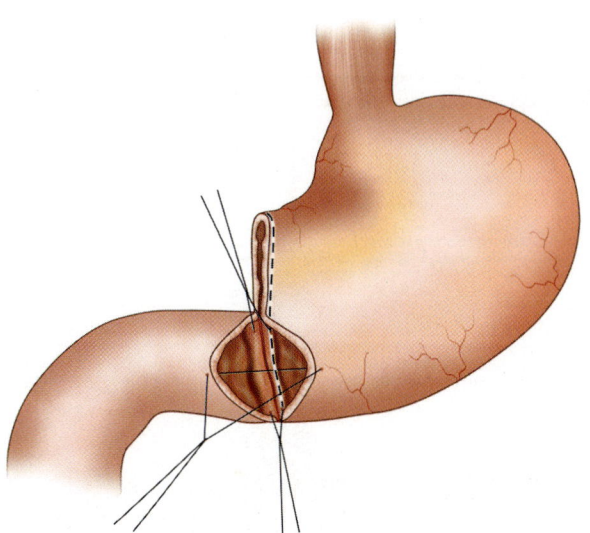

Placement of guide sutures

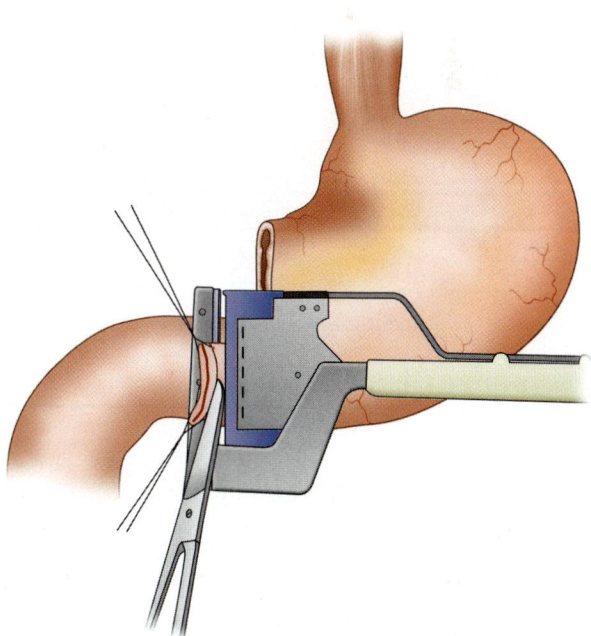

Posterior wall anastomosis using a TL60 linear stapler

Ego is a sword with two edges, the outer edge cuts your popularity while the inner edge cuts your purity.

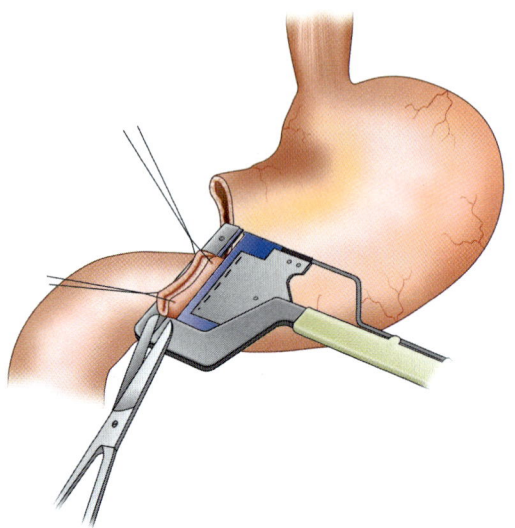

Anterior wall anastomosis using a TL60 linear stapler

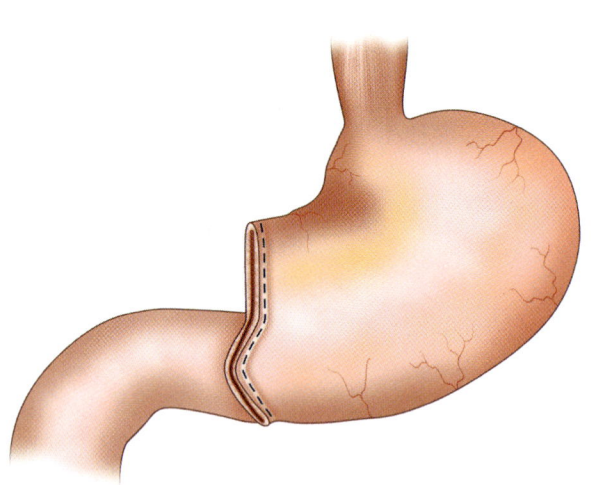

Completed procedure

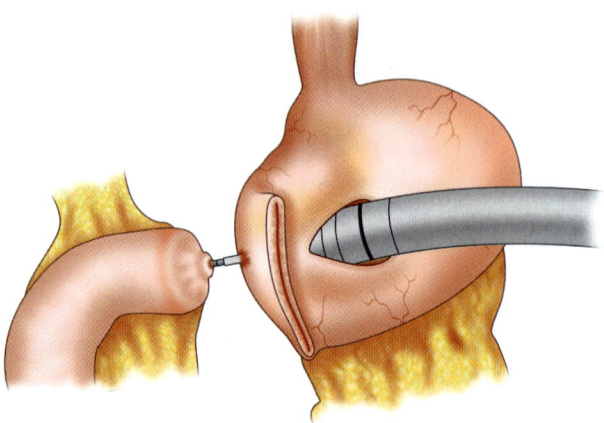

The divice is placed for firing

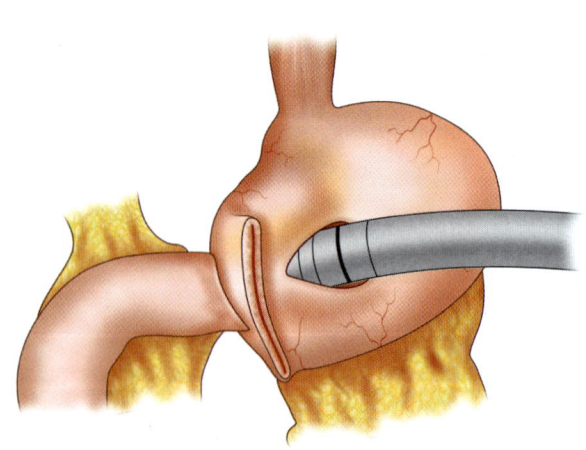

The divice is closed and fired

A negative thinker sees a difficulty in every opportunity, a positive thinker see an opportunity in every difficulty.

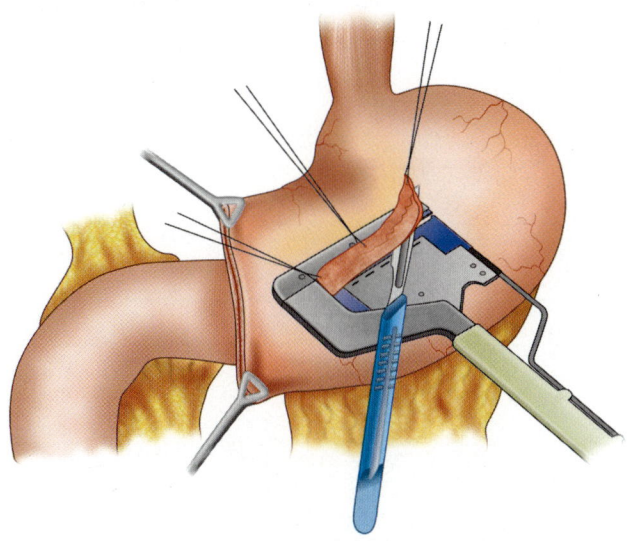

Closure of the gastrostomy with a TL60 linear stapler

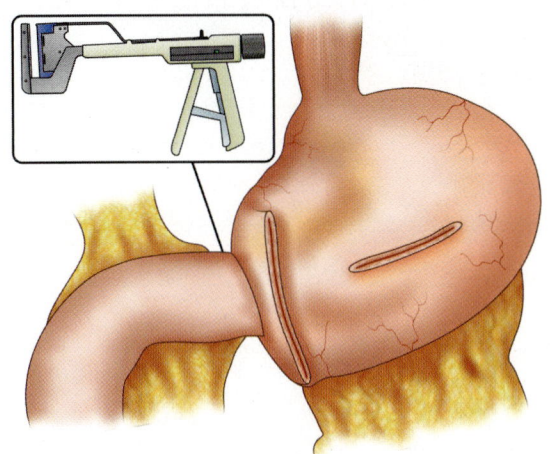

The procedure is completed

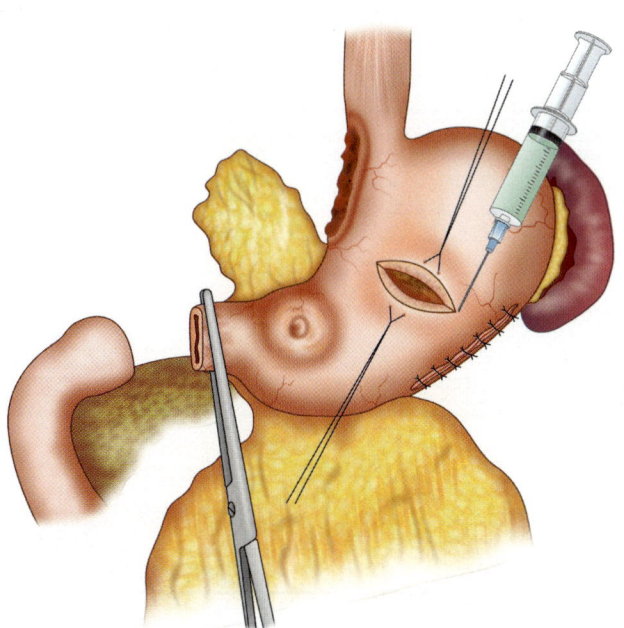

Alternative technique using a circular stapler

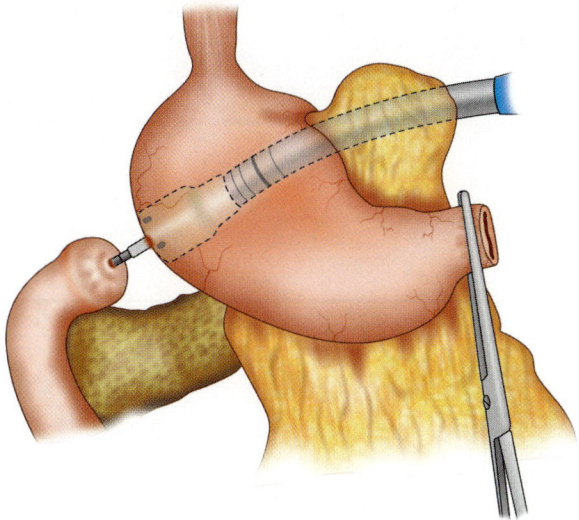

Use of CDH25 or CDH29 circular stapler through the gastrostomy

The nobility of a being is measured by its capacity of gratitude.

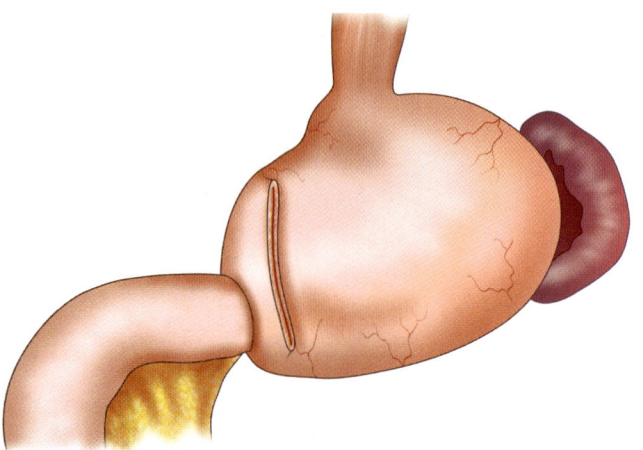

The procedure is completed

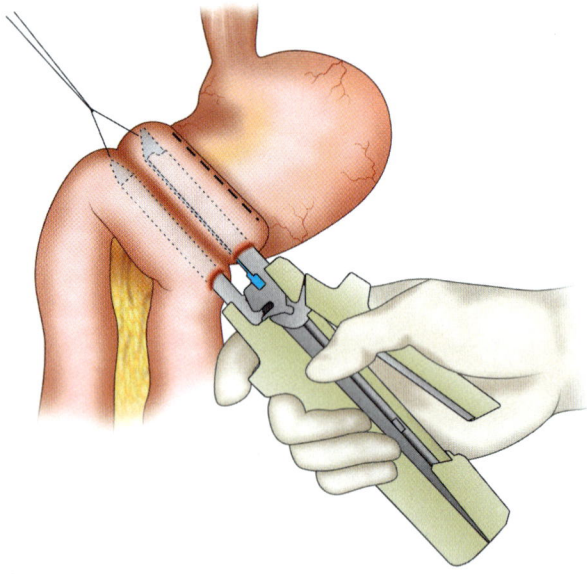

Gastrojejunal anastomosis with the firing of a TLC75 linear cutter

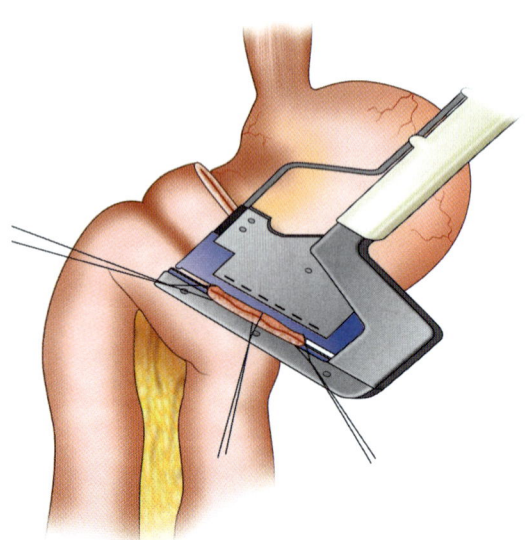

Closure of the common opening using a TL60 linear stapler

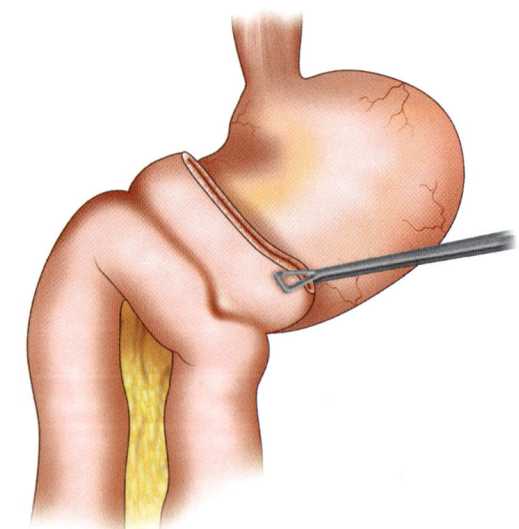

The procedure is completed

Get out of your sensations to have the true feelings.

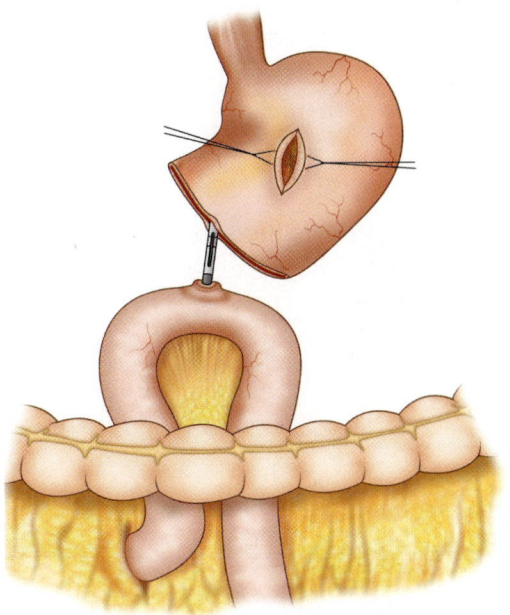

Alternative technique using a CDH25 or a CDH29 circular stapler

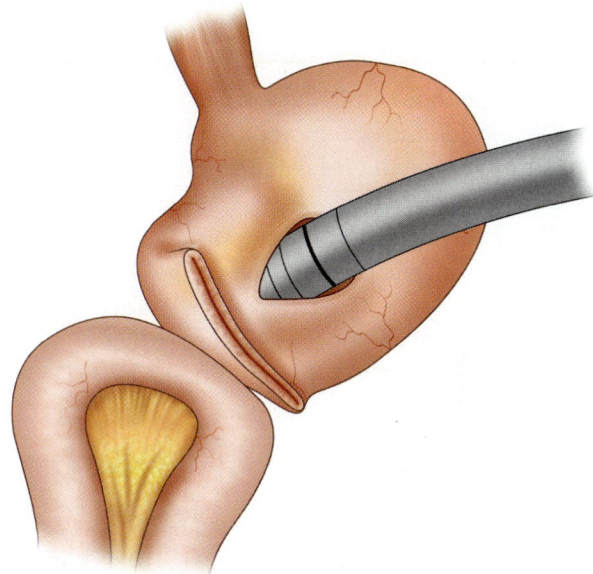

Introduction of the body of the stapler through the gastrostomy

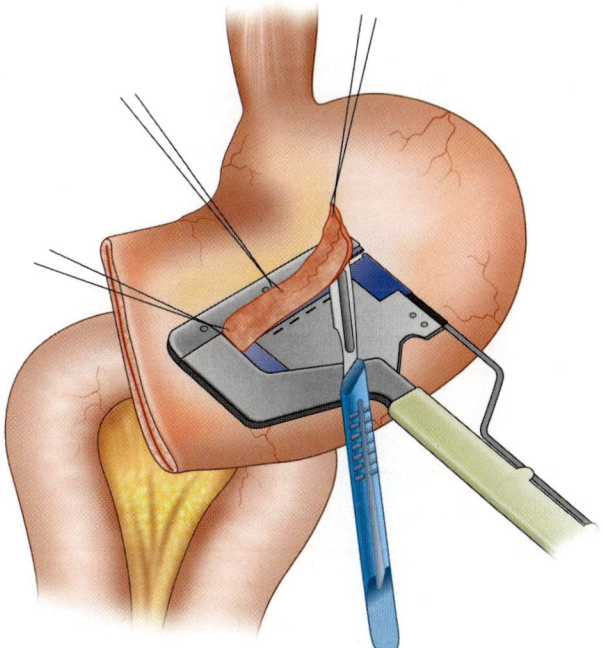

Closure of the common opening using a TL60 linear stapler

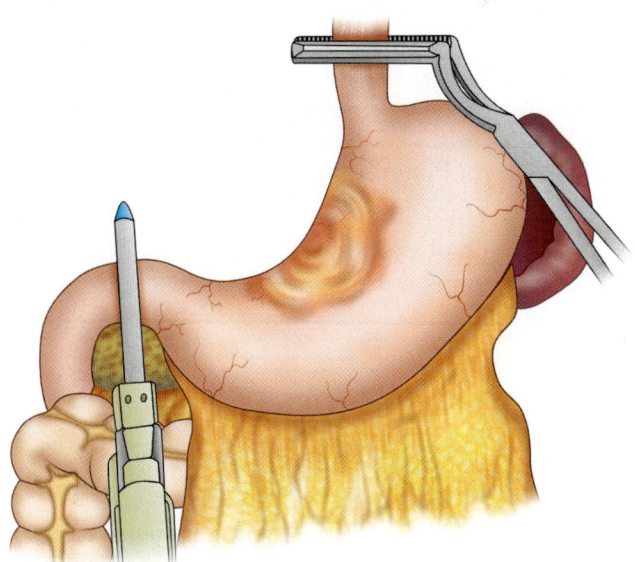

Duodenal transcetion with a TLC55 linear cutter

But, few are they who tread the sunlit path; only the pure in soul can walk in light.

TOTAL GASTRECTOMY WITH ROUX-EN-Y ANASTOMOSIS

- Skeletonization of the greater and lesser curvatures
- Duodenal transection with a TLC55 linear cutter
- Placement of a purse-string suture and esophageal transection
- Specimen retrieval
- Jejunal transection distal to the ligament of Treitz
- The jejunal loop is passed retrocolic and a purse-string suture is placed on its proximal end
- Placement of the anvil of a CDH21 or a CDH25 circular stapler in the esophagus
- Closure of a purse-string suture around the integral trocar and elimination
- Distal jejunostomy
- Retrograde introduction of the device through the jejunostomy
- Joining of the device components
- Firing of the device
- Check the integrity of the esophagojejunal anastomosis
- Antimesenteric jejunostomy in the distal end of the proximal jejunal segment
- The jejunojejunal anastomosis is made with one firing of a TLC55 linear stapler
- Placement of traction and guide sutures
- Closure of the common opening using a TL60 linear stapler
- Elimination of excess tissue.

Alternative Technique

- Placement of the anvil of a CDH25 circular stapler in the distal end of the proximal jejunal segment
- Placement of the anvil of a CDH21 circular stapler in the distal esophagus
- Closure of the purse-string sutures around the integral trocars and elimination of excess tissue
- Anterograde introduction of the device through the proximal end of the distal jejunal segment
- Joining of the components and firing of the device
- Jejunostomy and retrograde introduction of a CDH21 circular stapler
- Joining of the components and firing of the device.

Verification of the Integrity

- Closure of the jejunostomy with a TL60 linear stapler
- Elimination of excess tissue
- Completed procedure.

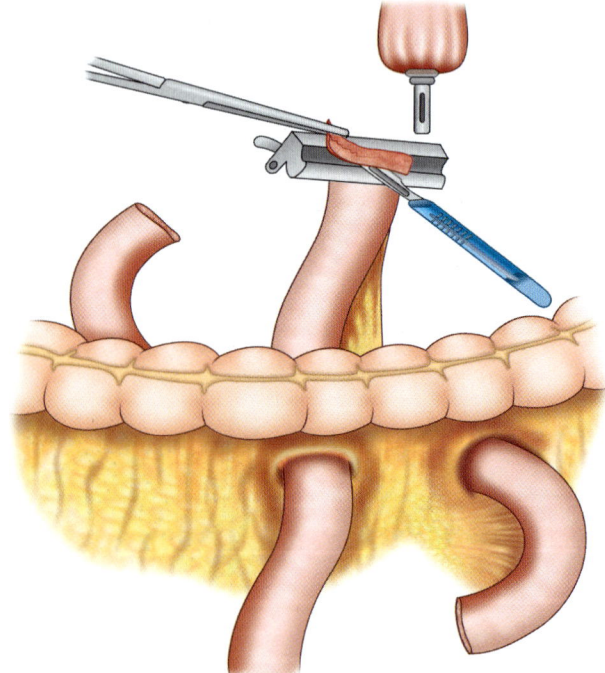

Placement of the anvil of a CDH21 or a CDH25 circular stapler in the esophagus

---

Our greatest weakness lies in giving up. The most certain way to succeed is always to try just one more time.

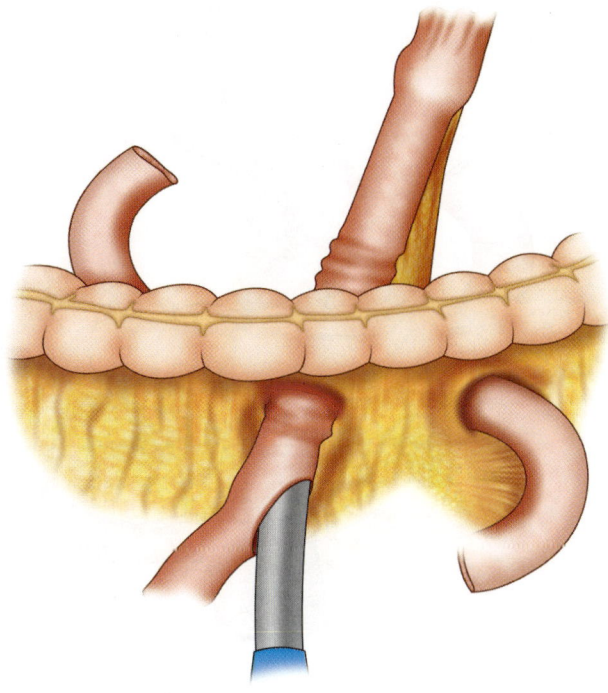

Retrograde introduction of the device through the jejunostomy

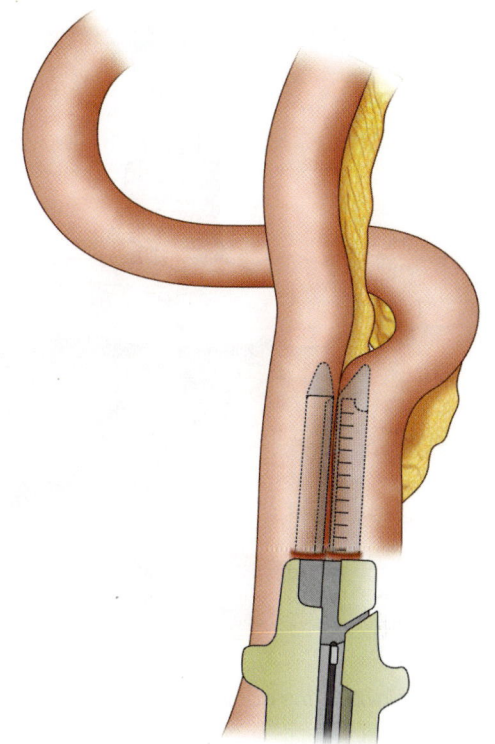

The jejunojejunal anastomosis is made with firing of a TLC55 linear stapler

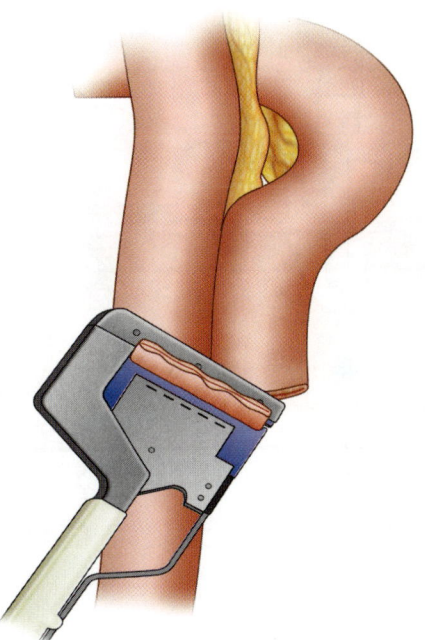

Closure of the common opening using a TL60 linear stapler

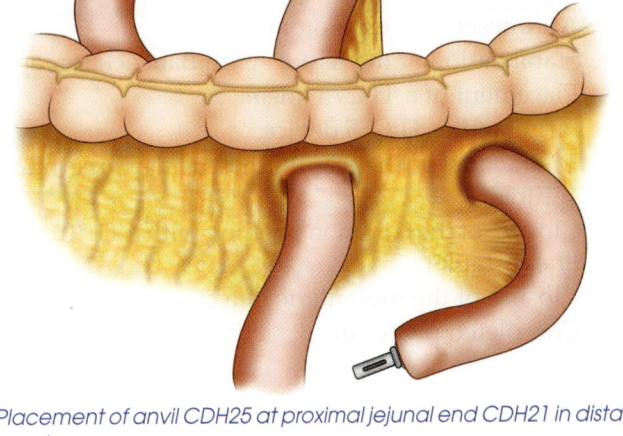

Placement of anvil CDH25 at proximal jejunal end CDH21 in distal esophagus

Get out of your mind to have the true intelligence.

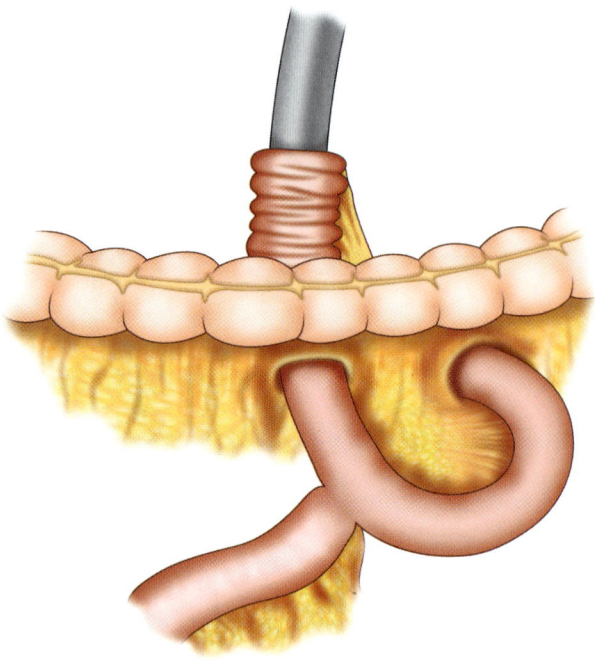

Joining of the components and firing of the divice

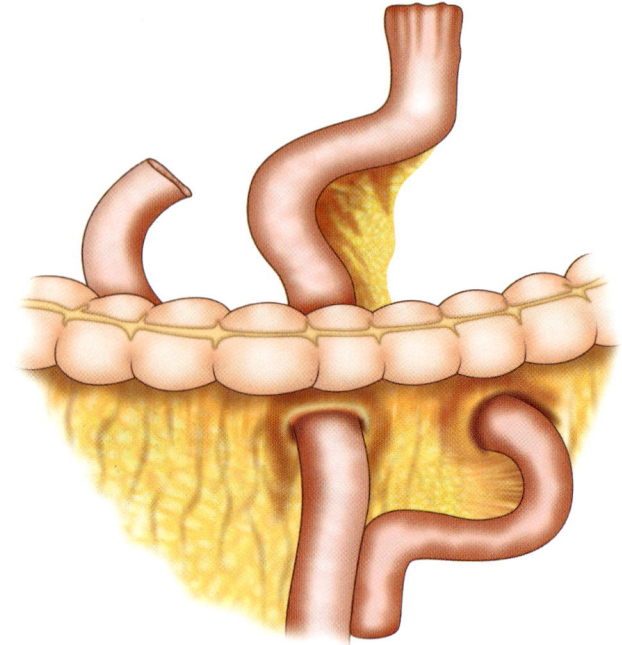

Closure of the jejunostomy and complete the procedure

COLORECTAL SURGERY

Right Hemicolectomy

Side-to-side Ileocolic Anastomosis

- Mobilization of the right colon
- Mobilization of the hepatic flexure
- Ileal transection with a TLC75 linear cutter
- The instrument is reloaded
- Transection of the transverse colon using the same device
- Antimesenteric enterotomies
- Stabilization of the tissues with Babcock forceps
- Placement of a TLC75 linear
- Firing of the TLC75 device
- Distraction of the staple lines using three traction sutures
- Closure of the common opening with a TL30 or TL60 linear stapler
- Closure of the mesenteric defect
- Completed procedure.

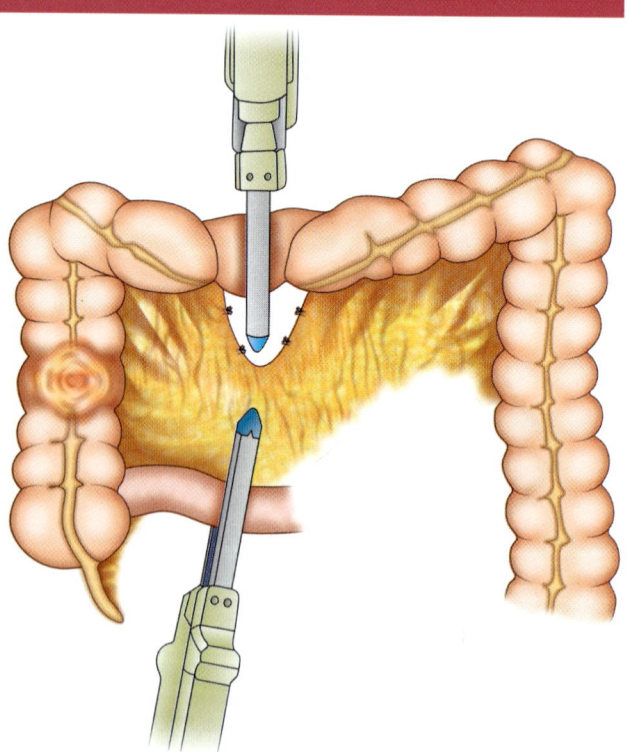

Ileal transection with a TLC75 linear cutter

There is no greater courage than to be always truthful.

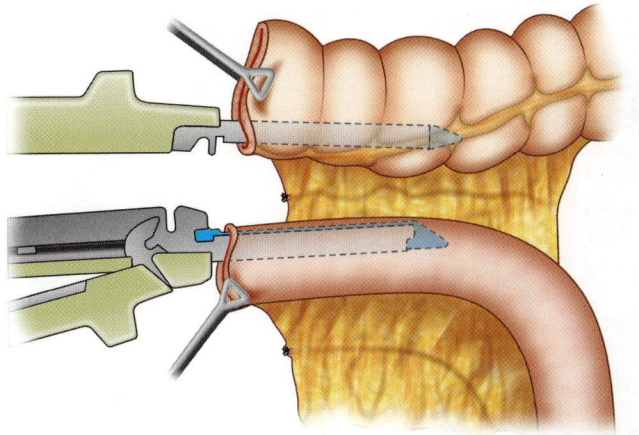

Placement of a TLC75 linear stapler

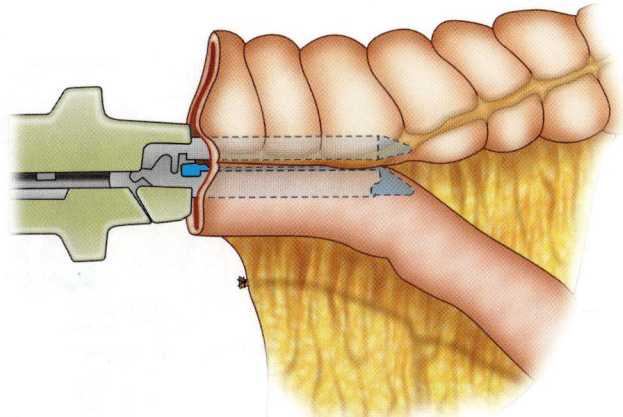

Firing of the TLC75 divice

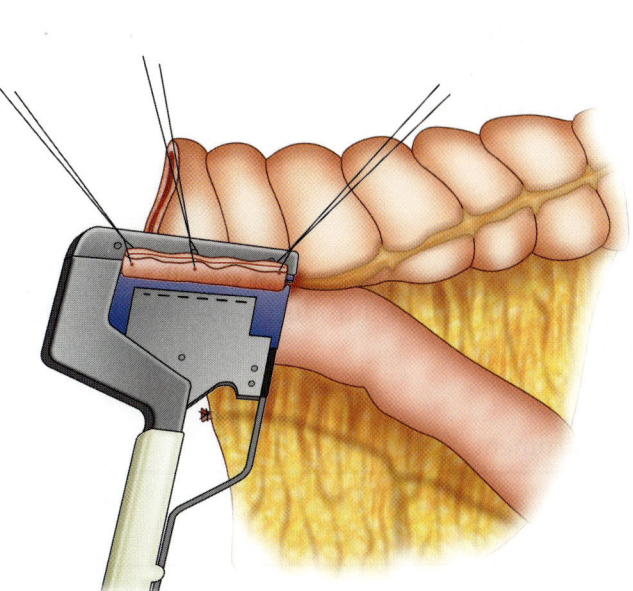

Closure of the common opening using a TL60 linear stapler

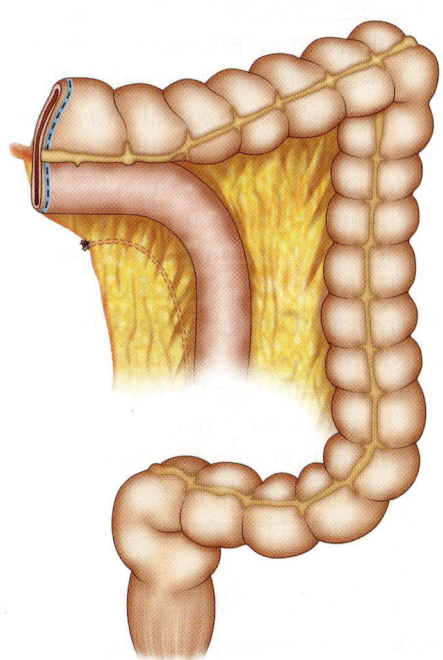

Closure of the mesenteric defect and complete the procedure

Talent is God given, be humble; fame is man given, be grateful; conceit is self-given, be careful.

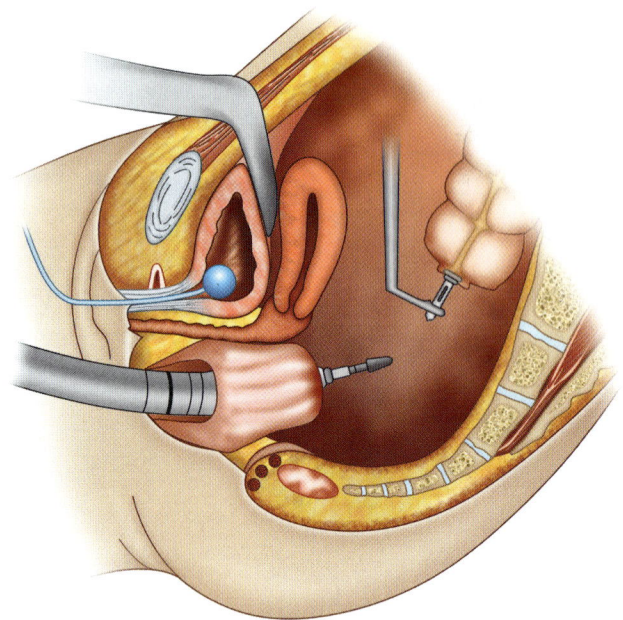

Transanal introduction of the body of the instrument

LOW ANTERIOR RESECTION WITH END-TO-END ANASTOMOSIS

- Colorectal mobilization
- Closed specimen extraction: Proximal and distal transections with a TLC55 linear cutter
- Placement of proximal and distal purse-string sutures
- Alternative: Use of a rigid or articulating linear stapler for the creation
- Removal of the proximal line of staples
- Placement of the anvil of a CDH29 or CDH33
- Closure of the purse-string suture over the integral trocar
- Elimination of excess tissue
- Transanal introduction of the body of the instrument
- Alternative: If a distal line of staples is present, then the integral trocar is introduced passing through it, thus eliminating the need for a distal purse-string suture
- Closure of the purse-string suture around the integral trocar
- Elimination of excess tissue
- The tissues must be taut over the anvil and body of the instrument
- Completed procedure.

COLOPROCTECTOMY WITH ILEAL "J"

Pouch and Ileoproctostomy

- Creation of the rectal stump
- Placement and firing of an ACCESS55 articulating linear stapler 2 cm superior to the line of the crypts
- Rectal transection using the instrument as a cutting guide

Happiness is the best revenge as nothing drives your enemies more insane than seeing you smiling and living a good life.

- Creation of the ileal pouch
- Distal enterotomy at the end of the "J" loop
- Introduction and firing of a TLC55 or TLC75 linear cutter
- The instrument is reloaded
- The instrument is introduced again, allowing the tissues to "bunch" over the shoulders of the device, and fired again
- A purse-string suture is placed on the enterotomy in preparation for the anastomosis
- Placement of the anvil of a CDH29 or CDH33 circular stapler in the enterotomy
- Closure of the purse-string suture and elimination of excess tissue
- Transanal introduction of the circular stapler body
- The integral trocar must perforate the rectal staple line
- The instrument is fired and the integrity of the staple line is verified
- Completed procedure.

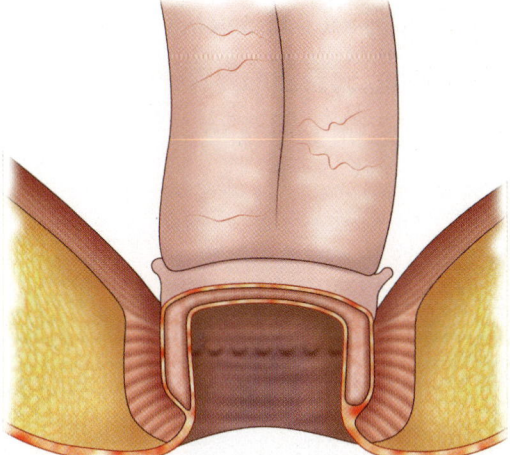

Coloproctectomy with ileal "J" pouch and ileoproctostomy

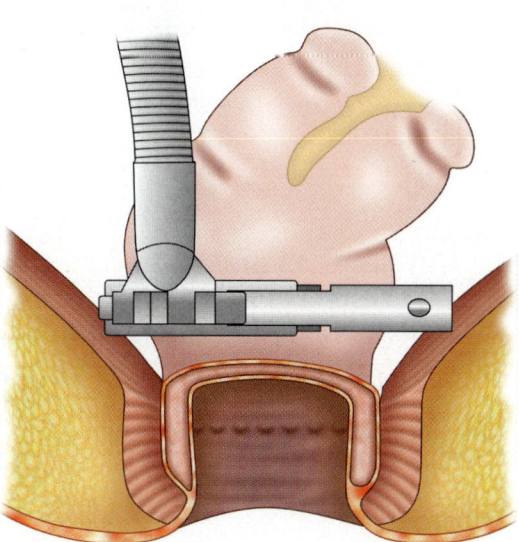

Placement and firing of an ACCESS55 articulating linear stapler

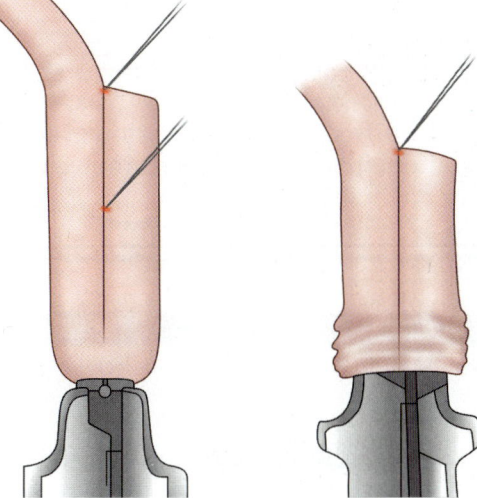

Introduction and firing of a TLC55 or TLC75 linear cutter and distal enterotomy at the end of the "J" loop

Keep the smile, leave the tear, think of joy and forget the fear. Hold the laugh, leave the pain, be joyous because it is only your day.

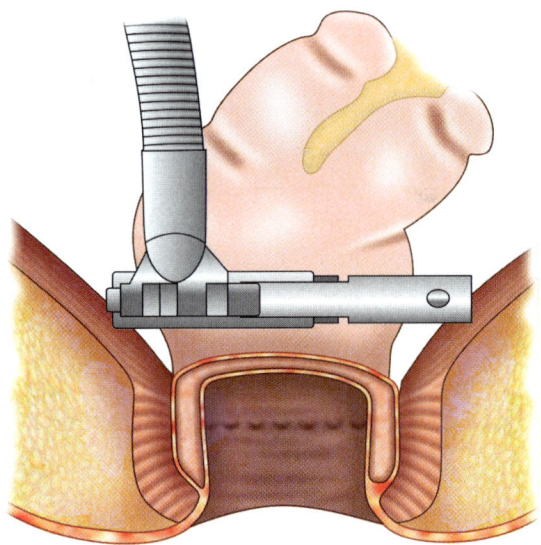

Placement of the anvil of a CDH29 or CDH33 circular stapler in the enterotomy

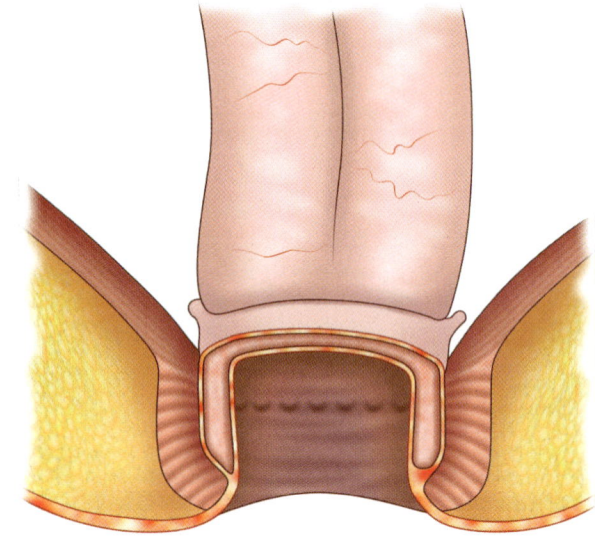

Ileoproctostomy completed

GASTROINTESTINAL STAPLING TECHNIQUES

Introduction

Until now in the course you have been using suturing techniques in different situations, however, the development of mechanical stapling devices means that there are alternative ways of performing many anastomoses.

Trials have not shown any benefit in terms of outcome for either a sutured or a stapled anastomotic technique. There is no doubt, however, that stapling techniques are quicker to perform, particularly in situations where access is difficult, such as a low colorectal anastomosis or an esophageal anastomosis. Stapling should, therefore, be part of the modern surgeon's armoury and you should be equally adapted with a staple gun as with a needle holder and suture.

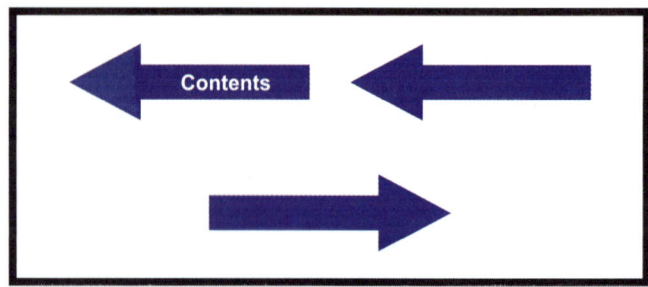

Challenges are what make life interesting and overcoming them is what makes life meaningful.

Historical Principles

There are many types of stapling devices that may be used on the bowel, but these may be broadly categorised into those which:

- Produce a linear staple line
- Cut between two linear staple lines
- Cut and result in a circular staple line.

In all cases, it is essential to be sure of what you wish to achieve with the mechanical stapler and to then select the appropriate instrument. In many cases, there are different sizes of instrument and the correct one must be chosen for the correct procedure. Similarly, the size of the staples may be different or may be changeable depending upon the instrument and the manufacturer—clearly this must be gauged by the surgeon, again depending upon the task in hand.

Because the actual anastomosis is performed with a mechanical device instead of the individual placement of sutures, it does not mean that you afford to be any less meticulous in the setting up of the anastomosis and in the performance of the procedure.

A stapled anastomosis will fail in the same way that

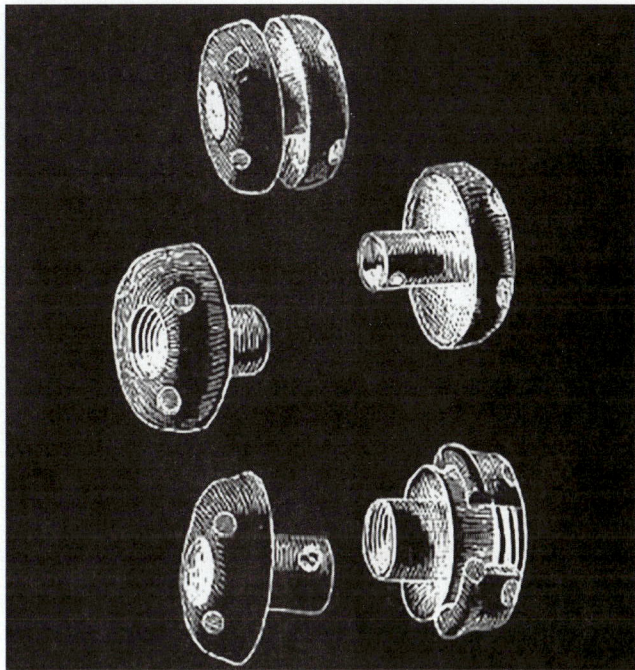

Murphy's Button in 1892 as an early mechanical device for gastrointestinal (GI) anastomoses

a sutured anastomosis will, i.e. if the bowel ends are not well vascularized are under tension or there is a technical failure in the performance of the anastomosis.

Clearly, the application of each of these points will be dependent upon the site of the anastomosis, i.e. whether this is a small bowel, a colorectal or esophagogastric anastomosis. For the purposes of this course, we will describe the reconstruction following a total gastrectomy using a stapling technique. Instead, emphasis will be given to stages of the reconstruction in which stapling devices are frequently utilized.

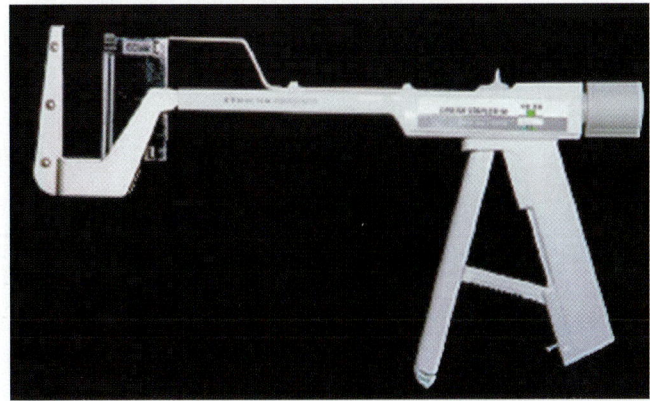

Linear stapling device

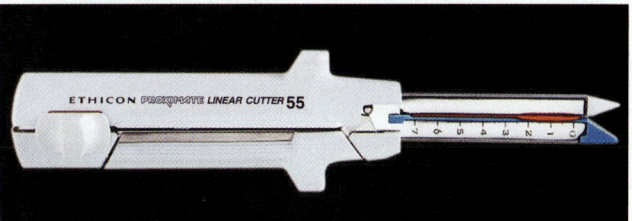

Linear stapler and cutting device

Help everyone so much that even God will wonder whether I "Created" this person in my heaven or he is the one who is "Recreating" me on the earth.

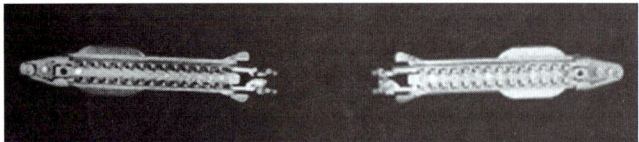

Note the two cartridge sizes

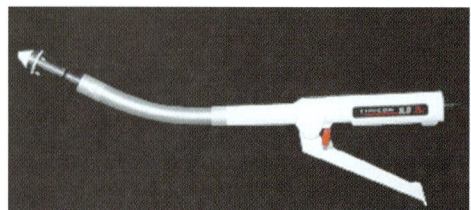

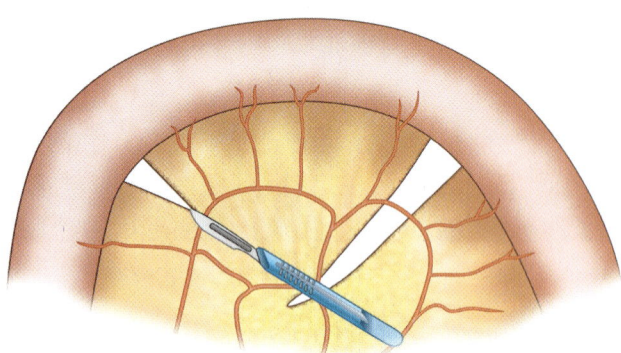

Division of the peritoneum covering the mesentery facilities visualization of the underlying vessels

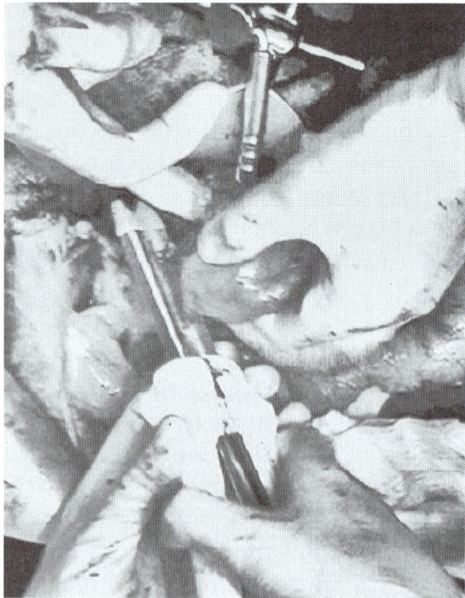

Division of duodenum

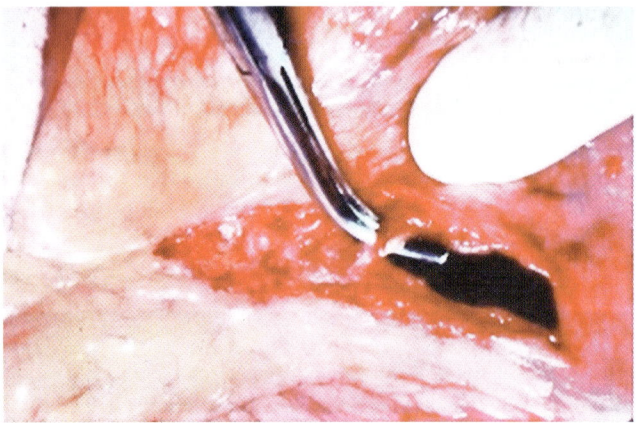
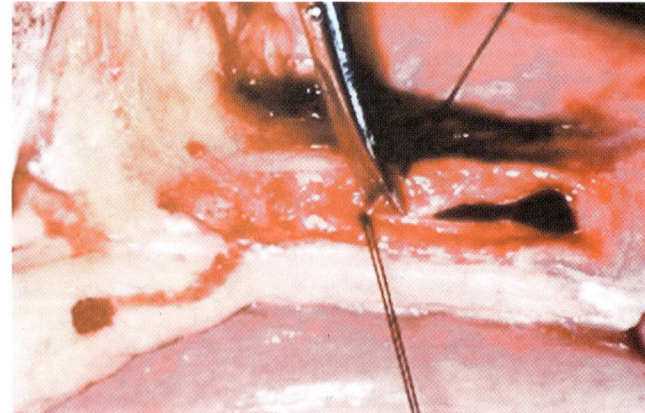

Ligation of mesenteric vessels in continuity

DIVISION OF THE DUODENUM

The duodenum is divided at least 2 cm distal to the proximal border of the tumor. Care should be taken in the mobilization of the duodenum to ensure that the small vessels between the first part of the duodenum and the

Life can be happier and stressless. If we remember one simple thought: "we can't have all that we desire, but God will give us all that we deserve".

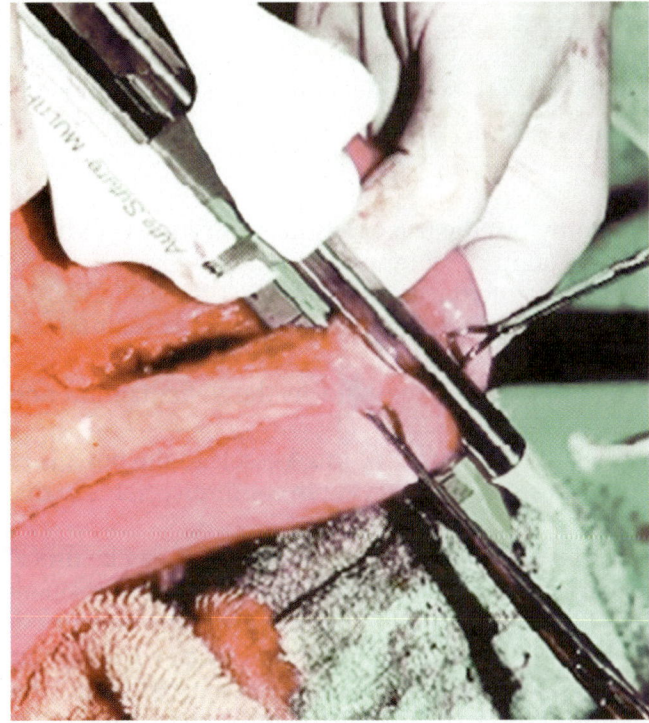

Division of the jejunum

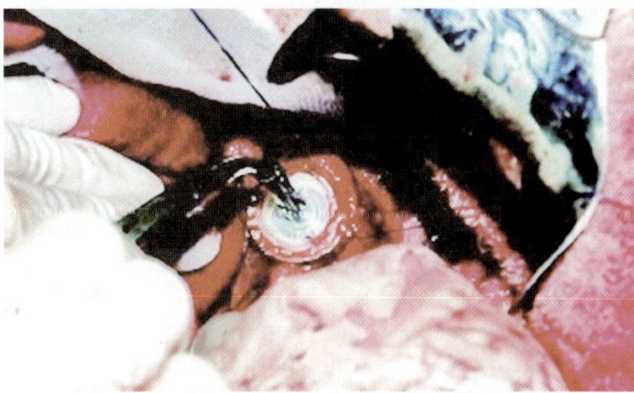

Insertion of the anvil of a circular stapler into the esophagus

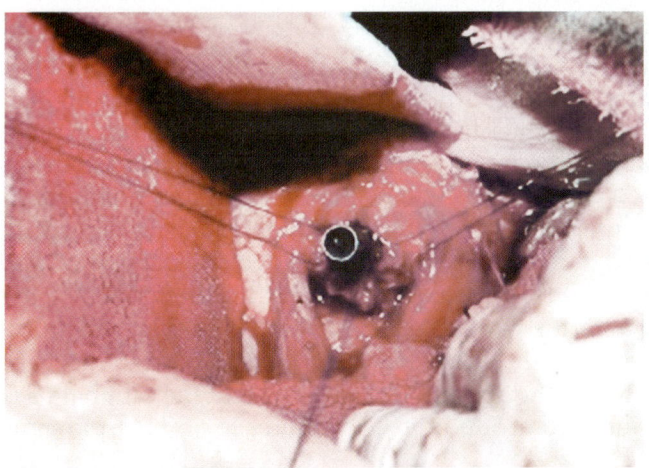

A purse-string suture has been tied around the anvil of a circular stapler in the esophagus

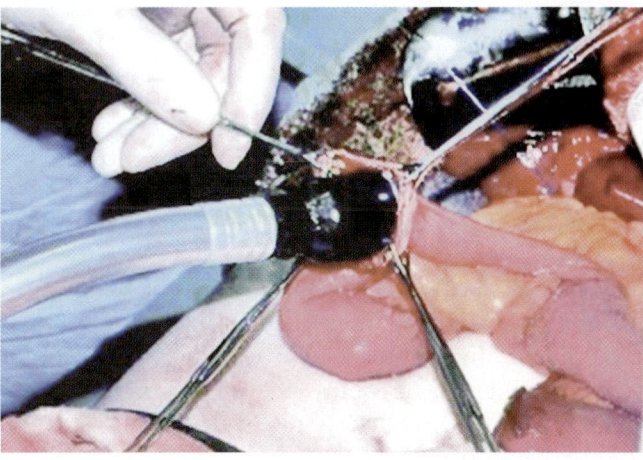

A circular stapling device is inserted into the jejunum

pancreas are ligated or coagulated as these may bleed profusely. When the site of the duodenal transection has been decided upon, ensure that the common bile duct will not be compromised.

A clean and reliable method of transection of the duodenum is to use a linear cutting stapler, such as the PLC (Ethicon, UK) or GIA (Autosuture, UK)

Fallen flowers cannot grow back on a tree, but if the root is strong new flowers certainly can, life is not about what you could not do so far, it is WHAT YOU CAN STILL DO.

Division of the Duodenum

The advantage of this technique is that the duodenum is divided cleanly and both the gastric and duodenal margins are sealed with a row of staples. Many surgeons will then invert the duodenal stump using a continuous 3-0 PDS suture although this may not be necessary.

Formation of a Roux-en-Y Loop

There are many ways of reconstruction after a total gastrectomy but the use of a Roux-en-Y loop is perhaps the most widely utilized. It has the advantage of providing a loop of jejunum without any tension on the anastomosis and at the same time reducing the risk of bile reflux into the esophagus. The preparation of the jejunal loop has to be undertaken with the utmost care always ensuring that the vascularity is maintained. There are certain technical aspects to this:

- The division of the peritoneum over the mesentery using a scalpel may aid in the visualization and subsequent division of vessels.
- Care must be taken in the application of ligatures to vessels such that the feeding vessels to the bowel are not compromised. The use of Lahey's forceps to place the sutures and then tying in continuity helps in this regard.
- Where a long loop of jejunum is required and several arcades of vessels have to be ligated it may be useful to apply a soft clamp to the vessels so that the vascularity of the bowel can be assessed prior to any permanent ligation and division.

Once the mesentery has been divided, the jejunum is divided. This is conveniently performed using a short linear cutting stapling device, the smaller size of staple being favored for most cases (blue cartridge). After firing the stapler, the jejunum is cut and sealed. However, the ends must be inspected to ensure that there is good vascularity or, alternatively, they are not bleeding.

The distal limb of the jejunum is now brought retrocolically to the level of the eventual esophagojejunal anastomosis.

Esophagojejunal Anastomosis

This can be a very difficult anastomosis to perform as access may be difficult, a long segment of jejunum may be required, and its vascularity may, therefore, be difficult to maintain so the esophagus may not be well vascularized. Care must be taken in your setup and preparation to circumvent these problems. The anastomosis can be performed using a sutured technique but a stapled anastomosis will be described in this situation.

The site of the anastomosis should be on the antimesenteric border of the jejunal loop at a site that easily reaches to the divided end of the esophagus, approximately 2–5 cm away from the divided end of the jejunum.

Prior to the division of the esophagus stay sutures should be placed at the right and left sides of the esophagus. After division, further stay sutures placed anteriorly and posteriorly will allow the anvil of a circular stapling device to be inserted into the esophagus.

Care must be taken at this stage to ensure that the anvil is of the appropriate size and that the esophagus is not split/torn by its insertion. A purse string suture is inserted around the circumference of the esophagus and tied snugly against the anvil.

Attention is now focused on the jejunal loop. At a distance 45–50 cm proximal to the intended site for the anastomosis, an enterotomy is made and the circular stapling gun is inserted into the jejunum.

It should be well lubricated and gently advanced, concertaining the jejunum over this until the chosen point for the anastomosis is reached. The jejunum is held taught over the end of the gun and an assistant advances the spike through the bowel wall. Care is taken not to tear the jejunum and often a small incision over the advancing spike is helpful.

Different staplers have different mechanisms but the anvil and stapler should be joined together.

The truth cannot be formulated, it cannot be defined – it is to be lived.

Now, the stapling gun should be tightened so that the jejunum and the esophagus are approximated. Ensure that the jejunum lies well, i.e. untwisted and with no other tissues interposed between the esophagus and the jejunum. Most devices will have an indicator as to when the anvil and stapling gun are close enough together; only when this is reached can the gun be fired. After the stapler has been fired, it should be loosened (usually two full twists of the tightening mechanism). The whole stapler is now gently rotated and then removed. Inspection of the cartridge should reveal two complete circles of jejunum and esophagus. The staple line should also be inspected to ensure that it is complete.

Jejunojejunostomy

The final stage of the reconstruction is to join the proximal divided jejunum to the jejunal loop. To ensure that there is adequate biliary diversion, this should be 45–50 cm distal to the esophagojejunostomy. The enterotomy site used for the insertion of the staple gun is a suitable site for the anastomosis. The proximal jejunal loop should be brought to lie adjacent to the existing enterotomy. It may be useful to insert stay sutures both at the site of the enterotomy and distally. An enterotomy is made on the proximal loop of jejunum and a linear stapling device inserted into the two limbs of jejunum.

Care must be taken to ensure that the two components of the stapler are correctly fitted back together and that the jejunum is held up against the proximal end of the stapler—thereafter the stapler can be fired. After removal of the stapler, the enterotomy wounds can be closed with a serosubmucosal continuous PDS suture as described previously.

Key Points

1. When using stapling devices ensure you are familiar with their assembly and function.
2. Careful preparation and meticulous setup of the anastomotic site is as essential when stapling as when suturing.
3. Ensure that you select the correct-sized instrument for the task required.

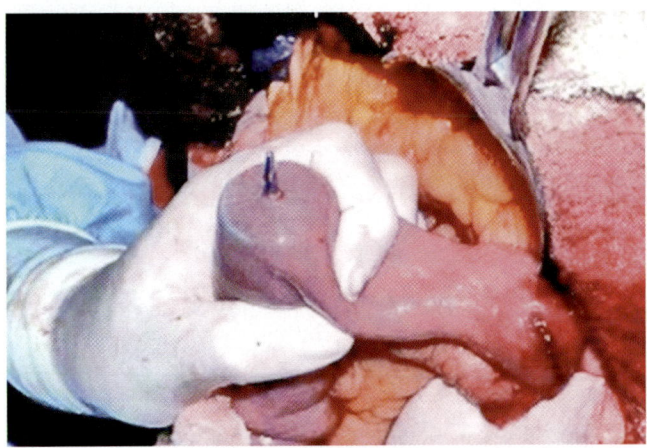

The spike of a circular stapling device is shown emerging through the antimesenteric border of the jejunum at the proposed site of an esophagojejunal anastomosis

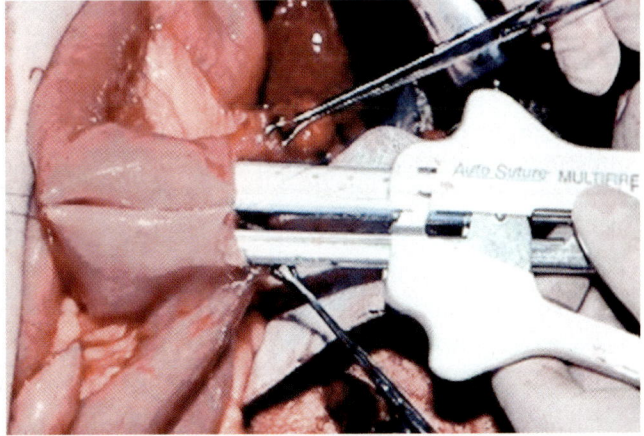

Side-to-side jejunostomy using a linear cutting stapler

Laughing faces do not mean that there is absence of sorrow, but it means that they have the ability to deal with it.

KNOW A FEW IMPORTANT THINGS ABOUT SUTURE MATERIALS

Ideal Suture Material—Criteria

- Adequate tensile strength
- Minimal tissue reaction
- Good knotting capacity
- Nonallergic, noncarcinogenic
- Easy handling quality
- Less memory
- Easily available
- Relatively cheaper.

Classification

A. Absorbable
  i. Natural
  ii. Synthetic
B. Nonabsorbable
  i. Natural
  ii. Synthetic

Examples of different sutures:
  i. Natural
    a. Plain catgut
    b. Chromic catgut
  ii. Synthetic
    a. Polyglactic acid (vicryl)
    b. Polyglycocolic acid (dexon)
    c. Polydioxanone suture (PDS)
    d. Polyglecaprone (monocryl)
    e. Glycomer (sisyn)
    f. Polyglyconate (maxon).

Note: Catgut is synthesized from the submucosa of sheeps' intestine or serosa of beefs' intestine, not cats', intestine. Plain catgut is treated with 20% chromic acid called chromic catgut.

Uses of Absorbable Suture

- In bowel anastomosis, cholecystojejunostomy, choledochojejunostomy, pancreas jejunostomy, etc.
- To suture mucosa, subcutaneous tissue muscle, fascia, peritoneum
- Base of the appendix, stump of the appendix
- Closure of subcostal incision rectus sheath, external oblique aponeurosis
- In ligating pedicles
- In circumcision.

Remember: Absorbable suture should not be used in vascular anastomosis, vessels, tendon and nerve.

Never forget that you are not alone. The divine is with you helping and guiding you.

Nonabsorbable suture:

a. Natural
   i. Silk
   ii. Linen
   iii. Cotton

b. Synthetic
   i. Polypropylene (prolene)
   ii. Polyethylene (ethylene)
   iii. Polyamide
   iv. Steel
   v. Polyester (ethibond)
   vi. Nylon, etc.

Uses of Nonabsorbable Suture

- Closure of abdomen
- In herniorrhaphy for repairing posterior wall of inguinal ligament
- Repair of incisional hernia
- In tendon injury
- Vascular anastomoses
- Suturing of skin
- Posterior seromuscular suture in small gut anastomosis, gastrojejunostomy, pancreaticojejunostomy, etc.

Monofilament and Polyfilament Suture

Monofilament

Suture is made of a single strand of fiber. So, the surface of this suture is smooth.

Usually, these sutures are strong and chances of bacterial contaminations are less but knot holding capacity is poor. So, 4 of 5 knot to be tied.

Examples: Polypropylene, polyamide catgut, poliglecaprone (monocryl), etc.

Polyfilaments: Suture is made of multiple strands of fibers.

Surface is not smooth but knot holding capacity is excellent chance of bacterial contaminations is more due to presence of crevices. So, infections: Silk, linen, polyglactin (vicryl), polyglycocolic acid (dexon), braided polyamide, braided polyester suture.

Numbering of Suture Materials

2-thick suture

1, 0, 1-0, 2-0, 3-0, 4-0, 5-0, 6-0, 7-0, 8-0, 9-0.

No. 2 is used usually for pedicle ligation

2-0, 3-0 for bowel suturing.

5-0, 6-0 for vascular anastomosis, nerve repair, etc.

9-0 is used under microscopic vision. Usually used in ophthalmic surgery.

The number indicates thickness of the suture. Higher the number, thicker is the suture.

When o is used suffixed, higher the number, finer the sutures.

Example: 4-0 is thinner than 3-0 sutures.

The most difficult phase of life is not when no one understands you. Its when you do not understand yourself.

Mechanism of Absorption of Suture

Absorbable Suture

These sutures get absorbed in the tissue, either enzymatic digestion or by phagocytosis except polyglactin (vicryl), poliglecaprone—which digested by (monocryl) hydrolysis. So, the sutures leave behind the scar mark over the skin. For this, why absorbable suture usually is not used in cosmetic area like face, neck, etc.

Nonabsorbable suture remain in the tissue for indefinite period for this why it is used for hernia repair. In body surface, it is removed at face at 4 days, neck 4–5 days, abdomen 7–10 days, upper limbs 10–12 days and lower limbs 12–14 days.

Example of Tensile Strenghth

	Tensile strength	*Absorbed by*
Polyglactin (vicryl)	28–30 days	80–90 days
Vicryl rapid	10–12 days	40–45days
Poliglecaprone (monocryl)	18–21 days	90–120 days

PDS (polydioxanone suture): It maintains tensile strength for a longer period, i.e, about 56 days

At 2 weeks tensile strength	75% maintained
At 4 weeks	50% maintained
At 6 weeks	25% maintained

At 8 weeks, it loses its all tensile strength.

Atraumatic Suture

When the suture is attached with an eyeless needle called atraumatic suture. Chance of tissue injury is less here.

SPECIMEN

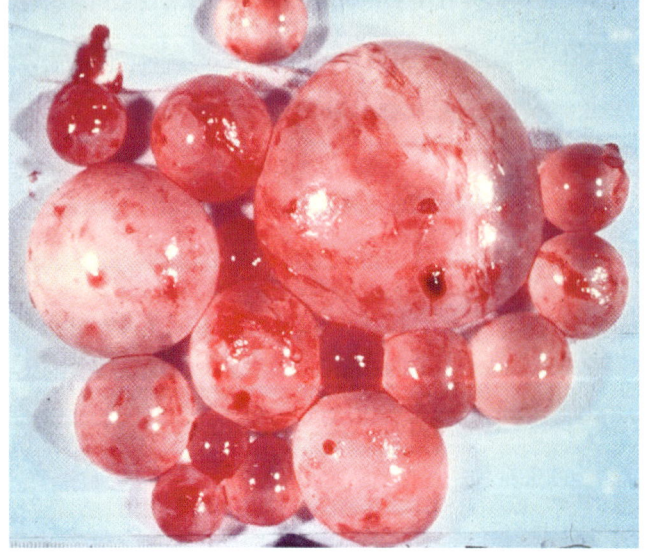 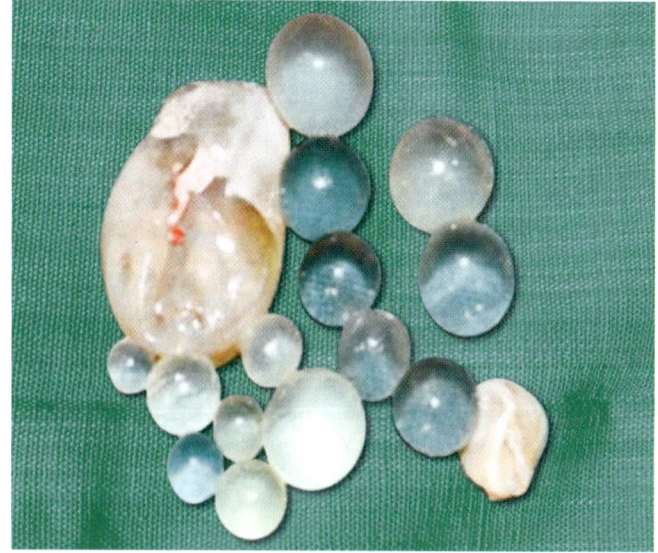

Hydatid cyst

A "Desire" changes nothing; A "Decision" changes something. But A "Determination" changes everything.

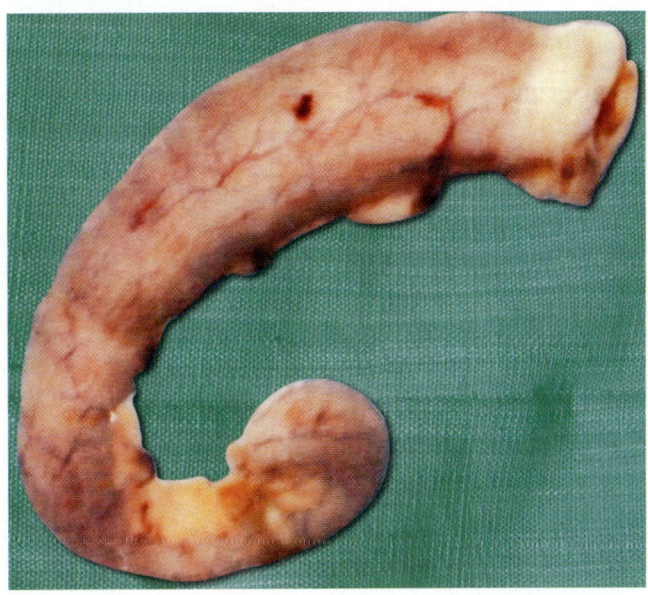

Acute appendicitis

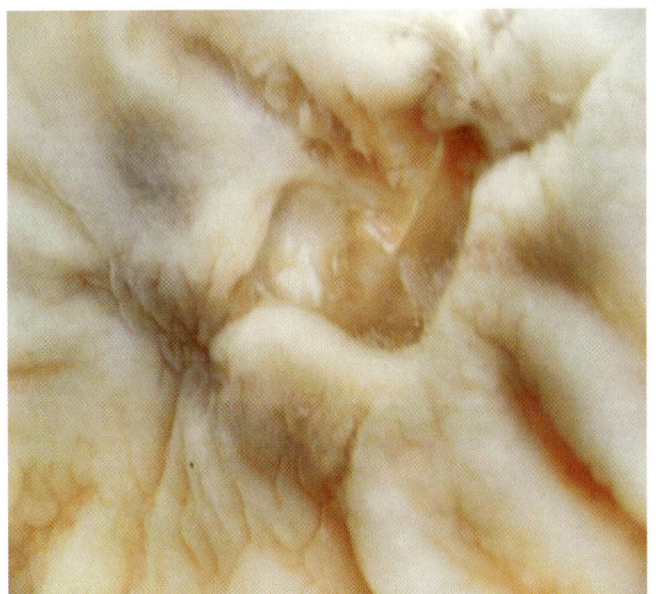
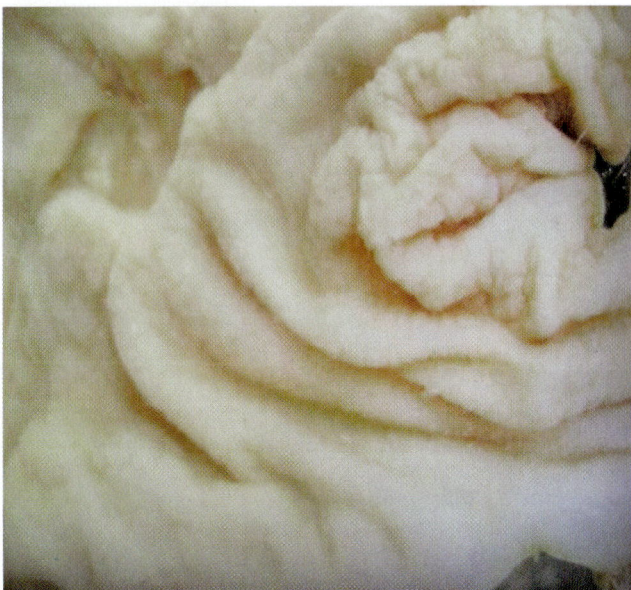

Large gastric ulcer—most probably benign

This is the specimen of stomach showing an ulcer. The margin is well defined. The mucosal folds are converged toward the margin of ulcer so most probably this is a benign gastric ulcer.

The specimen of stomach: One wall is cut open showing a proliferative growth. The margin of ulcer is rolled out and everted. There is a flattering of the mucosal folds around the ulcer. So most probably, this is a specimen of malignant ulcer of the stomach.

There is no greater victory than that of controlling oneself.

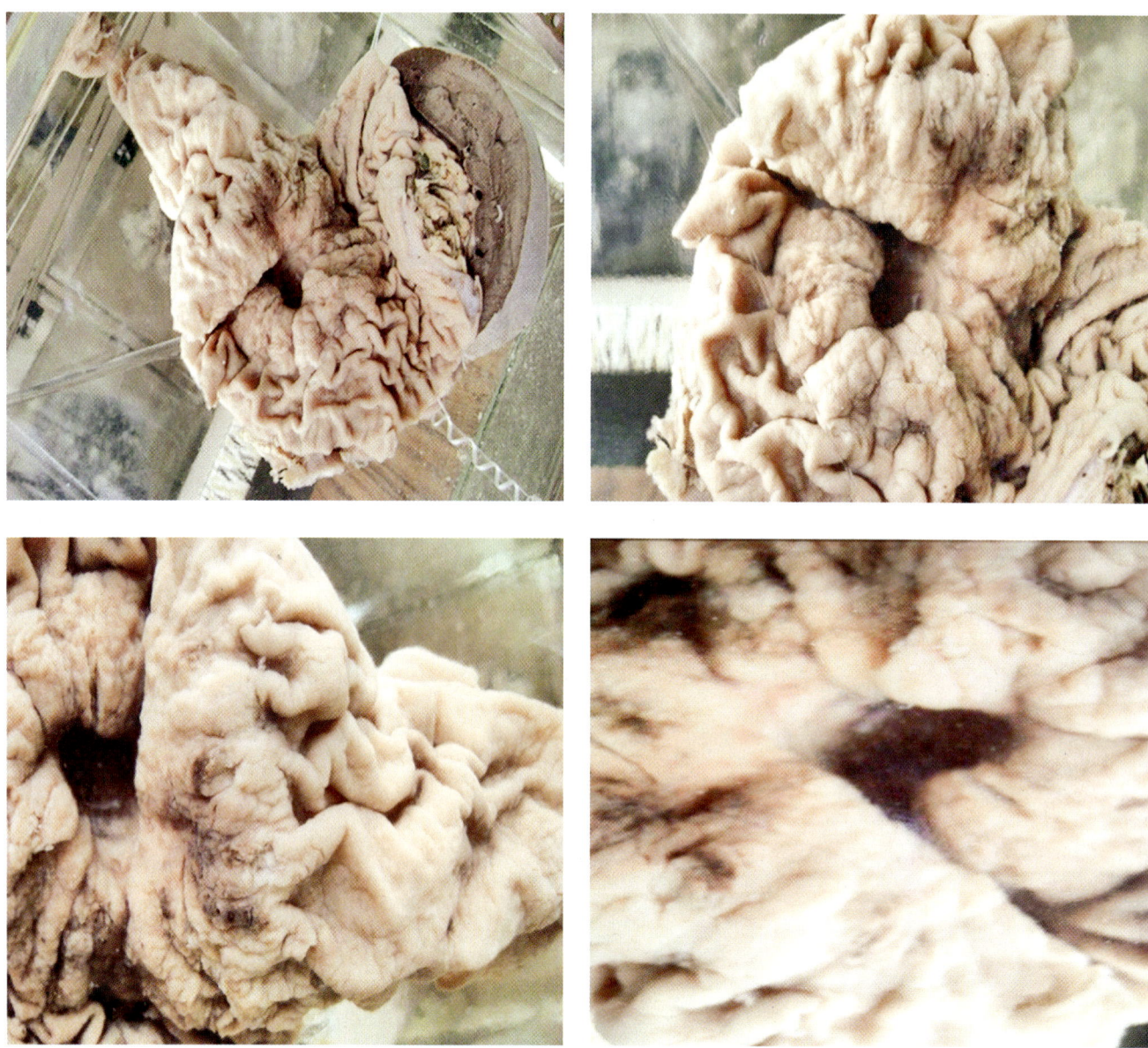

Gastric cancer

The specimen is showing the role of hair and indigestible vegetable fibers. So, this is a specimen of trichobezoar.

Collections of indigestible material found in the gastrointestinal tract (usually the stomach).

Risk of trichobezoar (eating of hair) is greater among mentally retarded or emotionally disturbed children, common in 10–19-year-old girls.

Phytobezoar is nothing but the rolled of poorly digested vegetable fibers, such as skin and seeds of fruits and vegetables.

The worms with long rounded body look, like spaghetti noodles and approximately 15 cm and it has got mouth, body and a curling tail. So, this nothing but the human roundworms, i.e. *Ascaris lumbricoides*.

Consecrate your life to the realization of something higher and broader than yourself and you will never feel the weight of the passing years.

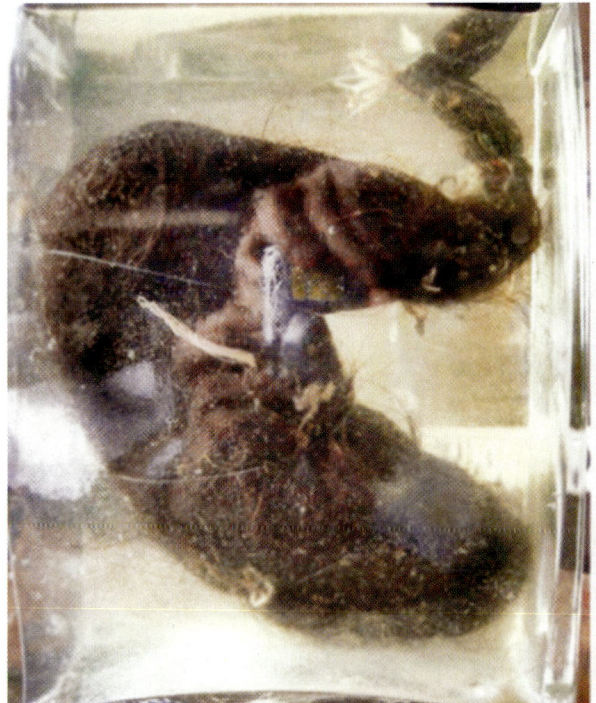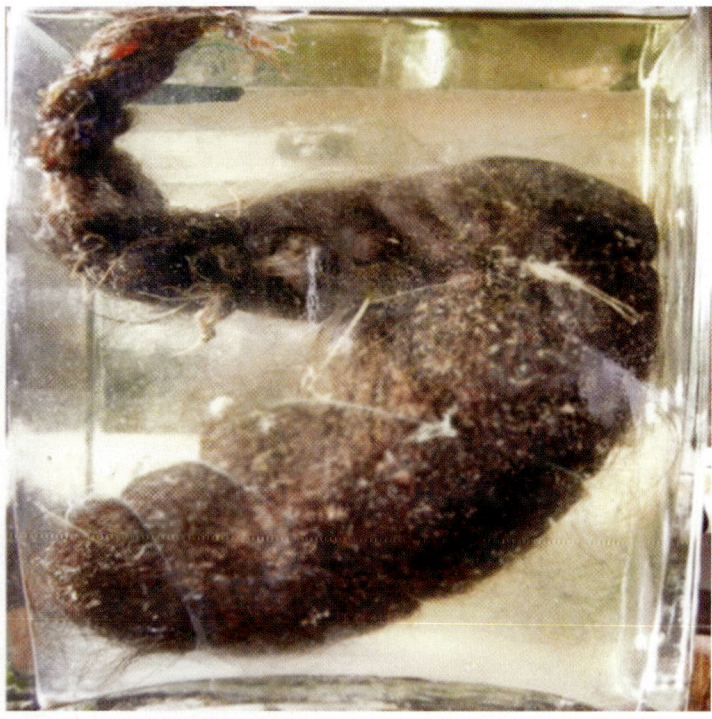

Trichobezoar

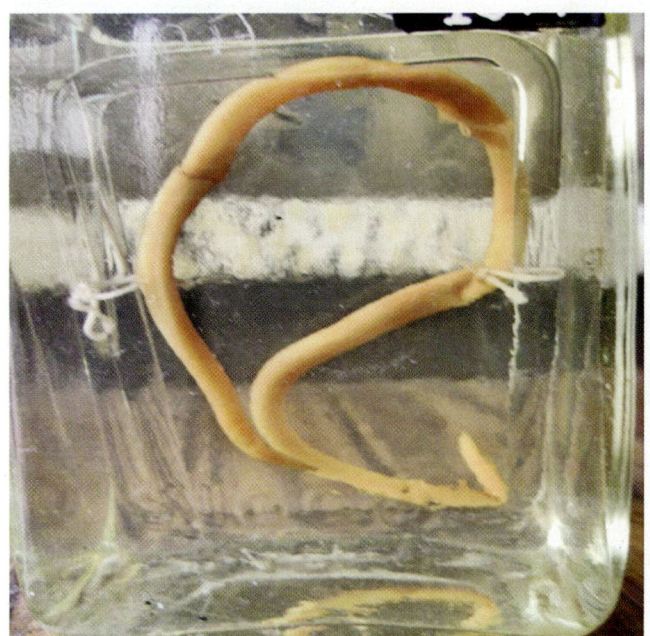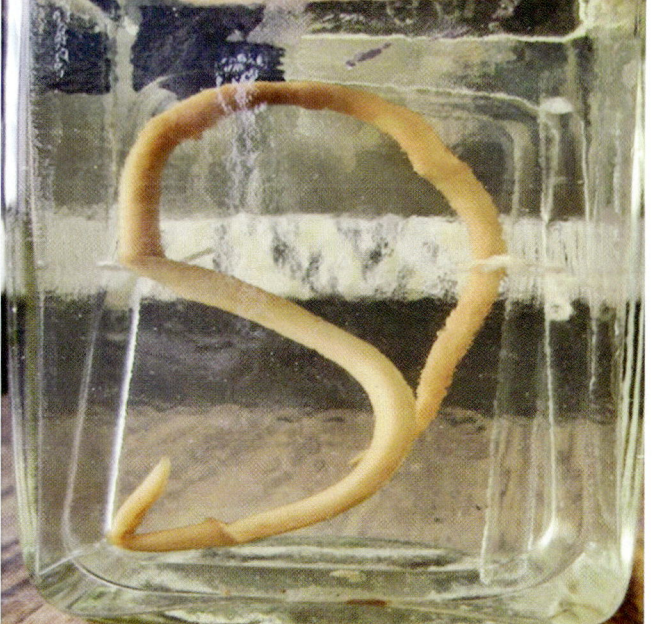

Roundworm—Ascaris lumbricoides

Darkness cannot drive out darkness; only light can do that. Hate cannot drive out hate; only love can do that.

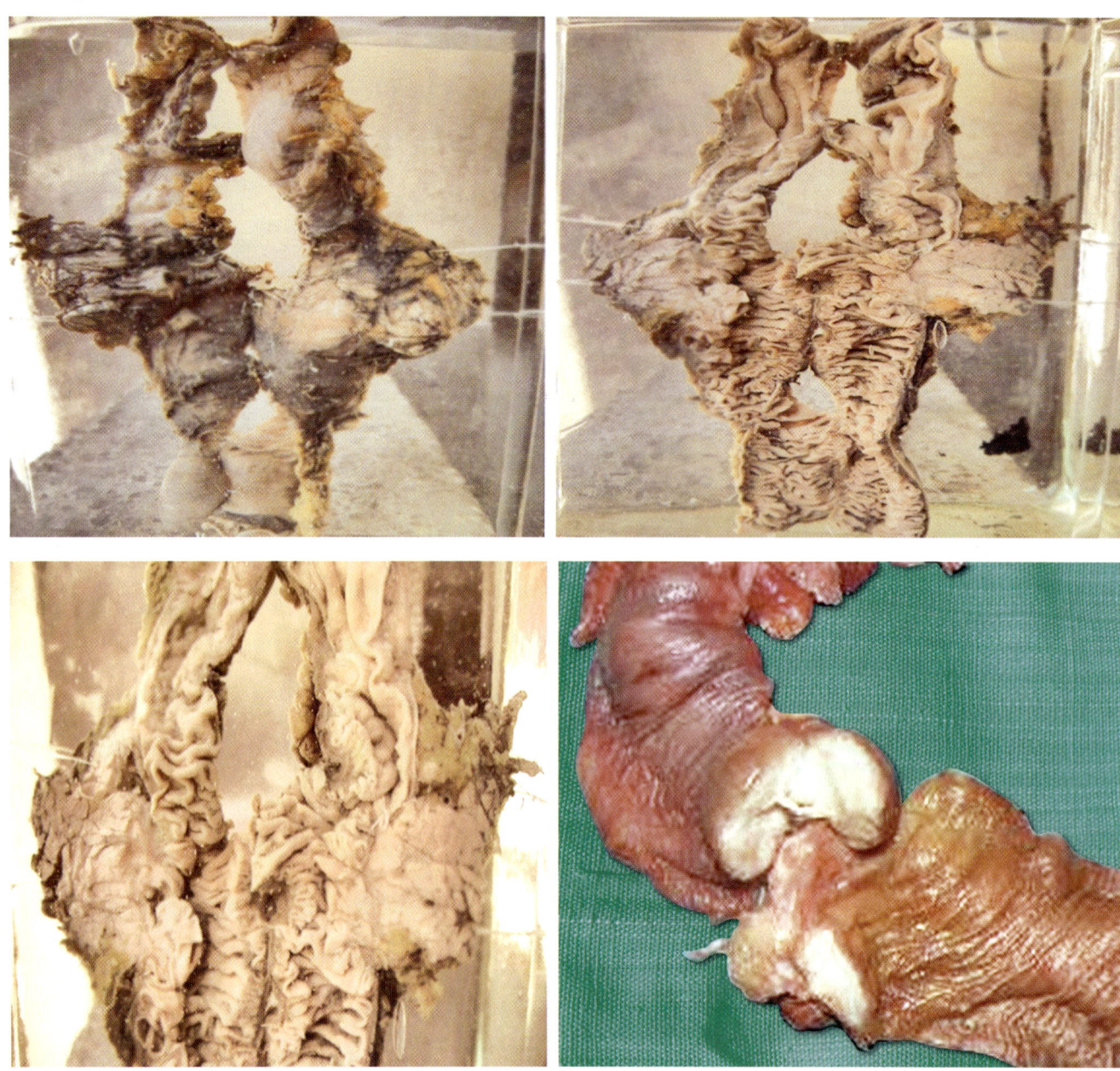

Jejunal mass

    This is a specimen of jejunum showing the multiple polypoidal lesions within the lumen. The intervening mucosa appears normal. The serosal surface of the jejunum appears normal. So, this is a specimen of jejunal polyps.

Donot choose such friends who have reached the heights! But, choose those friends who can hold you when you fall from heights.

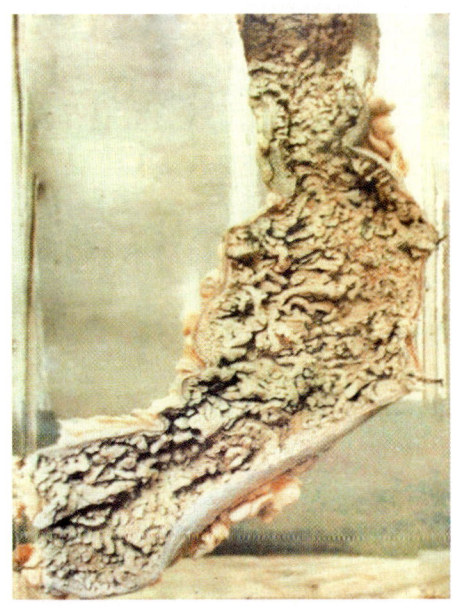

Polyposis of colon

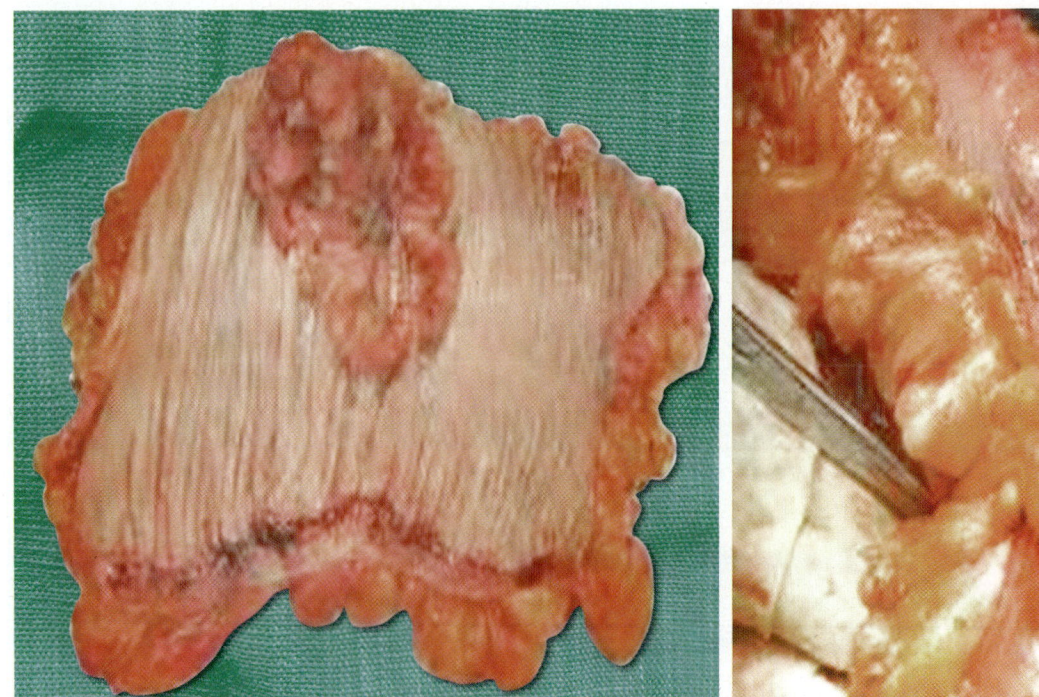

Carcinoma colon

Ulceroproliferative mass at the specimen of colon most probably carcinoma colon.

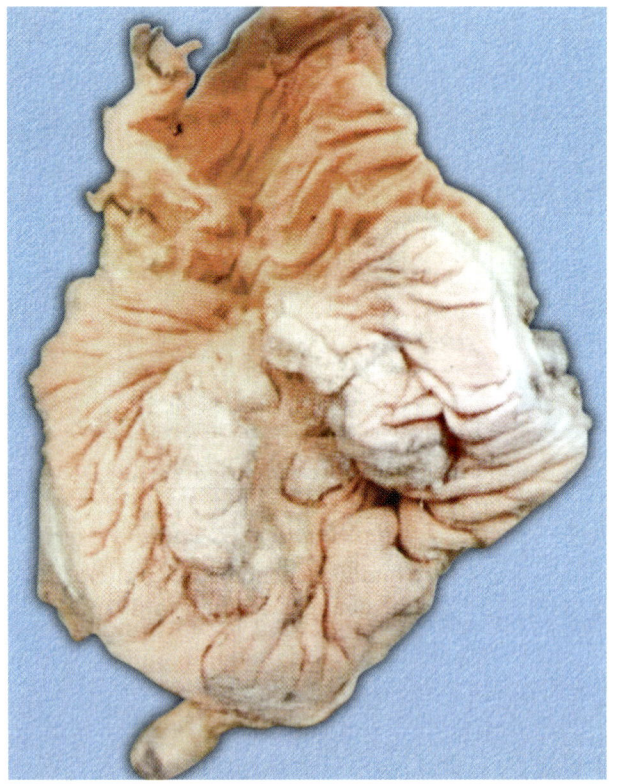

Carcinoma colon

This specimen is showing a mass at cecum. The mass is ulceroproliferative. The outer serosal surface is also involved by the tumor. This is a specimen of carcinoma cecum.

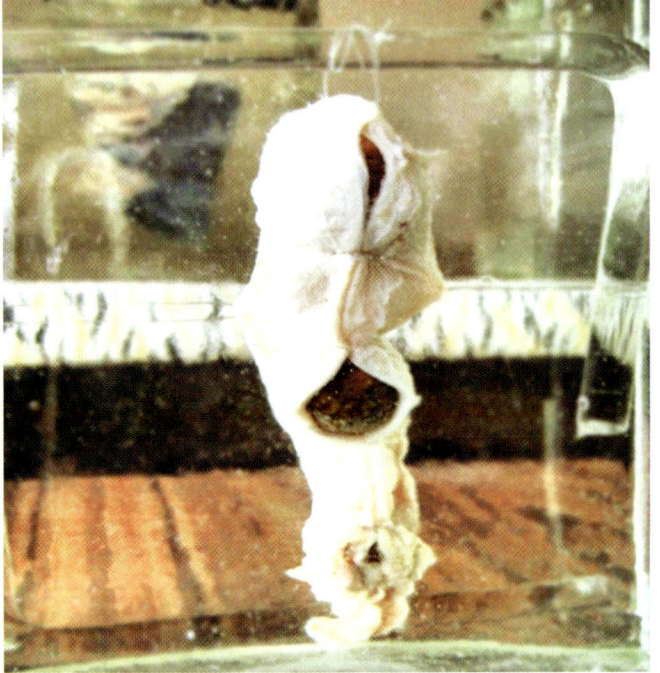
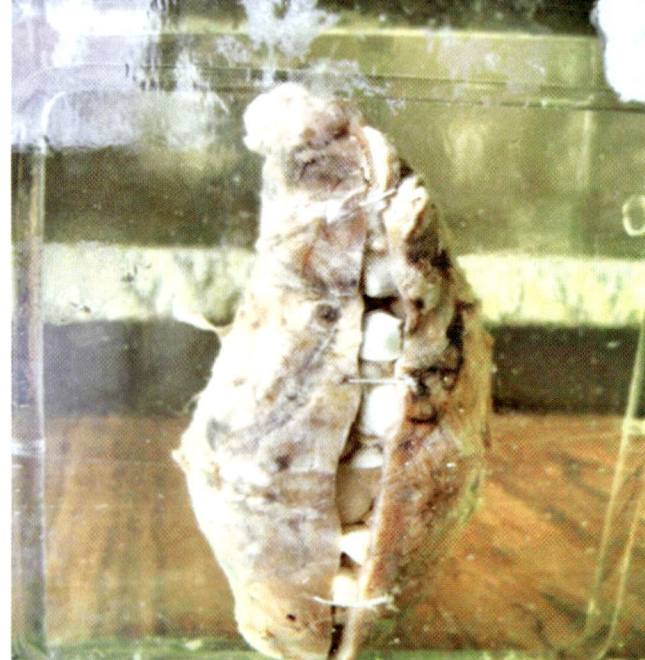

Specimen of gallbladder with multiple stones

Even if things are not as they ought to be, worry does not help to make them better. A quiet confidence is the source of strength.

This is a specimen of gallbladder which is white in color and will shrunken. The one-sided wall is cut open and the wall appears thicker. There is a stone/multiple stones looking inside the gallbladder. So, this is nothing but a specimen of chronic cholecystitis with cholelithiasis.

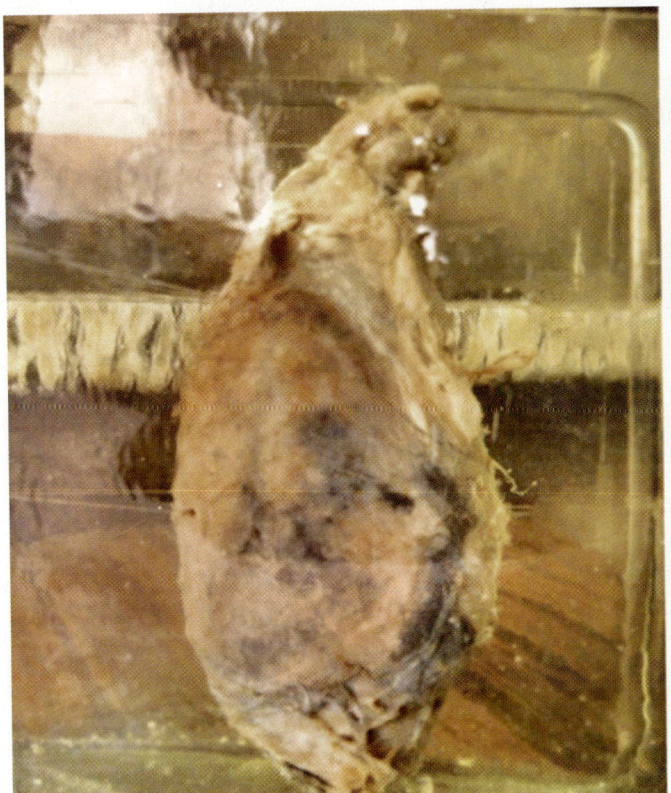 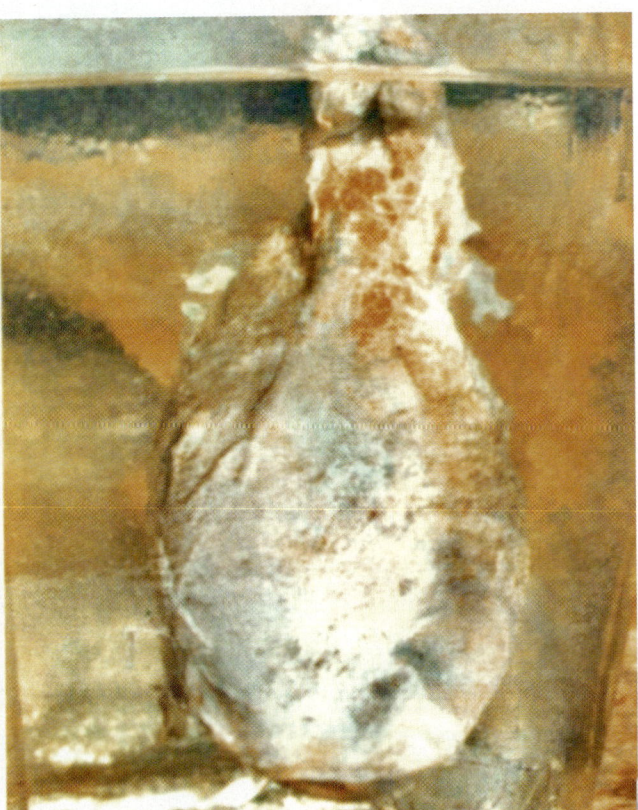

Specimen of empyema gallbladder

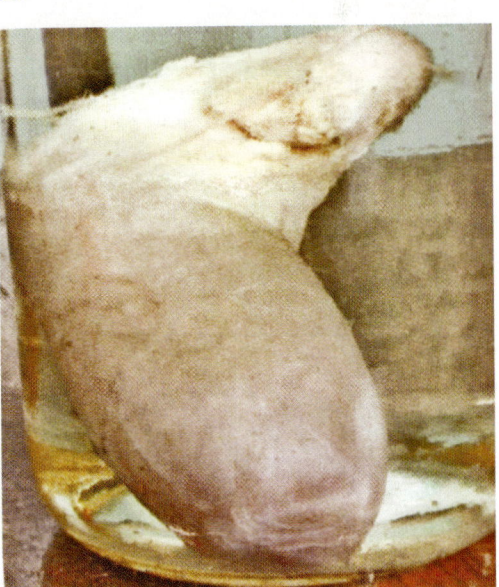

This is a specimen of gallbladder with distended appearance. The wall appears pale, irregular and shabby. So most probably, this is a specimen of empyema of gallbladder.

(In case of mucocele of gallbladder, the wall appears smooth and regular).

The specimen is showing the distended gallbladder with smooth surface. The gallbladder appears whitish (pale) and most probably there is a stone at the neck of the gallbladder. So most probably, this is a specimen of mucocele gallbladder.

Mucocele of gallbladder

Nowhere will you be able to find peace unless you have peace in your heart.

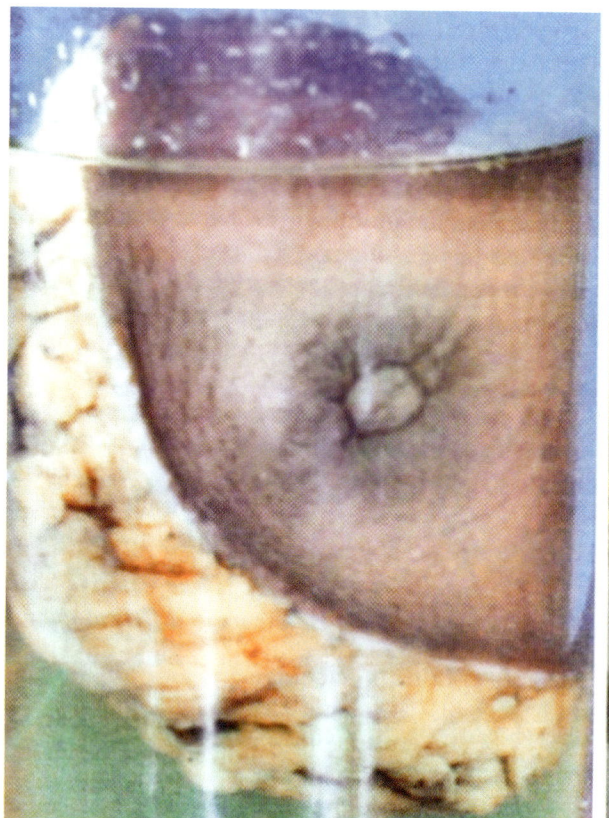 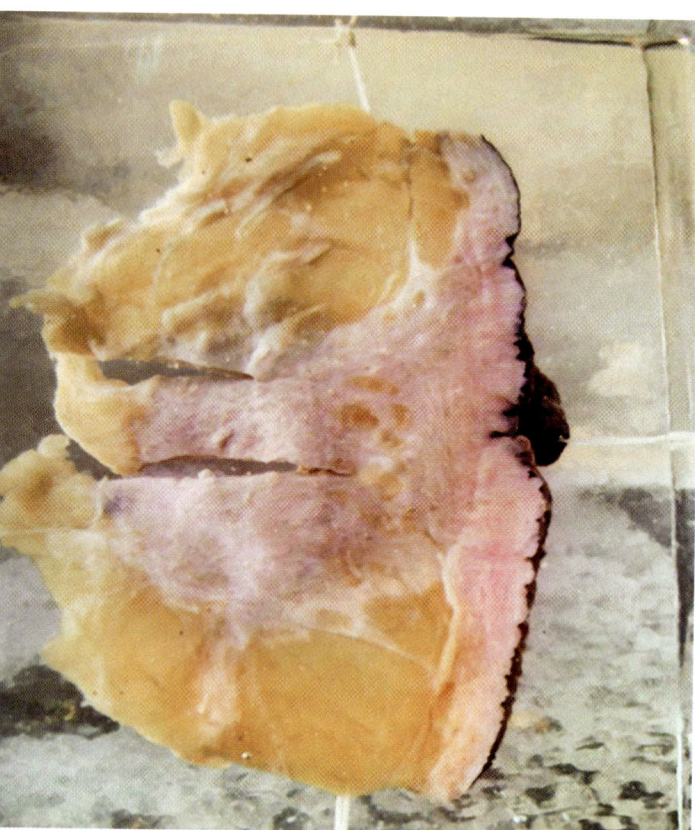

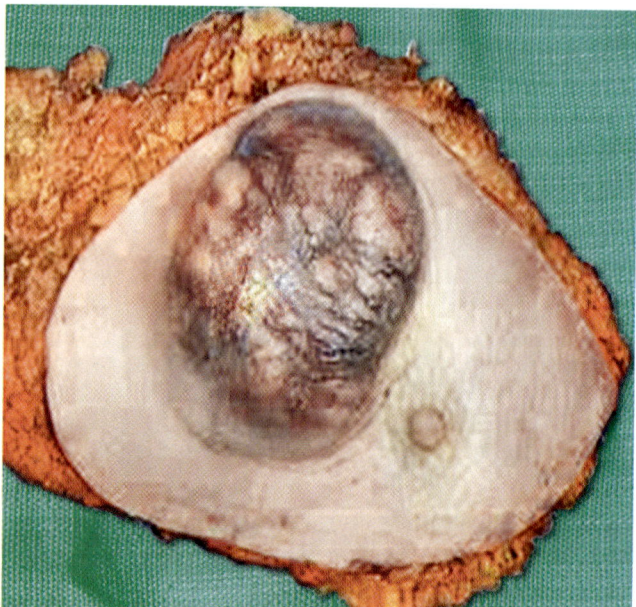

Carcinoma breast

This is a spcimen of breast showing an irregular mass within the breast parenchyma. There is no definite capsule all around the tumor. The nipple appears retracted. So, this is a specimen of breast lump most probably carcinoma breast.

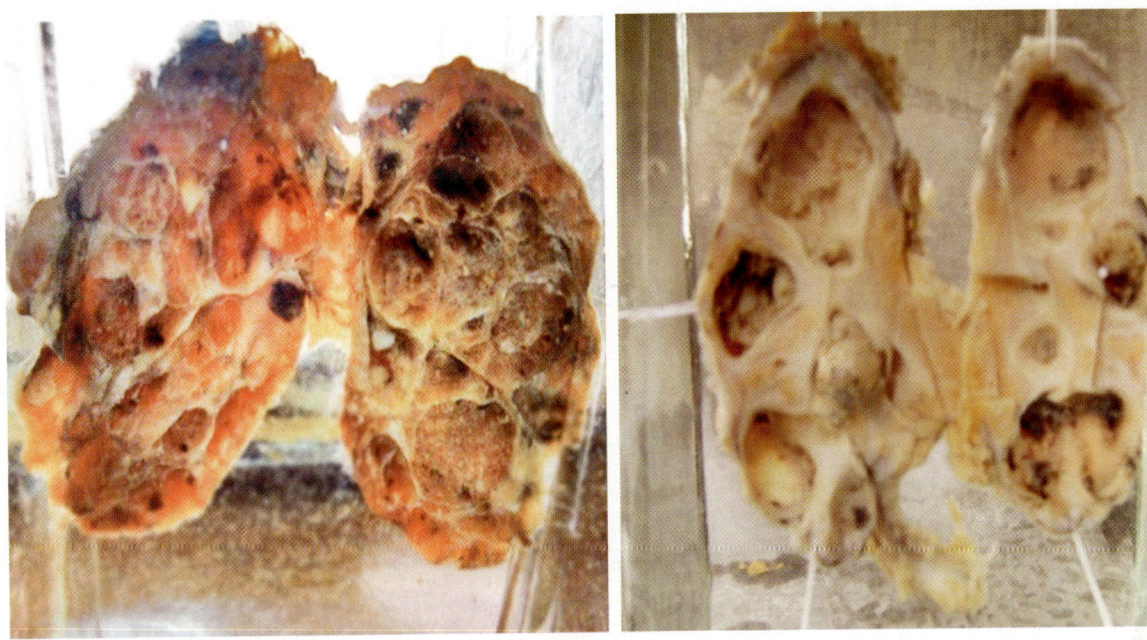

Hydronephrosis on cut section

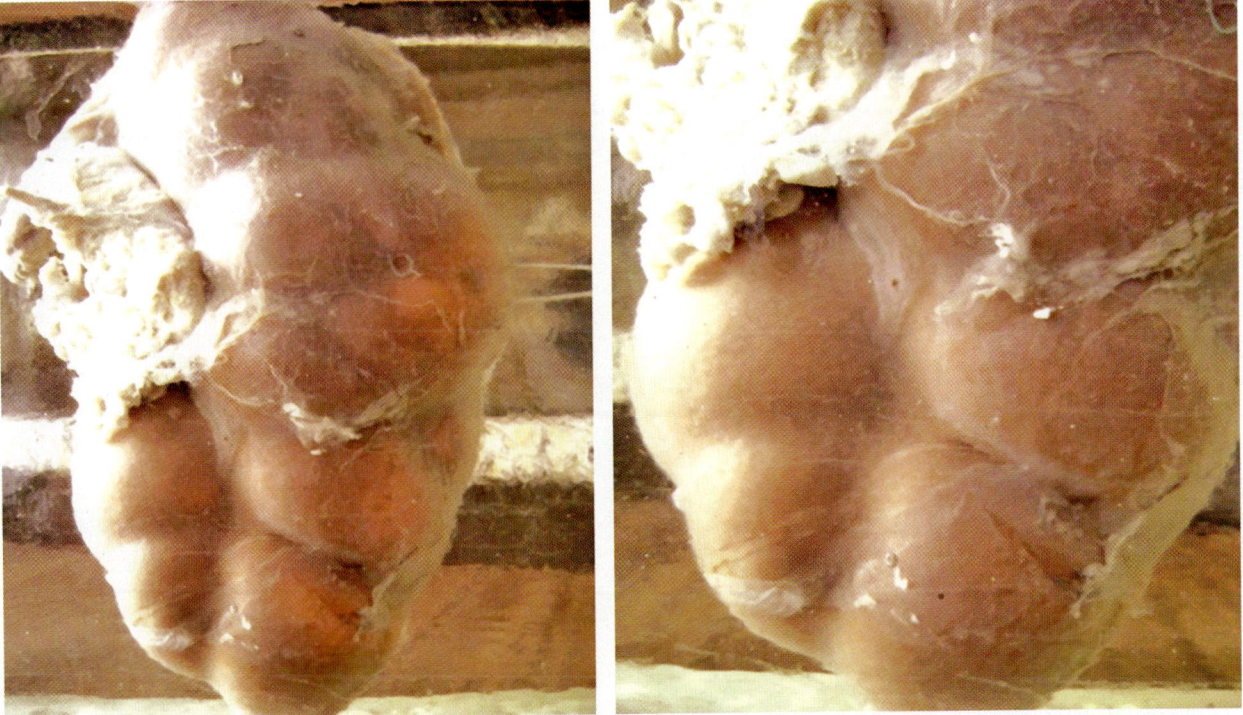

Hydronephrosis

This is a specimen of kidney along with the renal pelvis and which is grossly enlarged. The cortex of the kidney is thinned out and there are multiple cystic appearance in the substance of the kidney. So, this is a specimen of hydronephrosis of the kidney.

Relationships are like bird, if you hold tightly they die, if you hold loosely they fly, but if you hold with care they remain with you forever.

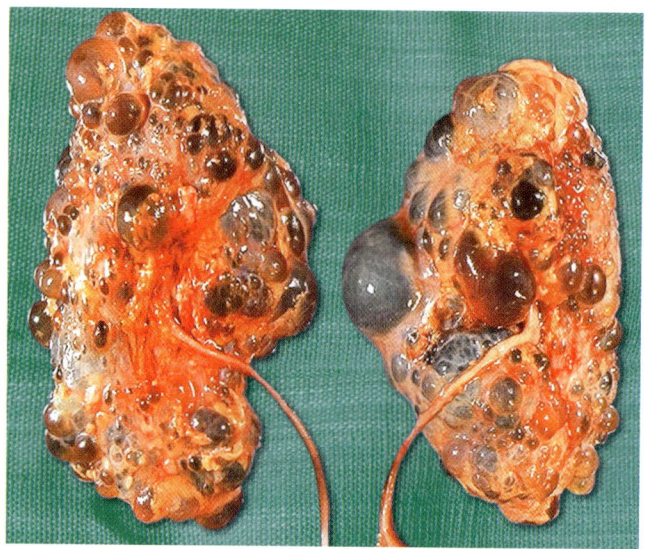

Polycystic kidney disease

This is a specimen of bilateral kidney showing enlargement of both kidneys and there are multiple cysts of different sizes all over the kidney parenchyma. Some of the cysts are filled with hemorrhagic material. The cysts are isolated and no communication with pelvis of the kidney. So, this is a specimen of polycystic kidney.

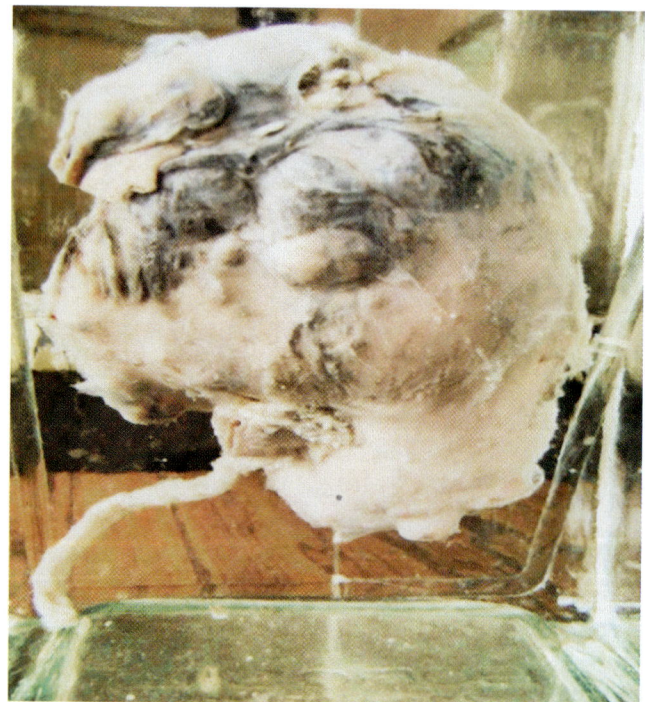 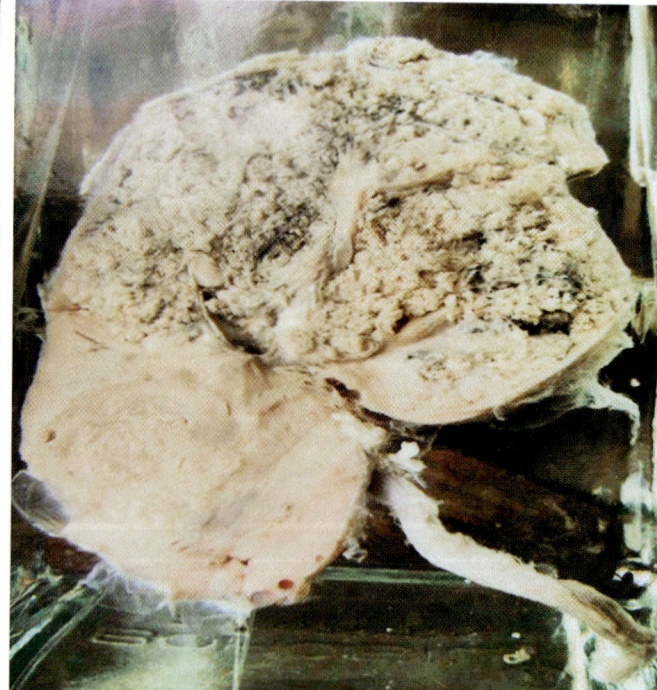

Kidney—upper pole tumor—renal cell carcinoma (RCC)

Every good and kind deed brings light, restfulness, joy—the sunshine in which flowers bloom.

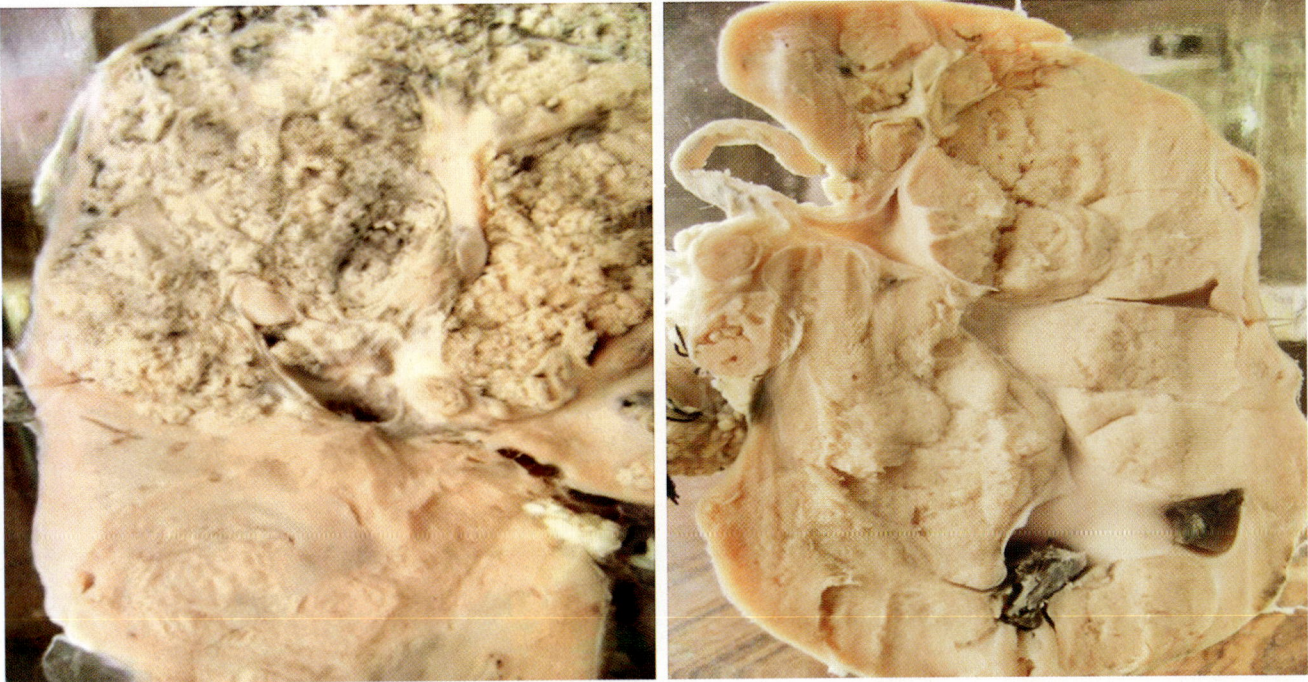

Kidney—upper pole tumor—renal cell carcinoma (RCC)

This is a specimen of kidney, cut open, showing a large mass in upper pole of the kidney. The mass is grayish in color and there are different areas of hemorrhage. There are also multiple lobules and septa within the mass, so this is a specimen of renal mass most probably renal cell carcinoma.

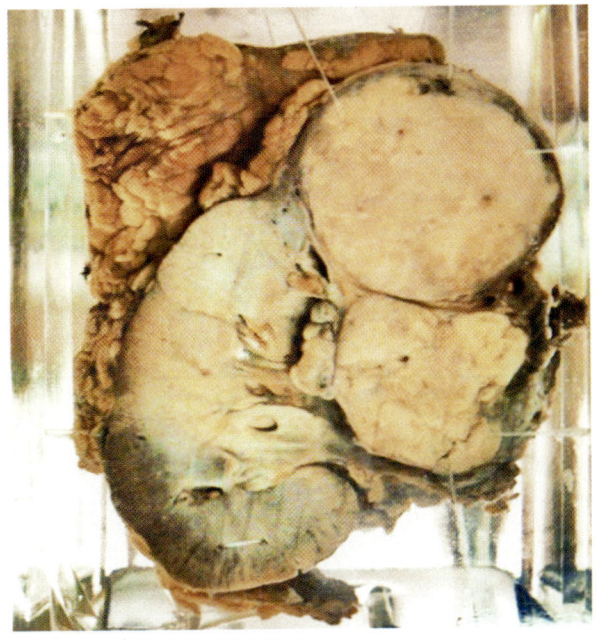

Adrenal tumor

The specimen showing grossly enlarged mass over the upper pole of the kidney showing multiple areas of hemorrhage, necrosis and calcifications.

What is easy, difficult and hard in life? Easy is to judge the mistakes of other. Difficult is to accept our own mistakes and hard is to correct those mistakes.

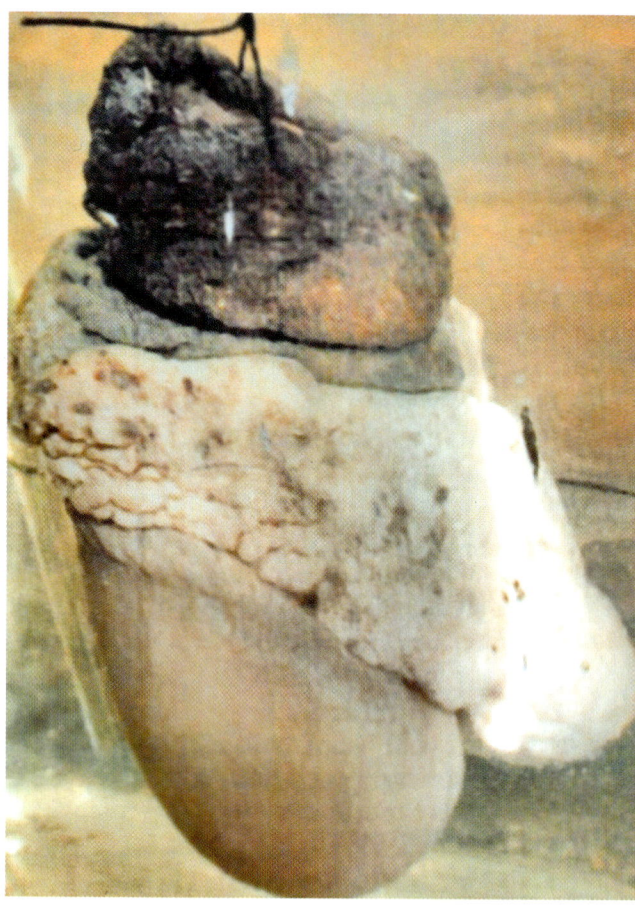

Carcinoma penis

This is a specimen of partially amputed penis showing a proliferative growth in the region of corona glandis. So, this is a specimen of carcinoma penis for which the partial penectomy done.

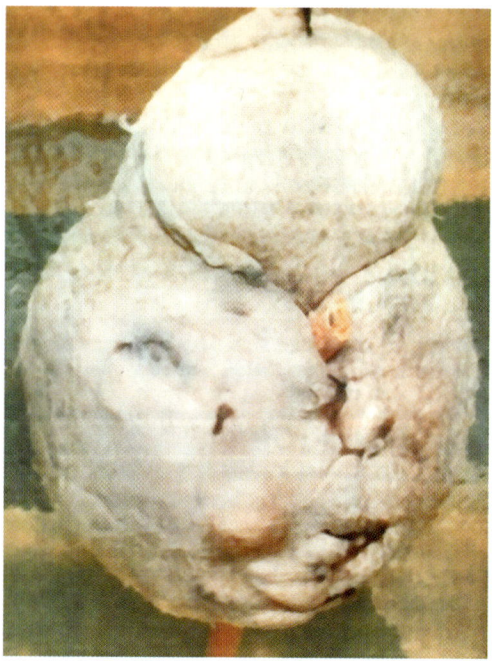

Benign prostatic hyperplasia (BPH)

This is a specimen of prostate showing enlarged two lateral lobes and the median lobe. So most probably, this is a specimen of BPH.

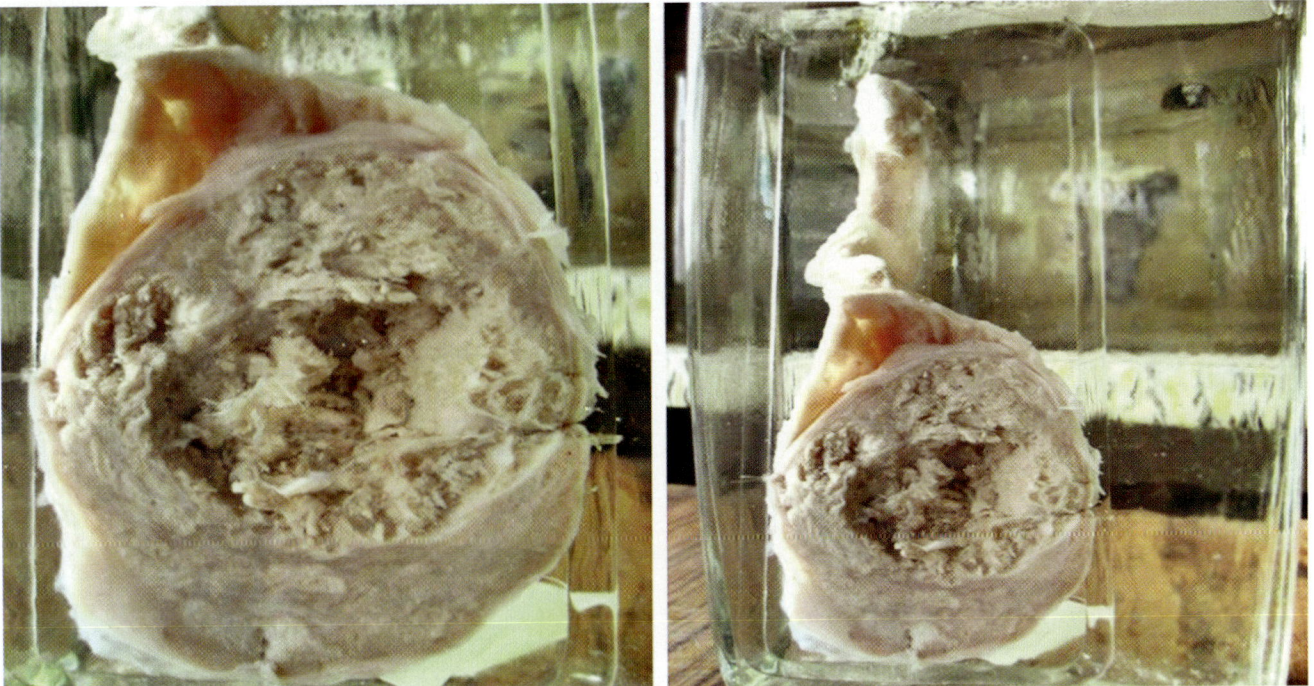

Nonseminomatous germ cell tumor (NSGCT) testis

This is a specimen of testis with part of spermatic cord. The cut open testis showing a tumor involved almost whole of the testis. The tumor has variegated appearance, nonhomogenous with areas of hemorrhage and necrosis. This is a specimen of NSGCT.

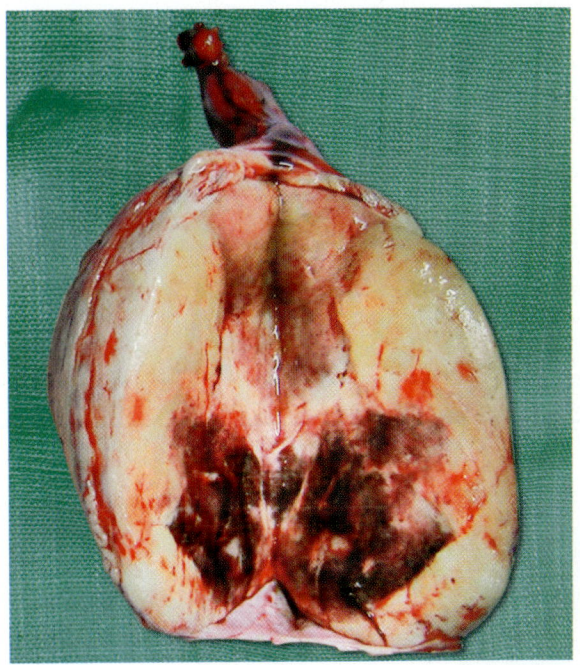

Cut section of NSGCT. The area of hemorrhage and necrosis is obevious

Progress: to be ready, at every minute, to give up all one is and all one.

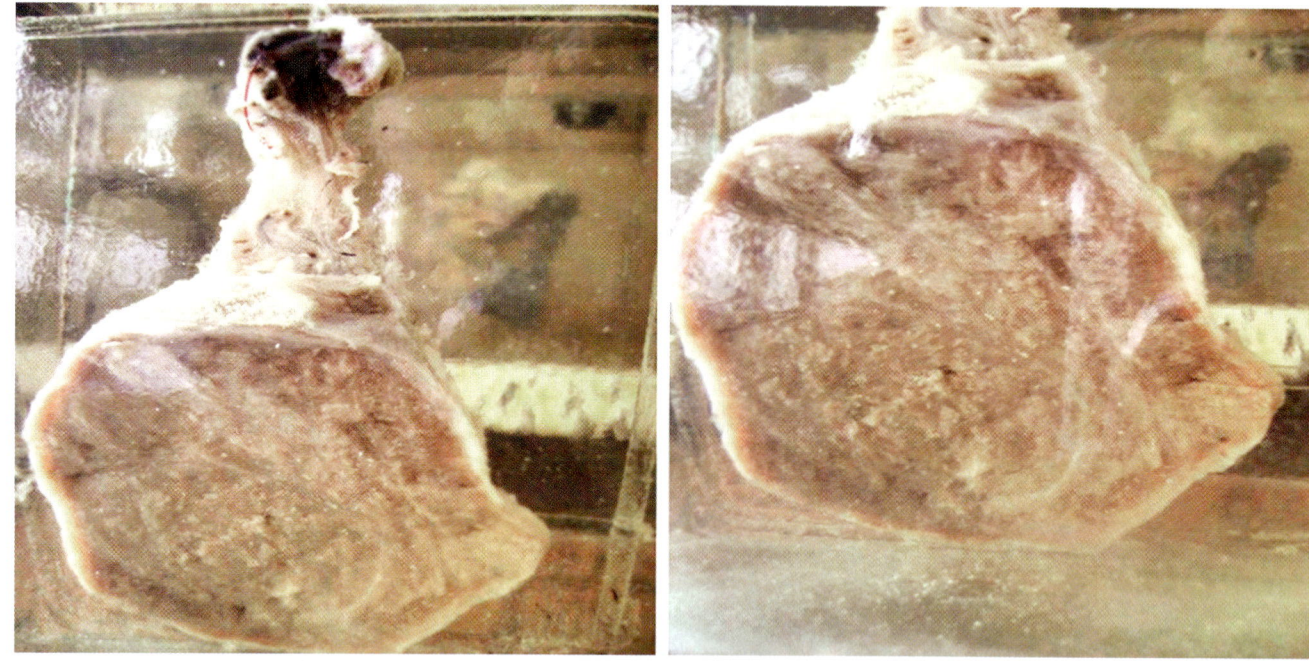

Seminoma testis

This is a specimen of testis with a part of spermatic cord. The tumor appears to be involved whole of the testis. The cut open testis is showing uniform in appearance. There is fine lobulation on the cut surface. So, this is a specimen of seminoma testis.

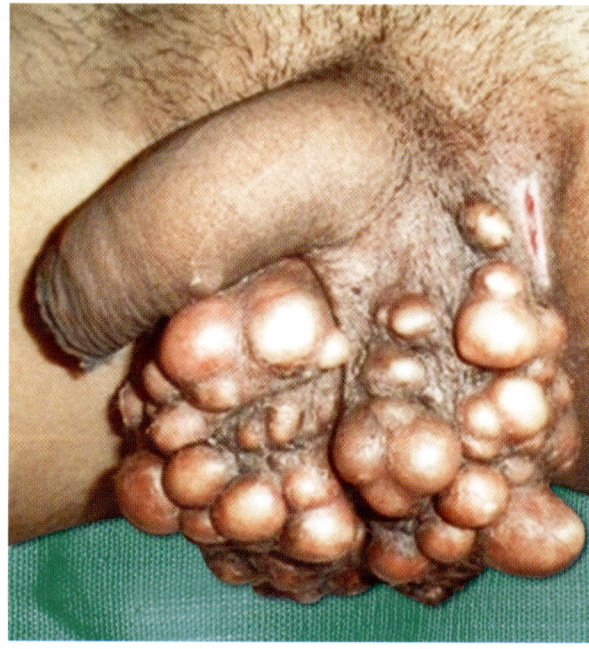

Sebaceous cyst scrotum

Life is like a camera – Just focus on what's important and capture the good ones, develop from the negatives and if things do not turn out, forget it just take another shot.

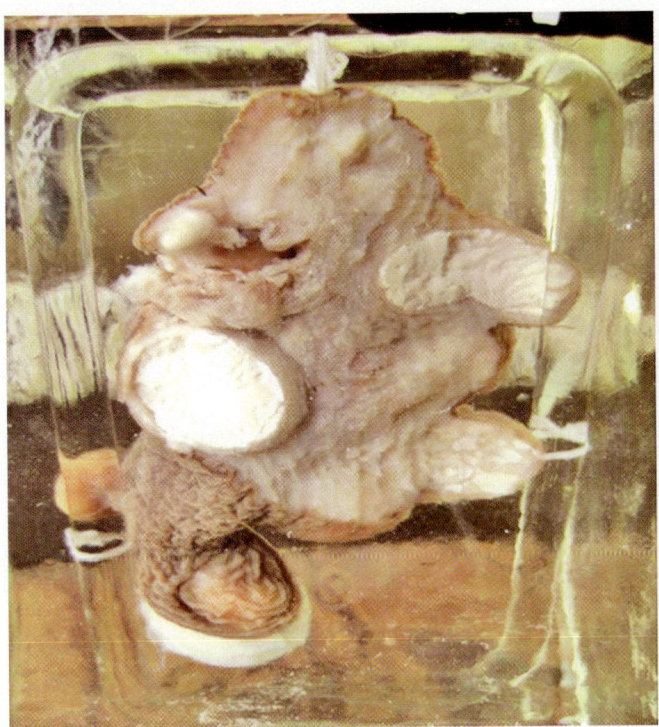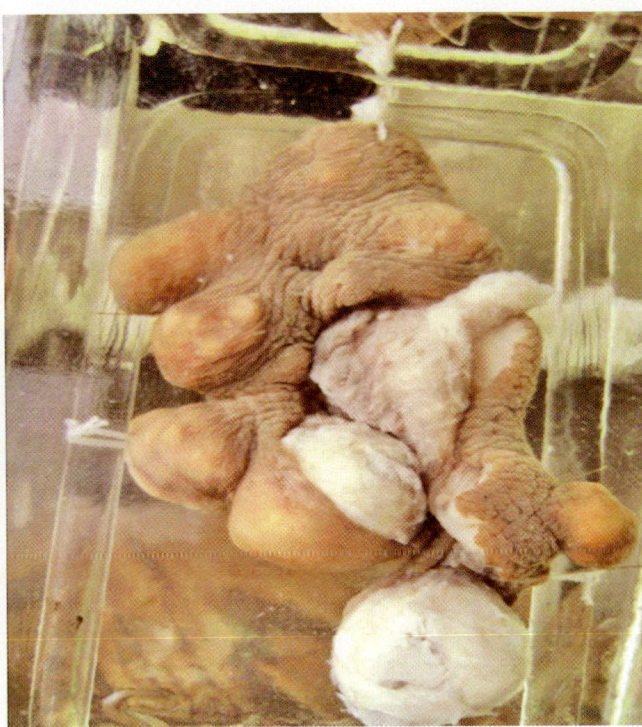

Multiple sebaceous cysts in scrotum

The specimen of scrotum showing multiple solid cystic lesion in scrotal skin. Multiple swellings are found arising from the scrotal skin largest measuring 1.5 cm. The swellings are pearly white in color as seen in the picture and are looking firm. This is a specimen of multiple sebaceous cyst scrotum.

AUTHOR'S IMAGINARY WORLD "THE CARE WORLD"

- Brings colors to life

Author's appeal to everybody to work, as per individual capability, on World Population Control (WPC) as Population growth is the change in population overtime and can be qualified as the change in the number of individuals in a population using "per unit time" for measurement.

Over population has a negative impact on the environment due to pollution and over crowding. The more people are there, more resources they use and the more pollution that results.

- Air pollution is due to increased fossil fuel emissions from vehicles.
- Land or water pollution due to increased amounts of waste.

Population increases as people are born or immigrate into a country and decrease as people die or emigrate. Rate of population growth, usually expressed as a percentage, vary greatly.

Our aim should be to control world population by preventing unwanted newborn and make the world a happier place forever.

Index